SAQs, MCQs, EMQs and OSCEs
for
MRCOG Part 2

SAQs, MCQs, EMQs and OSCEs for MRCOG Part 2

A comprehensive guide

Justin C. Konje MBA, MD, FMCOG (NIG), FRCOG
Professor and Honorary Consultant Obstetrician and Gynaecologist
Leicester Royal Infirmary
University of Leicester, UK

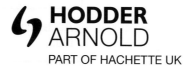

HODDER
ARNOLD
PART OF HACHETTE UK

First published in Great Britain in 2003 by Hodder Arnold.

This second edition published in 2009 by
Hodder Arnold, an imprint of Hodder Education, part of Hachette UK, 338 Euston Road, London
NW1 3BH

http://www.hoddereducation.com

Whilst the advice and information in this book are believed to be true and accurate at the date of going
to press, neither the author nor the publisher can accept any legal responsibility or liability for any
errors or omissions that may be made. In particular (but without limiting the generality of the
preceding disclaimer) every effort has been made to check drug dosages; however it is still possible that
errors have been missed. Furthermore, dosage schedules are constantly being revised and new side-
effects recognized. For these reasons the reader is strongly urged to consult the drug companies'
printed instructions before administering any of the drugs recommended in this book.

British Library Cataloguing in Publication Data
A catalogue record for this book is available from the British Library

Library of Congress Cataloging-in-Publication Data
A catalog record for this book is available from the Library of Congress

ISBN   978 0 340 941 683

1 2 3 4 5 6 7 8 9 10

Commissioning Editor: Gavin Jamieson
Project Editor: Francesca Naish
Production Controller: Joanna Walker
Cover Designer: Helen Townson

Typeset in 10 on 12pt Minion by Phoenix Photosetting, Chatham, Kent
Printed and bound in India

What do you think about this book? Or any other Hodder Arnold title?
Please visit our website: www.hoddereducation.com

Contents

CONTENTS

Preface

The MRCOG Part 2 examination has evolved over the past decade. The impetus for the various changes has come from a desire to make the examination reflect its aims. The overall objective of the examination is to assess clinical competencies, most of which are pitched at the trainee at the end of year 4 (ST4).

The examination consists of short-answer questions (SAQs), multiple-choice questions (MCQs), extended matching questions (EMQs) and an oral examination otherwise known as the objective structured clinical examination (OSCE). The structure of examination, especially the compartmentalisation of the short-answer questions, has minimised the previous problems of candidates regurgitating chapters from textbooks, especially *Progress in Obstetrics and Gynaecology*, but many candidates continue to experience difficulties with the written examination. This is not because of lack of knowledge but owing to a poor approach to the short essays. Experience from various revision courses, and from the examination itself, suggests that given the correct points required for each question, candidates still find difficulties in presenting the facts in a way that will convince examiners.

This book aims to provide candidates with a different approach to preparing for the examination, especially the short-answer questions. It is based on the experience gained from running one of the most successful MRCOG Part 2 revision course at Leicester and also from examining. The aim is not to provide a prescriptive format for answering questions, but to guide candidates in the right direction and, more importantly, to show them how to avoid the path to failure. The book is divided into five sections: the first focuses on how to approach the examination; the second concentrates on SAQs in obstetrics and gynaecology; the third section on MCQs; the fourth on EMQs; and the fifth section on the oral examination itself.

Individual chapters in Section Two consist of several questions. Each question is followed by common mistakes made by candidates, the important points required for a good answer and, lastly, a sample of a good answer. Some of the sample answers may be much longer than would be expected from candidates within the time allocated for each question. This is deliberate to ensure that as much as possible is covered. Candidates must appreciate that the answers are by no means definitive. Indeed, some points may not be discussed. Their absence does not imply that they are irrelevant.

Section Three contains 225 MCQs in the format of the examination. They are included to encourage the candidates to practise.

Section Four contains 40 EMQs in the format of the examination. Again, this is for practice only. An explanation to the questions is provided as an aide-memoire.

Section Five introduces the objective structured clinical examination (OSCE). Candidates should practise answering the questions during their preparation for the examination. More sample questions for practice may be found in other examination books available from the RCOG bookshop.

I know that most candidates preparing for the MRCOG Part 2 examination are terrified, but good clinicians should have no difficulties in passing – provided their approach to the short essays is the correct one. I hope that this book will provide all the ingredients you need for the examination and I wish you the very best of luck.

I would like to thank my children Justin (Jr), Monique and Swiri, and my wife Joan Kila Konje for their support and encouragement during the writing of this second edition.

Justin C. Konje

This book is dedicated to my grandmother Mambotoh Tabe,
who died in August 1969

Abbreviations

AC	abdominal circumference	CTG	cardiotocograph(y)
ACE	angiotensin-converting enzyme	CVA	cerebrovascular accident
		CVP	central venous pressure
AEDs	antiepileptic drug	CVS	chorionic villus sampling
AFP	alpha-fetoprotein	CXR	chest X-ray
AID	artificial insemination by donor	DOCA	deoxyhydrocorticosterone acetate
AIH	artificial insemination by husband	DNA	deoxyribo nucleic acid
		DHEA	dehydroepiandrosterone
AIS	adenocarcinoma *in-situ*	DHEAS	dehydroepiandrostendione sulphate
AR	autosomal recessive		
ARM	artificial rupture of fetal membranes	DIC	disseminated intravascular coagulation
AST	alanine aminotransferase	DVT	deep vein thrombosis
βhCG	beta-human chorionic gonadotrophin	ECG	electrocardiograph(y) *or* electrocardiogram
BBI	blood-borne infection	ECV	external cephalic version
BCG	bacille Calmette–Guérin	EMQ	extended matching question
BMI	body mass index	EUA	examination under anaesthesia
BP	blood pressure	FAS	fetal alcohol syndrome
BPP	biophysical profilometry	FBC	full blood count
BSO	bilateral salpingo-oophorectomy	FBS	fetal blood sampling
		FDP	fibrinogen degradation product
CAH	congenital adrenal hyperplasia		
CDH	congenital diaphragmatic hernia	FGR	fetal growth restricted
		FGR	fetal growth restriction
CIN	cervical intraepithelial neoplasia	FISH	fluorescent *in situ* hybridisation
CJD	Creutzfeldt–Jakob disease	FSE	fetal scalp electrode
CMV	cytomegalovirus	FSH	follicle-stimulating hormone
CNS	central nervous system	FT4	free thyroxine
COCP	combined oral contraceptive pill	FVS	fetal varicella syndrome
		GA	general anaesthesia
CPA	cyproterone acetate	GnRH	gonadotropin-releasing hormone
CPP	chronic pelvic pain		
CT	computerised tomography	GP	general practitioner

ABBREVIATIONS

GUM	genitourinary medicine
HAAT	highly active antiretroviral therapy
Hb	haemoglobin
HbAlc	glycosylated haemoglobin
HBIG	hepatitis B immunoglobulin
hCG	human chorionic gonadotropin
HDU	high dependency unit
HIV	human immunodeficiency virus
hMG	human menopausal gonadotropin
HRT	hormone replacement therapy
HPV	human papillomavirus
HRT	hormone replacement therapy
HSG	hysterosalpingography
HSV	herpes simplex virus
HVS	high vaginal swab
HyCoSy	hystero-contrast-sonography
ICSI	intracytoplasmic sperm injection
ICU	intensive care unit
i.m.	intramuscular
INH	isoniazid
IUD	intrauterine contraceptive device
IUFD	intrauterine fetal death
IUGR	intrauterine growth restriction
i.v.	intravenous
IVF	*in vitro* fertilization
IVF-ET	*in vitro* fertilisation with embryo transfer
IVU	intravenous urogram
LA	local anaesthesia
LARC	long-acting reversible contraceptive
LFT	liver function test
LH	luteinising hormone
LLETZ	large loop excision of the transformation zones
LMP	last menstrual period
LMWH	low-molecular-weight heparin
Lng-IUCS	levonorgestrel intrauterine contraceptive system
LUNA	laparoscopic uterosacral nerve ablation
LVS	low vaginal swab
MAP	mean arterial pressure
MCA	middle cerebral artery
MCQ	*Multiple-choice* question
M/C/S	microscopy, culture and sensitivity
MDT	multidisciplinary team
MRI	magnetic resonance imaging
MSU	midstream specimen of urine
NHS	National Health Service
NICE	National Institute for Health and Clinical Excellence
NICU	neonatal intensive care unit
NSAID	non-steroidal anti-inflammatory drug
NT	nuchal translucency
NTD	neural tube defect
OCSE	objective structured clinical examination
OD450	optical densitometric analyses at wavelength of 450 nm
ODP	operating department practitioner
OHSS	ovarian hyperstimulation syndrome
PAPP1	pregnancy-associated plasma protein-1
PCOS	polycystic ovary syndrome
PCR	polymerase chain reaction
PE	pulmonary embolism
PET	pre-eclampsia
PFE	pelvic floor exercise
PID	pelvic inflammatory disease
PMS	premenstrual syndrome
POP	progestogen-only pill
POPQ	pelvic organ prolapse quantification
PUO	pyrexia of unknown origin
RCOG	Royal College of Obstetricians and Gynaecologists
RDS	respiratory distress syndrome
SANDS	Stillbirth and Neonatal Deaths Society

SAQ	Short-answer question	TVS	transvaginal ultrasound scan
SERM	selective oestrogen receptor modulator	TVS	transvaginal ultrasound scanning
SCJ	squamocolumnar junction	TVT	transvaginal tape
SHO	senior house officer	TVT	tension-free transvaginal tape
SSRI	selective serotonin reuptake inhibitor	U&Es	urea and electrolytes
STI	sexually transmitted infection	USI	urodynamic (genuine) stress incontinence
TAH	total abdominal hysterectomy		
TB	tuberculosis	USS	ultrasound scan
TED	thromboembolic deterrent	UTI	urinary tract infection
TENS	transcutaneous electrical nerve stimulator	VAIN	vaginal intraepithelial neoplasia
TOT	trans-obturator tape	VE	vaginal examination
TPR	temperature, pulse and respiratory rate	VTE	venous thromboembolism
		VZV	varicella zoster virus
TSH	thyroid-stimulating hormone	WCC	white cell count
TST	tuberculin skin test	WHO	World Health Organization
TTN	transient tachypnoea of the newborn		

Section One

How to approach the Part 2 examination

1

The structure of the MRCOG Part 2 examination

The examination consists of two parts:

1. The written examination – consisting of a multiple-choice question (MCQ) paper, an extended matching question (EMQ) paper and the two short-answer question (SAQs) papers.
2. The oral examination.

The MCQ paper consists of 225 true or false questions. There is no negative marking. Although there may be several 'twigs' to a statement, each statement should be read independently. The EMQ paper is made up of 40 questions. It is a modified multiple-choice examination. The answer to each question has to be selected from an option list which is often thematic and varies from 10 to 25. Occasionally, the number of options may be less than 10 or more than 25. There are two short-answer question papers – one consisting of four obstetric questions and the other of four gynaecology questions.

There is no set pass mark for the written examination; however, the minimum total that a candidate must obtain to progress to the oral part of the examination is determined by a process known as 'Standard Setting'. This ensures that there is consistency in the standard of the examination with difficult examinations more likely to have a lower pass mark and vice versa for easier examinations. A candidate does not have to pass the three parts of the written examination to proceed to the oral stage. Progression is determined by the total score – hence one part could compensate the other. Experience has shown that very few candidates actually compensate. The mark distribution for the written examination is as follows – EMQs (15 per cent), MCQs (25 per cent) and SAQs (60 per cent).

The oral or objective structured clinical examination (OSCE) consists of 12 stations each lasting 15 minutes. Two of these stations are preparatory stations. Details of this part of the examination are provided under the appropriate section in this book.

2

How to fail the examination

I am certain that no candidate will willingly enter an examination to fail. However, if you fail to prepare properly, then you have indirectly opted for this rather unpleasant experience. There are a few tips on how to fail and I hope that you will not waste your time reading this book if it was your intention to fail. The following tips will be extremely useful to those who want to have a go at the examination just for the fun of it.

1. Do not prepare for the examination.
2. Do not read the recommended book.
3. Read only CRASH Course Books and undergraduate textbooks.
4. Spend more time on your books rather than with patients.
5. Do not consult the Royal College of Obstetricians and Gynaecologists education materials and journals, especially *Green-top Guidelines*, the *British Journal of Obstetrics and Gynaecology* and *The Obstetrician & Gynaecologist*.
6. Memorise answers in books and regurgitate them in the exams for questions that look similar.
7. In the examination itself, do not bother understanding the questions; dump down everything you know about the subject and hope that the examiner will be kind enough to filter; do not answer all the questions; make sure that your handwriting is illegible, etc.
8. When you are sitting the multiple-choice questions and the extended matching questions papers, only answer the questions you know and leave the others.
9. In the oral examination, be opinionated, condescending and offer the views of your senior colleagues.

Section Two

Short essay questions

How to approach short-answer questions

There are many textbooks on multiple-choice questions (MCQs) in obstetrics and gynaecology. All candidates sitting the MRCOG Part 2 examination will have had the experience of this type of examination from Part 1. The short-answer questions (SAQs) are different and require a completely new approach. The questions are clinical and require logic and structure. Most questions require a matured and well-reasoned approach – a personal rather than a generic one. Although the questions may appear straightforward, candidates fail to provide the correct answers because of their lack of understanding of the key issues within them. It is expected that these questions will be approached from a clinical perspective rather from a theoretical basis. The MCQs test theory, whereas the SAQs and the oral or objective structured clinical examination assess clinical competencies. Here, some guidance is provided on how to approach the SAQs. Always remember that the question is asking what *you* would do rather than what your consultant, another colleague or the textbook would do. If in doubt, imagine that you are faced with a patient in the clinic, on the wards or in theatre and you have to explain to your consultant how and why you would manage that patient in a particular way. Below are some guiding principles for the short essays.

Important questions to ask before starting any question

- What does the examiner want (what is the question asking)?
- What does the question not ask?
- Have you read and understood the question?
- What do I have to write to convince the examiner that I am clinically competent?
- What exactly do I need to write and how do I need to argue my point?
- Do I need an introduction and a conclusion? This is often unnecessary.

Answering the questions

- Do you have a plan?
- What are the relevant issues and have you written them down?
- What is the logical approach to the question?
- Do you have to make many sentences to get your point across?

- Is it in essay form or bullet points, lines, notes, short phrases, etc.?
- How easy is it to read your handwriting?

Understanding the wording in the question (commonly used instructions)

- Evaluate
- Critically appraise
- Consider the options
- Justify
- Summarise
- Compare
- What steps will you take?
- Debate
- Outline
- Consider the options

Read the question and underline the key words or phrases first

Evaluate

- Place a value on – literally what price will you place on something?
- No need to place a price on what you put down
- Need to have some order or preferencing in your answer

Critically appraise

- Two words – *critical* and *appraise*
- *Critical* – fault-finding, discerning, decisive, skilled in judgement
- *Appraise* – estimate value of
- *Critically appraise* – combine fault-finding and estimation of value

Justify

- Prove right, vindicate – you must give reasons for your answer

Debate

- Argue – advantages and disadvantages (similar to *critically appraise*, except more structured)

Suggested approach to the short-answer papers

- First, read through the whole paper very quickly
- Go through each question and underline the key words
- Jot down a rough plan for each question – starting with the difficult ones
- Wipe your hands before you start writing if they are sweaty
- Start with the easy questions – builds confidence
- Do not finish with the difficult question (may not have enough time)
- Time yourself – and be disciplined
- Read through your answers if possible

You do not need to fill the two pages to pass the examination. In fact, most candidates score most of their marks from the first two paragraphs of their answer. It is better to have a concise and well-structured answer than a lengthy, meaningless one. If you present your work neatly, examiners will find it easier to read and assess. If you create extra lines on the answer sheet, write across the paper and fail to paragraph your essay, you run the risk of losing marks. Remember that persistent factual errors and incorrect and dangerous statements are penalised by deduction of marks (you could lose up to 4 marks out of 20 for this). Candidates are in the habit of quoting figures to impress examiners. It is dangerous to quote incorrect figures. You are advised not to quote figures unless you are very sure of them. You may lose marks for incorrect figures.

You must aim to complete all 8 questions. If you concentrate on five, six or seven and hope to make up for the one(s) you do not know, you are very unlikely to pass. It is better to spend your time equally on each question, as this strategy will offer you a better chance of passing. Each question should take 26 minutes. My advice is for candidates to spend the first 10 minutes of the examination writing a plan for the four SAQs (of each paper) and the last 10–15 minutes reading through each answer to correct spelling mistakes. Some of these mistakes may alter the content of your answer.

Section Two

Part One: Obstetrics

1

Epidemiology, social obstetrics, drugs in pregnancy

1. An alcoholic is seen at 6 weeks into her first pregnancy. (a) Outline the maternal and fetal risks associated with her alcoholism. (6 marks) (b) How will you modify her antenatal care to reduce these risks? (14 marks)

2. An 18-year-old books for antenatal care and confirms that she smokes marijuana and 30 cigarettes per day. (a) Briefly outline the adverse effects of these on her pregnancy. (12 marks) (b) Justify the steps you will take in persuading her to give up smoking in pregnancy. (8 marks)

3. A 22-year-old mother of two attends for antenatal care at 30 weeks' gestation with her partner and their two children. You observe that the children are rather subdued and also, during your examination, you elicit tenderness over the left lower loin, which is also bruised. You suspect domestic violence. (a) How will you confirm your suspicion? (6 marks) (b) Briefly outline your immediate management. (8 marks) (c) Discuss your subsequent management of the rest of pregnancy. (6 marks)

4. During a routine antenatal care a well-informed woman at 24 weeks' gestation wishes to seek information about drugs in pregnancy from the internet. (a) Explain the benefits and disadvantages of obtaining information from the internet. (12 marks) (b) What advice will you give her? (8 marks)

1. An alcoholic is seen at 6 weeks into her first pregnancy. (a) Outline the maternal and fetal risks associated with her alcoholism. (6 marks) (b) How will you modify her antenatal care to reduce these risks? (14 marks)

Common mistakes

- Discussing details of the management of the patient in pregnancy
- Identification of fetal alcohol syndrome (FAS) by ultrasound or other means
- An alcoholic – no need to ask how much she drinks
- Why are you an alcoholic? Why do you have to drink so much? (Be sensitive in your approach)
- Advice to consult general practitioner (GP), social workers, etc. for information on how to stop drinking. How realistic is this?
- You need to be specific – not just say alcohol is associated with features of FAS, etc.

A good answer will include some or all of these points

(a) Outline the maternal and fetal risks associated with her alcoholism. (6 marks)

- Fetal risks:
  - Miscarriages
  - Congenital malformations
  - FAS
  - Fetal growth restriction (FGR)
  - Preterm labour
- Maternal risks:
  - Malnutrition
  - Vitamin deficiency
  - Encephalopathy
  - Anaemia – especially folate and B12
  - Liver failure
  - Heart failure

(b) How will you modify her antenatal care to reduce these risks? (14 marks)

- Education on lifestyle modifications – smoking, alcohol, other drugs
- Counselling and detoxification programmes
- Multidisciplinary team (social worker, psychologists, detoxification units)
- Removal of precipitating factors, e.g. domestic violence, etc.
- Book in consultant-led unit
- Management pathways for intrapartum and postnatal care
- Fetal monitoring – detailed ultrasound scan in tertiary unit, normal labour and delivery

- Ensure that other substances are not abused
- The approach must be sensitive, supportive, empathic and non-judgemental
- The problems of teratogenicity and alcohol ≥15 units/week
- Involvement of social workers
- Social and other background information (from patient or other people) – problems possibly associated with the drinking will be identified and, once resolved, are more likely to be associated with success in stopping drinking
- Organisations – Alcoholics Anonymous, other support/help groups, pamphlets about alcohol and pregnancy
- Staff – GP, midwives, family, friends, social workers
- Maternal dangers of alcohol – liver failure, heart failure, encephalopathy, anaemia, vitamin B12 deficiency

Sample answer

(a) Outline the maternal and fetal risks associated with her alcoholism. (6 marks)

These problems arise where alcohol intake is more than 80 g/day (eight units per day = eight glasses of wine or four pints of lager/day). The adverse effects of excessive alcohol intake in pregnancy could be fetal or maternal. The fetal risks include spontaneous miscarriages, congenital malformations such as cardiac anomalies, microcephaly, skeletal anomalies and microophthalmia. Some of the malformations including microcephaly and FGR form part of the FAS. Other risks to the fetus are impaired intellect and neurodevelopmental delay. In addition, the pregnancy is at risk of preterm delivery. These consequences are often compounded by lifestyle factors such as smoking and drugs (which tend to be more common in alcoholics). The consequences of alcohol on the mother include liver failure, heart failure, encephalopathy, anaemia, vitamin B deficiency – leading to Wernicke–Korsakoff's encephalopathy and gastrointestinal disturbances, such as gastritis and pancreatitis.

(b) How will you modify her antenatal care to reduce these risks? (14 marks)

Her antenatal care should be provided by a multidisciplinary team in a consultant unit. The team should include a consultant with an interest in alcohol in pregnancy if available, a specialist midwife, a social worker and a member of the alcohol unit or detoxification unit, depending on which is available. This team will ensure that appropriate sensitive, supportive, empathic and non-judgemental counselling and support are provided. It is important that she is not antagonised from the outset. Once she develops confidence in the clinician, the process becomes easier and the results are much better. The first stage in counselling is to make sure that the patient is aware of the existence of a problem. There may be initial denial but persistence and supportive counselling will eventually result in acknowledging that there is, indeed, a problem. The next stage in the counselling will be to educate the patient on the possible consequences of excessive alcohol on the fetus.

An important step in the counselling is to ensure that she seeks expert support and help.

This will be from social workers who may provide home support for her and any children she may have. Her partner also needs to be counselled. Often, he too is alcoholic and failing to involve him in the counselling process will be counterproductive. It is important to obtain some social and other relevant background information about the patient. This may provide clues as to why she drinks. For example, it may be related to childcare, abuse from partner or family, rejection by society or other deep-seated problems. Identification and resolution of these problem(s) may suddenly result in a change in attitude.

Organisations such as Alcoholics Anonymous or other support groups locally or nationally and contact with other women who have had similar problems may provide support. These organisations may also provide information pamphlets about alcohol and pregnancy, which will reinforce the discussion on teratogenicity and the consequences of alcohol on the mother. The GP, midwife, friends and family should be involved if possible. It may be easier for the patient to relate to them than to doctors at the hospital. Once a breakthrough has been achieved, this has to be followed up by frequent positive reinforcement and encouragement. Relapse is easy and therefore the counselling must not only concentrate on pregnancy but must also make provisions for continuing support after delivery.

In view of the risks to the fetus, a detailed ultrasound scan, preferably at the tertiary level, including a fetal echo would be offered at 20 and 23–24 weeks respectively. Regular ultrasound scans from 24 weeks to monitor fetal growth will be essential. It may be useful to involve a paediatrician and an anaesthetist in her care antenatally. Such a multidisciplinary approach will ensure that clear management pathways for labour and postnatal care both for the mother and baby are clearly documented in her notes.

2. An 18-year-old books for antenatal care and confirms that she smokes marijuana and 30 cigarettes per day. (a) Briefly outline the adverse effects of these on her pregnancy. (12 marks) (b) Justify the steps you will take in persuading her to give up smoking in pregnancy. (8 marks)

Common mistakes

- Take a history and examine patient
- Refer to physician
- Offer alternative cigarettes
- Discussing the diagnosis and management of FGR
- Advantage – reduce the risk of pre-eclampsia (PET)
- Failure to justify the steps in part (b)
- Discussing the effects of recreational drugs on pregnancy in general

A good answer will contain some or all of these points

(a) Briefly outline the adverse effects of these on her pregnancy. (12 marks)

- Smoking produces nicotine and carboxyhaemoglobin. These cross the placenta and circulate within the fetus
- Smoking affects the baby and the mother
- Education/counselling about the side-effects on the pregnancy and mother:
  - Pregnancy:
    - Miscarriages
    - FGR
    - Placental abruption
    - Intrauterine death/hypoxia
    - Preterm labour
  - Newborn/infant:
    - Neonatal death:
      - Cot death
      - Early neonatal death
      - Reduced intelligence
      - Short attention span and hyperactivity
      - Increased neonatal morbidity and mortality
  - Maternal complications:
    - Chronic lung disease
    - Venous thromboembolism (VTE)
    - Maternal death
    - Arterial disease
    - Cancer of the lungs
    - Chronic obstructive airway disease

(b) Justify the steps you will take in persuading her to give up smoking in pregnancy. (8 marks)

- Fetal:
  - Miscarriage
  - Preterm labour
  - Intrauterine fetal death
  - Placental abruption
  - Intrauterine hypoxia
  - Prolonged pregnancy
- Maternal:
  - Chronic respiratory lung disease
  - Malnutrition
  - Addiction
  - Consequence of other drugs of addiction

Sample answer

(a) Briefly outline the adverse effects of these on her pregnancy. (12 marks)

Smoking produces nicotine and carboxyhaemoglobin, which cross the placenta into the fetal circulation. The consequences of this combination include miscarriages, intrauterine hypoxia, FGR, preterm labour, long-term neurodevelopmental disability, poorer intellect, short attention span and hyperactivity and cot death. In addition, the fetus may develop polycythaemia, which may be complicated by neonatal venous thrombosis (VTE) and associated mortality.

The consequences of smoking for the mother include chronic lung disease, placental abruption, hypertension and VTE. Long-term consequences include lung cancer and arterial disease, heart failure, heart attacks, chronic malnutrition and chronic obstructive airway disease. Although not a direct effect, the cost of purchasing cigarettes is high and this affects the patient's expenditure on other more important household goods.

(b) Justify the steps you will take in persuading her to give up smoking in pregnancy. (8 marks)

The first step in persuading this woman to give up smoking is to educate her on the consequences of smoking, first on her baby, and then on herself. The next step will be to offer support and alternative means of giving up smoking. Counselling on these consequences may not be enough to stop her from smoking. Even if she is motivated enough, she may occasionally lapse. It is therefore important to consider the use of nicotine patches and gum, which may provide some fallback whenever there is a craving for a cigarette. The patient's partner or family members who smoke must also be counselled and their role in supporting her highlighted to them. The dreaded problem of sudden infant death syndrome (cot death) has been associated with smoking during and after pregnancy. Providing this information to the patient may persuade her to stop smoking.

It must be remembered that patients will cite friends who have smoked and then had normal pregnancies. The definition of 'normal' is vague and the patient must be informed that the absence of a congenital abnormality does not mean a healthy baby. Often, smoking will have important but less obvious consequences that only manifest later in life.

Lastly, the process must involve experts who are devoted to supporting and counselling such patients. These may be support groups, midwives or social workers whose role is to counsel women to give up smoking in pregnancy.

3. A 22-year-old mother of two attends for antenatal care at 30 weeks' gestation with her partner and their two children. You observe that the children are rather subdued and also, during your examination, you elicit tenderness over the left lower loin, which is also bruised. You suspect domestic violence. (a) How will you confirm your suspicion? (6 marks) (b) Briefly outline your immediate management. (8 marks) (c) Discuss your subsequent management of the rest of the pregnancy. (6 marks)

Common mistakes

- Take a history about domestic violence from the patient and her partner
- Involve social workers, so that the children can be taken away to safety
- Confront the husband and ask him to stop
- Offer more frequent visits to the hospital and ensure that the midwife sees patients weekly

A good answer will include some or all of these points

(a) How will you confirm your suspicion? (6 marks)

- History and physical examination – from patient on her own (i.e. without the partner). Hospital admission may be necessary to get this information
- Positive indicators:
  - Repeated unexplained hospital admissions
  - Self-harm history
  - Depression or unexplained psychiatric problems
  - Non-compliance with recommended treatment
  - Self-discharge from hospital
  - Vague symptoms and history
- Physical examination:
  - Unexplained bruises
  - Unexplained scars
  - Unexplained burns
- History from social worker/midwife – this may be necessary if the above information is not forthcoming

(b) Briefly outline your immediate management. (8 marks)

- Reassurance and gain confidence – may be frightened about partner finding out about disclosure
- Remove from threatening environment (home) – most likely admission
- Provide support – social and psychological

- Safety of other children – involve social workers to assess them at home and remove them if indicated. If not, require constant vigilance

(c) Discuss your subsequent management of the rest of the pregnancy. (6 marks)

- Treat or remove cause(s) of violence if possible:
  - Financial
  - Drugs and alcohol
  - Unemployment, etc.
- Education of partner and providing support/counselling
- Long-term hospitalisation/remove to safer environment (sometimes without the knowledge of the partner)
- Child protection – assess whether child needs to be on the at-risk register
- Consider involvement of the police if criminal actions (liaise with social services for this)

Sample answer

(a) How will you confirm your suspicion? (6 marks)

The only way the suspicion may be confirmed will be from interviewing the woman. Certainly, this cannot be done in the presence of her partner. However, it may be possible to create an opportunity to interview the patient on her own in the clinic, but this must be done carefully as the partner may be suspicious. In fact, in most cases, the partner dominates and is commonly the one who speaks for the patient. If there is sufficient evidence to make this most likely, an alternative could be to admit the patient and interview her during the admission. During the interview, the patient needs to be certain that information provided will be treated in the strictest confidence and such an assurance should be provided voluntarily, otherwise the patient may not volunteer any information.

Additional information should be obtained from the patient during the interview. The aim of this is to identify other risk factors for domestic violence, such as alcohol, drugs, depression, stress – especially at work (this is more likely if the partner has just lost his job), if the pregnancy was unplanned or if there are extraneous factors, such as impending separation or divorce.

The physical examination should be meticulous and all suspicious areas documented carefully as they may be used as evidence. It will be difficult to examine the children in the clinic but social workers should be involved. They will visit the family and use their special skills to acquire the information.

(b) Briefly outline your immediate management. (8 marks)

Domestic violence is a difficult problem to diagnose and manage. It requires sensitivity, tact, confidence-building with the patient and professional advice from those with expertise in the management of these patients. Once this is suspected, the management must be tailored to confirming this diagnosis before appropriate counselling can be offered.

If the children are considered to be at risk, attempts must be made to protect them. Social workers will explore the possibility of the unborn child being at risk. It may also be that the children are on an at-risk register. If so, steps must be taken by social workers to either remove the children from the care of the parents or remove the violent partner from the home.

If the suspicion is confirmed, various authorities need to become involved. The obstetric complications of domestic violence are preterm labour and placental abruption (if there is trauma to the abdomen). The patient must be educated on the warning signs of these two complications. She should also be educated on the need to report early if there is any trauma to the anterior abdominal wall.

Domestic violence is difficult to manage and unless the patient is willing to co-operate, it may be difficult to diagnose and managed properly. It is also important to remember that although the violence may be coming from the partner, it may also stem from the patient.

(c) Discuss your subsequent management of the rest of the pregnancy. (6 marks)

The pregnancy should be monitored closely as compounding factors such as smoking and alcohol abuse will increase the risk of preterm labour, FGR and placental abruption. In addition, all efforts must be made to remove the possible causes or precipitating factors (such as financial constraints, drugs and alcohol, unemployment, lack of support at home, etc.) of the domestic violence. The partner needs to be educated and support provided where appropriate. Where the life of the woman or her children is at risk, she/they will have to be removed from home and therefore danger. The children and the unborn child may have to be placed on the child protection register and appropriate supervision instituted. Finally consideration must be given to involving the police if the violence involves criminal actions. No special measures will be required for the labour but follow-up must continue after delivery.

4. During a routine antenatal care a well-informed woman at 24 weeks' gestation wishes to seek information about drugs in pregnancy from the internet. (a) Explain the benefits and disadvantages of obtaining information from the internet. (12 marks) (b) What advice will you give her? (8 marks)

(a) Explain the benefits and disadvantages of obtaining information from the internet. (12 marks)

- Benefits:
  - Easy access
  - Readily available
  - Different sources (medical and layperson's)
  - Website specific – subject based
  - Individual experiences – shared
- Disadvantages:
  - Unvetted
  - Provided by individuals who may not necessarily be experts
  - Unavailability of help and explanations
  - Lack of opportunity to ask questions and seek clarification
  - May increase anxiety
  - Biased information
  - Difficulties unravelling content and explanations

(b) What advice will you give her? (8 marks)

- Recognise the limitations of the information
- Best from web-specific sites, not individual sites
- Sites for laypersons better
- Presentation in question and answer forms
- Beware of forums – open forums where experiences are shared
- Remember that there are never two similar cases in all aspects
- Bring back information to experts for further clarification and discussion

Sample answer

(a) Explain the benefits and disadvantages of obtaining information from the internet. (12 marks)

The internet has become an important source of information for both clinicians and patients. There are several advantages for the patient with regards to seeking information from this source. First, the information is freely available. It can be accessed in the home and from several sources which are medical and non-medical. More importantly, there are specific web sites for different conditions which often contain well-researched and well-presented information for the layperson. Another advantage is the opportunity to learn from others' experiences and yet retain anonymity.

However, there are disadvantages in seeking information from the internet. This information, especially that from non-medical websites, can be biased and poorly presented. There is the risk of the information reflecting individuals' views or practices. Since the information can be from any part of the world, it may be misleading with respect to practices in particular parts of the world (e.g. there are differences between UK and USA practice). The patient may struggle with understanding the information especially that from professional sites. If she is not medically trained, there is the risk of uncommon problems generating significant anxiety in the patient. One other problem is the potential difficulty deciding where to find the information.

(b) What advice will you give her? (8 marks)

The patient will be counselled on the limitations of information obtained from the internet. This will include the advantages and disadvantages outlined above. Where she has a specific problem, for which she is sorting information, advice may be provided on which websites to visit for information. Websites that deal with specific problems and are run by special bodies are a better source of information. She would benefit more from sites that provide information in question and answer form. Obtaining information from the internet could result in obtaining information that is loosely associated with the original problem and consequently can cause more distress. The unbounded nature of the information, the limitless time available to explore this and the lack of direction pose a potential challenge to such a means of obtaining information. Finally, she would be advised to seek medical opinion on information she obtains from the internet.

2

Infections in pregnancy

1. Universal screening for human immunodeficiency virus (HIV) is better than selective screening. (a) Briefly outline the advantages and the disadvantages of universal screening. (14 marks) (b) Comment briefly on selective screening. (6 marks)

2. A 19-year-old primigravida books for antenatal care at 12 weeks' gestation and is found to be hepatitis B positive on screening. (a) What steps will you take in her management during pregnancy? (12 marks) (b) She then presents in spontaneous labour at 39 weeks' gestation with intact membranes. How will you manage her from now onwards? (4 marks) (c) What advice will you give her prior to discharge from the hospital? (4 marks)

3. A 28-year-old presents at 37 weeks' gestation with a diagnosis of herpes simplex type II vulval infection. (a) What advice will you give her in the antenatal clinic? (8 marks) (b) How will this infection modify her antenatal care? (4 marks) (c) She presents in labour at 40 weeks' gestation. How will you manage her? (8 marks)

4. A schoolteacher in her first pregnancy at 6 weeks' gestation has been informed that one of her pupils has chickenpox infection. She is extremely worried. (a) What are the risks of the infection to her and the pregnancy? (6 marks) (b) How will you confirm that she has the infection? (8 marks) (c) If she has been confirmed to have acquired the infection, outline the steps you will take in her management. (6 marks)

5. A 28-year-old is diagnosed with HIV at 20 weeks' gestation. (a) What steps will you take to minimise the risk of transmission of HIV to the baby? (15 marks) (b) How would your management differ if the mother presented in labour having received no treatment? (5 marks)

1. Universal screening for HIV is better than selective screening. (a) Briefly outline the advantages and the disadvantages of universal screening. (14 marks) (b) Comment briefly on selective screening. (6 marks)

Common mistakes

- Discussing details of the criteria for a screening test
- History of HIV and its course once infection has occurred
- Benefits of screening
- Various laboratory test for the diagnosis of HIV
- Treatment of HIV

A good answer will include some or all of these points

(a) Briefly outline the advantages and the disadvantages of universal screening (14 marks)

- A viral infection that is increasingly becoming more common in the pregnant population
- All screening (including at-risk and not-at-risk population)
- Screening – why advantageous – ensures better outcome for the mother and fetus
- Universal screening:
  - Difficulties – resources – manpower for counselling
  - Disclosure of results and consequences of a positive test
  - Benefits – all of those infected are identified
  - Treatment offered and therefore outcome for the baby and mother better
- Two types of universal screening – testing everyone or offering test to everyone and encouraging take-up (current approach in the UK)
- Decrease in risk of missing cases
- Removes stigma of selective screening
- Reduces spread of HIV to staff and unsuspecting partners
- Ensures identification of all babies at risk
- Education of staff to support
- Resources – funding is essential
- Manpower – required to provide the screening, counselling and discussion of results and follow-up
- Less attention to high-risk population
- Treatment of all babies at risk

(b) Comment briefly on selective screening. (4 marks)

- High-risk populations targeted

- Limited resources (manpower and other) better used:
  - Misses out others who are infected; danger of spreading the disease
  - Cost – probably more effective
  - Risk of alienating at-risk groups who may not attend for screening

Sample answer

(a) Briefly outline the advantages and the disadvantages of universal screening (14 marks)

Human immunodeficiency virus is a retrovirus whose incidence is increasing in the sexually active population. It has significant consequences on patients and their unborn fetuses. It is recognised that early identification, institution of treatment and modification of the method of delivery and postnatal feeding significantly minimises the risk of vertical transmission. Screening and identifying those who are HIV positive therefore affords the opportunity to deliver the strategy outlined above to improve outcome.

Universal screening can be achieved by testing everyone or offering testing to all. The first approach ensures that all pregnant women are screened for HIV. The problem of marginalising a particular group, either on the basis of lifestyle or race, does not arise. The difficulty with this approach is the large population that has to be screened. Appropriate screening must be accompanied not only by staff but by financial resources to support tests. Although laboratory tests may not be expensive, the need for adequate manpower for counselling before screening, and after identification of positive cases, will impose considerable strain on the limited resources within the National Health Service.

The second approach, which operates at the moment in the UK, offers all patients an opportunity to be screened. Uptake of screening is increasing, but patients still have to opt in. There is the danger that with this approach, those who are at high risk may fear that they are infected and not take up the testing. It is clear that a large proportion of infected women is missed during pregnancy, as has been demonstrated by anonymous pilot testing. Therefore, on balance, the best approach is likely to be universal screening, resources permitting. The argument of cost is unlikely to be tenable considering the implications for a positive diagnosis not only for the woman and her unborn child but also for society as a whole. Until the stigma of testing is removed by offering universal screening, many people will continue to be reluctant to come forward for testing for fear of being stigmatised.

(b) Comment briefly on selective screening. (4 marks)

Selective screening targets at-risk groups, such as intravenous drug abusers, bisexuals, those from geographical areas with endemic rates of the disease and their consorts. This approach may result in better use of limited resources. It will also ensure that testing is concentrated in those likely to be HIV positive. The problem with this approach is that the infection is spread through heterosexual contact and therefore a significant proportion of those infected will be missed. In addition, by targeting the at-risk population there is always the danger of the screening programme being perceived as discriminatory.

2. A 19-year-old primigravida books for antenatal care at 12 weeks' gestation and is found to be hepatitis B positive on screening. (a) What steps will you take in her management during pregnancy? (12 marks) (b) She then presents in spontaneous labour at 39 weeks' gestation with intact membranes. How will you manage her from now onwards? (4 marks) (c) What advice will you give her prior to discharge from hospital? (4 marks)

Common mistakes

- Outline the management of hepatitis B positive patients
- Outline the management of HIV
- Discuss lifestyle and risk factors for hepatitis B

A good answer will contain some or all of these points

(a) What steps will you take in her management during pregnancy? (12 marks)

- Hepatitis B – blood-borne and/or sexually transmitted infection (STI)
- May therefore coexist with other STIs:
  - Screening for other STIs should be discussed and offered
  - Consider referral to genitourinary medicine (GUM) clinic – counselling about transmission, risks, etc.
- Infectivity important, especially as regards staff: HbS, Hbc, Hbe antibodies and antigen. Presence of e antigen and absence of e antibody indicates very high infectivity
- Risk of transmission to the fetus, fetal growth restriction (FGR) (not associated with congenital anomalies, therefore termination not an issue)
- Mother:
  - Acute symptoms – supportive treatment
  - Chronic – usually asymptomatic
  - Long-term consequences – counselling from physician (hepatologist)
- Monitor:
  - Fetal growth
  - Liver function tests (LFTs)
  - Inform paediatrician and infective disease counsellor
- Follow unit protocol on how to identify patients with blood-borne infection (BBI) who at risk to staff and their babies

(b) She then presents in spontaneous labour at 39 weeks' gestation with intact membranes. How will you manage her from now onwards? (4 marks)

- Delivery – anticipate a normal vaginal delivery

- Delay rupture of membranes as long as possible
- Ensure all (universal) precautions are followed about risk of infections
- Avoid invasive procedures such as fetal blood sampling, fetal scalp electrodes (FSEs)
- Care of the neonate:
  - Administer hepatitis B immunoglobulin (HBIG) within 12 hours
  - Vaccinate within 7 days; second dose 1–6 months later
  - Hbs antigen (HbsAg) tested at 12–15 months
- Contraceptive advice before discharge

(c) What advice will you give her prior to discharge from the hospital? (4 marks)

- Family members counselled
- Recommend continue monitoring antigen levels:
  - Carrier status
  - Risk of liver cirrhosis

Sample answer

(a) What steps will you take in her management during pregnancy? (12 marks)

Hepatitis B is a BBI, which may also be sexually transmitted. It may therefore coexist with other STIs. The first step in the management of this patient will therefore be to exclude other STIs, especially HIV from serology and swabs taken from the endocervix, the urethra and rectum. Before initiating these investigations, appropriate counselling must be offered. In the presence of other STIs, the GUM physician should be involved in her care.

This patient is at risk of transmitting the infection to hospital staff. This depends to a large extent on infectivity; therefore this must be ascertained. If not already requested, hepatitis serology consisting of hepatitis B surface antigen and antibodies, hepatitis core antigen and antibodies, and e antigen and antibodies should be checked. The infectivity state is high if the patient has hepatitis e antigen but no e antibodies. If the patient has e antibodies, her infectivity is not high. However, whatever her state of infectivity, she remains a risk to the hospital staff. A means of identifying this patient as carrying a BBI should be instituted. This may take the form of a label on the notes but such a label should be placed in such a way that the patient does not feel singled out or discriminated against. Most units will have a protocol for such patients and this should be followed.

There is currently no recognised treatment for hepatitis during pregnancy. However, there is a risk of the virus being transmitted to the fetus *in utero*. Such a fetus is at risk of FGR. There are no recognised congenital malformations associated with hepatitis B and therefore the infection is not generally considered an indication for termination of pregnancy.

If the mother has acute symptoms, treatment will be mainly symptomatic and supportive. This is usually in the form of analgesics and ensuring that she is generally well nourished and rests properly. In view of the risk of FGR, the fetus must be monitored with growth scans serially from 24 weeks' gestation. In most cases, fetal growth is normal and delivery is normal at term.

The course of the disease in the mother is unpredictable. There may be progression with significant deterioration in LFTs. In most cases, there are no alterations in these. The mother should, therefore, be monitored by means of serial LFTs, probably every month.

(b) She then presents in spontaneous labour at 39 weeks' gestation with intact membranes. How will you manage her from now onwards? (4 marks)

This infection is not an indication for a Caesarean section. Her labour should be managed as normal. If the membranes are intact, rupturing them should be delayed as long as possible. In addition, invasive procedures such as the application of an FSE and fetal blood sampling should be avoided. Prolonged labour should also be avoided especially if there is rupture of fetal membranes. It would be expected that all staff managing the patient will adopt universal precautions to reduce the risk of being infected and any samples sent to the laboratory should be identified as such. The neonatologist should be informed that she is in labour although there is no need for delivery to be attended by paediatricians. Ideally, this should happen antenatally so that a management plan is agreed and documented in the patient's notes. The infection-control counsellor must also be notified to initiate screening for other infections after appropriate counselling.

(c) What advice will you give her prior to discharge from the hospital? (4 marks)

Although the fetus may not be infected *in utero*, the mother may transmit the disease to her newborn child. In addition, fetal infection acquired *in utero* may progress if appropriate steps are not taken after delivery to minimise this. After delivery, therefore, the neonate should be given HBIG within 12 hours. Appropriate hepatitis vaccination should be offered 7 days later. A second dose is offered within 1–6 months of the first immunisation. At 12–15 months of age, the child should be tested for HbsAg. Breastfeeding is not contraindicated since the baby will be immunised at birth.

Since this infection may be transmitted to other members of the family, appropriate counselling and screening should be discussed and offered. Expert counsellors need to be involved. There is also the need to continue monitoring the antigen levels in the mother long after delivery, as chronic carrier status may persist and increase her risk of liver cirrhosis. Prior to her leaving hospital, appropriate contraception must be offered and counselling against other STIs discussed. The intrauterine contraceptive device is not an appropriate method but hormonal contraceptives can be offered provided there is no demonstrable effect on the liver.

3. A 28-year-old presents at 37 weeks' gestation with a diagnosis of herpes simplex type II vulval infection. (a) What advice will you give her in the antenatal clinic? (8 marks) (b) How will this infection modify her antenatal care? (4 marks) (c) She presents in labour at 40 weeks' gestation. How will you manage her? (8 marks)

Common mistakes

- Take a good history and perform a physical examination
- Detail sexual history
- Viral screen HIV – without counselling
- Treat for other STIs – without having screened for these
- Deliver by Caesarean section
- If membranes ruptured, Caesarean section immediately
- No place for vaginal delivery

A good answer will include some or all of these points

(a) What advice will you give her in the antenatal clinic? (8 marks)

- Common viral infection – sexually transmitted
- Need to exclude other STIs as they tend to coexist
- Risk of infection – transmission to the fetus greatest for primary infections occurring within 6 weeks of delivery, usually during labour
- Consequences – pneumonia, meningitis, poor feeding, chorioamnionitis, mental retardation, neonatal seizures and death
- Is it a recurrent (chronic) or primary (acute infection) diagnosis?
- Immunosuppression of pregnancy may result in systemic symptoms, such as fever, myalgia, malaise and aseptic meningitis

(b) How will this infection modify her antenatal care? (4 marks)

- Screen for other STIs, especially HIV and hepatitis
- Refer to GUM clinic or involve GUM physician for counselling
- Initiate treatment with aciclovir if primary infection
- Treat any symptoms – pain, difficulties passing urine
- Counsel about the risk of disseminated disease – unlikely unless immunocompromised
- Screen for herpes simplex virus (HSV)-specific antibodies – herpes simplex type I (HSV-1) and type 2 (HSV-2)
- Presence will influence mode of delivery and counselling
- Counsel about mode of delivery
- Intrapartum plan – when to rupture membranes, use of FSEs and when to perform scalp pH

(c) She presents in labour at 40 weeks' gestation. How will you manage her? (8 marks)

- Main problem is how to deliver:
  - Intact membranes – active disease – Caesarean section
  - Recurrent (chronic) disease – allow vaginal delivery – why?; ruptured membranes – less than 4 hours – Caesarean section, more than 4 hours – vaginal delivery; chronic (recurrent) – no lesions at the time of delivery – can active lesions really be excluded?
- Monitor the fetus – notify the neonatologist and watch out for early signs of infection in the neonate (localised – skin, eyes and/mouth, central nervous system – or disseminated herpes)

Sample answer

(a) What advice will you give her in the antenatal clinic? (8 marks)

Genital herpes infection is commonly due to HSV-2 although it can also be caused by HSV-1. It is a common viral infection transmitted sexually. The main problem with this infection in pregnancy, especially at this gestation, is that of transmitting the infection to the fetus and its consequences on the neonate. This risk is greatest with primary infections especially within 6 weeks of delivery. This patient is 37 weeks and therefore falls in this category and should be counselled as such.

The diagnosis of herpes infection in this patient will alter the management of her pregnancy, especially the method of delivery. It is important to establish whether this is a primary or recurrent infection. A history of previous infection(s) may be unreliable and therefore HSV-specific antibody testing should be discussed and offered. This should aim to relate the type of antibody present to the type of virus isolated from the genital tract.

If she has recurrent herpes, her management will be different. In this case, a vaginal delivery is possible. It has been argued that in these patients, because of the antibodies that they produce, the baby is offered some protection and therefore acquiring the virus during delivery does not pose significant consequences for the neonate. Others argue that since there is no guarantee that the neonate would have received the antibodies from the mother *in utero*, in the presence of active lesions, the baby should be delivered by Caesarean section. Nowadays, those with chronic infections are allowed to deliver vaginally.

The risk of her being infected with other STIs is increased. She should therefore either be offered screening in the obstetric unit or referred to the GUM unit for appropriate counselling and testing.

The risk of severe disease at this stage is higher than in early pregnancy. She must therefore be counselled about the systemic symptoms such as fever, myalgia, malaise and those of aseptic meningitis and to report to the hospital if she develops any of these symptoms.

(b) How will this infection modify her antenatal care? (4 marks)

The first modification of her antenatal care is to offer screening and counselling for other STIs, especially HIV and hepatitis. This may be provided by a GUM physician within the maternity setting or following a referral to the GUM unit. Investigating for herpes specific antibodies should be undertaken. This will determine whether the specific type (HSV-1 or -2) is an acute or recurrent infection. For the acute infection she would be started on aciclovir at a dose of 400 tds or 200 mg five times per day for 5 days. If there are features of disseminated herpes, then this should be intravenous.

Counselling about mode of delivery will depend of several factors, including the presence or absence of the antibodies. If the type of HSV isolated from the lesions in the genital tract is different from the antibody present or there are no antibodies, then delivery should be by Caesarean section. Appropriate counselling about delivery should be offered and a plan documented in her notes. It would be advisable to involve the neonatologist who would provide counselling about the risks of neonatal herpes, its clinical manifestations and how the baby would be monitored.

(c) She presents in labour at 40 weeks' gestation. How will you manage her? (8 marks)

If the patient had been diagnosed for the first time, she would have been booked for an elective Caesarean section, in which case an emergency Caesarean section would be offered especially if the membranes are intact or have ruptured less than 4 hours before presentation. If the membranes ruptured more than 4 hours before the baby is delivered, there are no obvious benefits from delivery by Caesarean section on the basis that the virus would have ascended into the uterus and infected the fetus.

If she is considered to be a recurrent case, then by the time of delivery the presence of active lesions from the genital tract may influence the mode of delivery. A vaginal examination should therefore be performed to locate active lesions before a decision is made about the mode of delivery. In the presence of active lesions and intact membranes, or rupture within 4 hours of presentation, a Caesarean section should be performed. The diagnosis of active disease by such a method is unreliable. The absence of lesions does not exclude active disease. If she is allowed to labour with intact membranes, rupturing them should be delayed for as long a possible. In addition, during labour, a FSE should be avoided as well as fetal blood sampling. The neonatologist must be notified and the newborn observed closely for early signs of infection. These may manifest as feeding difficulties, clinical features of pneumonia or meningitis. Since this is an STI, all efforts must be made to exclude other STIs and, where possible, contact screening and treatment should be considered and offered.

4. A schoolteacher in her first pregnancy at 6 weeks' gestation has been informed that one of her pupils has chickenpox infection. She is extremely worried. (a) What are the risks of the infection to her and the pregnancy? (6 marks) (b) How will you confirm that she has the infection? (8 marks) (c) If she has been confirmed to have acquired the infection, outline the steps you will take in her management. (6 marks)

Common mistakes

- Take a good history and do a physical examination
- Screen for risk factors for varicella
- List the possible congenital malformations associated with chickenpox infection
- Offer termination of pregnancy
- Refer to a virologist
- Admit and treat with aciclovir

A good answer will include some or all of these points

(a) What are the risks of the infection to her and the pregnancy? (6 marks)

- Maternal risks:
  - Morbidity such as:
    - Pneumonia – occurs in up to 10 per cent of women in pregnancy, severity greater with advancing gestation
    - Hepatitis
    - Encephalitis
  - Mortality
  - Long term – risk of developing shingles and neuralgia
- Fetal risks:
  - Risk of spontaneous miscarriage is not increased (in this trimester)
  - Risk of fetal varicella syndrome (FVS) is minimal if seroconversion occurred after 4 weeks (first 28 days of pregnancy)
  - Does not occur at the time of initial fetal infection but results from a subsequent herpes zoster reactivation *in utero*
  - Occurs only in a minority of fetuses
  - If seroconversion occurred before, then the risk of FVS is increased and this includes:
    - Skin scarring in a dermatological distribution
    - Eye defects (microphthalmia, chorioretinitis, cataracts)
    - Hypoplasia of the limbs
    - Neurological abnormalities (microcephaly, cortical atrophy, mental restriction, dysfunction of bowel and bladder sphincters
  - FGR

(b) How will you make a diagnosis of this infection in this woman? (8 marks)

- History:
  - Type of infection – shingles (e.g. unexposed thoracolumbar – no risk)
  - If disseminated or exposed (e.g. ophthalmic) or in immunocompromised individual, where viral shedding may be greater, then risk of infection higher until lesions are crusted
  - Timing of exposure – from the time of active lesions (2 days before the rash appears) until they are encrusted
  - Type of contact – this has to be significant – defined as being in the same room for at least 15 minutes, face-to-face contact and setting of an open ward
- Susceptibility of woman:
  - Definite history of infection or shingles? If positive, assume immune
  - Uncertain immune status – no obvious history or doubts of previous infection – test for varicella zoster virus (VZV) IgG (24–48 hours for results). Approximately 80–90 per cent of women would have antibodies and therefore be reassured
- Definite diagnosis:
  - Culture of virus from vesicles
  - IgM
  - Viral DNA detected by polymerase chain reaction (PCR)

(c) If she has been confirmed to have acquired the infection, outline the steps you will take in her management. (6 marks)

- Counselled to avoid contact with other susceptible individuals until lesions have crusted – other pregnant women and neonates
- Symptomatic treatment and hygiene to prevent secondary bacterial infection of lesions
- Aciclovir should be used cautiously at this gestation (UK Advisory Group on Chickenpox recommend that oral aciclovir should be prescribed if the woman presents within 24 hours of the rash and is more than 20 weeks' gestation)
- Counsel about the potential risk and benefits of treatment with aciclovir – no reported congenital malformations but data are limited (small numbers of women studied)
- Aciclovir has no benefit once rash has developed
- Management should be in the community but consider referral to hospital if:
  - Chest symptoms
  - Neurological symptoms
  - Haemorrhagic rash
  - Dense rash with or without mucosal lesions
  - Immmunosuppressed women

Sample answer

(a) What are the risks of the infection to her and the pregnancy? (6 marks)

Chickenpox is a viral infection that is common among children. It is highly infective and transmitted by droplets. It may cause severe morbidity and occasional mortality in pregnant mothers. The morbidity associated with this infection includes pneumonia, which may affect up to 10 per cent of women, hepatitis and encephalitis. These complications tend to be more severe in the immunocompromised. Since this virus can lie dormant and be reactivated, the woman is at risk of developing shingles and its associated neuralgia.

Although spontaneous miscarriages were initially thought to be increased with first trimester infections, there is evidence to suggest that this is not the case. Since this infection is at 6 weeks' gestation, the fetus is at risk of FVS. This is more likely if seroconversion occurs within the first 28 days of pregnancy (within which this patient falls). The features, which include skin scarring in a dermatological distribution, eye defects (microphthalmia, chorioretinitis, cortical atrophy, cataracts), hypoplasia of the limbs and neurological abnormalities (microcephaly, cortical atrophy, mental restriction, dysfunction of the bladder and anal sphincters), occur only in a minority of cases and usually not at the time of the primary fetal infection but with subsequent herpes zoster reactivation *in utero*. Fetal growth restriction may result from this early infection.

(b) How will you confirm that she has the infection? (8 marks)

The diagnosis will be confirmed first from an appropriate history and investigations. The history must investigate the type of infection to which she was exposed and her susceptibility. Exposure to someone with thoracolumbar shingles that is likely to be unexposed will not pose any risk to the woman. This is unlikely to be the scenario with a pupil. Although disseminated infection is more common in immunocompromised adults, it may occur in children and such individuals shed greater amounts of the virus and therefore increase the risk of infection. If the infected child had disseminated disease, especially one involving the eyes, then viral shedding would have been higher.

The time of exposure to the infected child should be ascertained as infectivity is from 2 days before the rash until encrustation. Finally, the type of contact should be established. Infection is more likely with significant contact, defined as spending at least 15 minutes in the same room as the infected individual, face-to-face contact and in the setting of an open ward. If the pupil is in the teacher's class, then she would most likely have had significant contact.

The susceptibility of the patient is important. Has she had VZV infection in the past? If her immune status is uncertain, IgG antibodies should be measured in her serum. The results should be available within 24–48 hours.

The definite diagnosis is made from culture of the virus from vesicular fluid by PCR identification of viral particulate DNA from the fluids. The presence of IgM antibodies will also indicate an acute infection but a negative does not exclude infection.

(c) If she has been confirmed to have acquired the infection, outline the steps you will take in her management. (6 marks)

The first step will be counselling on the symptoms of severe disease and the risk of infecting others. She must be removed from school and needs to avoid contact with other susceptible individuals, such as pregnant women and neonates. Symptomatic treatment should be instituted where appropriate, e.g. antipyretics and pain killers. If aciclovir is to be prescribed at 6 weeks' gestation, it must be with extreme caution. Although there are no reports of associated malformations, the UK Advisory Group on Chickenpox recommends commencing oral treatment within 24 hours of the rash appearing and if presentation is after 20 weeks (RCOG, 2007).

The benefits of treatment versus the uncertain risks to the fetus at this gestation should be discussed with the patient and treatment commenced if she desires. She should also be counselled about the risk of congenital malformations and plans should be made for an early ultrasound scan to date the pregnancy and for subsequent scans to exclude anomalies (preferably at a tertiary level) and for growth monitoring. Her management should be in the community with the proviso that with the development of chest symptoms, neurological symptoms, a haemorrhagic rash, a dense rash with or without mucosal lesions or if she is immunocompromised, then hospital care would be mandatory.

Reference

RCOG (2007) *Green-top Guideline No 13. Chickenpox in Pregnancy*. September 2007. London: Royal College of Gynaecologists.

5. A 28-year-old is diagnosed with HIV at 20 weeks' gestation. (a) What steps will you take to minimise the risk of transmission of HIV to the baby? (15 marks) (b) How would your management differ if the mother presented in labour having received no treatment? (5 marks)

Common mistakes

- Take a history and do a physical examination
- Exclude other STIs
- Counsel about protective sexual intercourse (use condoms)
- Barrier nursing

A good answer will include some or all of these points

(a) What steps will you take to minimise the risk of transmission of HIV to the baby? (15 marks)

- Transmission to the fetus – vertical – transplacental, during delivery and breastfeeding
- Transmission influenced by viral load, CD4 count and other genital tract infection, immune statues and comorbidities such as tuberculosis
- Procedures which increase the risk of fetomaternal haemorrhage will increase the risk of transmission:
  - Avoid invasive procedures such as amniocentesis, chorionic villus sampling (CVS) and external cephalic version (ECV). May be a place to offer first trimester nuchal translucency (NT) and biochemical screening
- Antiviral treatment – monitor by viral load and CD4
- Offer Caesarean section
- Avoid breastfeeding
- Treat neonate

(b) How would your management differ if she presented in labour having received no treatment? (5 marks)

- Vertical transmission occurs in >90 per cent of cases
- Start treatment with antiretroviral treatment
- Offer Caesarean section
- Avoid breastfeeding
- Test baby at birth and 6 weeks after
- Treat baby with antiviral drugs for at least 6 weeks
- Counsel about screening for other STIs
- Offer contraception – preferably barrier methods
- Arrange follow-up with GUM to ensure that partner is screened and adequate screening offered

Sample answer

(a) What steps will you take to minimise the risk of transmission of HIV to the baby? (15 marks)

Human immunodeficiency virus infection is a blood-borne viral infection, which is transmitted sexually, via blood products or by shared needles. It is more common in homosexuals, intravenous drug users and those from endemic areas. The disease is transmitted vertically to the fetus during pregnancy, transplacentally, during labour and in the neonatal and infant periods through breastfeeding.

If untreated, this HIV-positive woman has approximately a 25–30 per cent risk of transmitting the virus to her fetus *in utero*. During breastfeeding, the risk is of the order of 50–60 per cent. Once the fetus or baby is infected, there is a high morbidity and mortality. Transmission is greatest with a high viral load, a low CD4 count, comorbidity and genital tract infections.

Reducing the transmission risks *in utero* and after delivery must therefore minimise these risk factors. The first step to minimise the risk of transmission is to reduce the viral load in the mother. This is done by offering the mother combination antiviral treatment. The most commonly used antiviral treatment is AZT. However, other highly active antiretroviral therapy (HAART) may be used. Treatment should be commenced at 20 weeks, but if the mother is reluctant to accept this, it must be commenced at 34 weeks at the latest, since >90 per cent of vertical transmission occurs after 34 weeks. Given during pregnancy, it reduces the viral load in the mother and therefore the risk of transmission to the fetus from 25–30 per cent to 8 per cent. The treatment must be offered with expert advice from an HIV specialist – usually a GUM consultant. She should also be screened and treated for other STIs and comorbidities such as tuberculosis. The treatment should be monitored with the patient's viral load and her CD4 count.

In this patient, any procedure that may increase the risk of fetomaternal haemorrhage should be avoided, unless it is not practicable to do so. Procedures such as amniocentesis, CVS and ECV should therefore be kept to a minimum. If the patient requires prenatal diagnosis, the least invasive test should be offered. It is in precisely this type of patient that prenatal diagnosis by a combination of NT and biochemistry in the late first trimester may be more appropriate. This will reduce the numbers being exposed to invasive testing.

Delivery by Caesarean section has been shown to significantly reduce the risk of vertical transmission to the fetus. The patient should therefore be offered an elective Caesarean section. Intravenous antiretroviral therapy should be given to the mother prior to delivery of the baby. In addition, she should avoid breastfeeding. The baby should be offered antiviral drugs for 6 weeks starting 8–12 hours after the birth. These measures will significantly reduce the risk of vertical transmission.

(b) How would your management differ if the mother presented in labour having received no treatment? (5 marks)

Most vertical transmission of HIV occurs after the 36th week; hence the baby is at a significantly greater risk of vertical transmission. Treatment should be instituted either before or

39

after delivery. This will not make a significant difference to the risk of transmission to the fetus. The patient should have a Caesarean section and avoid breastfeeding. The baby should have a blood test for viral count and antibody measurements. However, a negative antibody test does not exclude vertical transmission. This antibody test should be repeated after 6 weeks.

It is important that all labour ward staff take the necessary universal precautions to minimise the risk of cross-infection. Screening for other STIs needs to be discussed and offered before discharge from the hospital. Arrangements should be made follow-up in the community, including screening of her partner.

3

Hypertensive disorders in pregnancy

1. A primigravida presents with hypertension and proteinuria at 35 weeks' gestation. (a) Justify the investigations you will undertake on the patient. (8 marks) (b) How will you manage her pregnancy? (12 marks)

2. A 32-year-old primigravida with pre-eclampsia (PET) at 39 weeks' gestation has just had a fit in labour. (a) What complications may ensue if she is poorly managed? (7 marks) (b) Justify the steps you will take in her management. (13 marks)

3. A 27-year-old known hypertensive, in her first pregnancy, books for antenatal care at 10 weeks' gestation. (a) Discuss the complications that she may have and how you will diagnose them. (6 marks) (b) What steps will you take to improve the outcome of pregnancy? (14 marks)

4. A 26-year-old books for antenatal care at 8 weeks' gestation. (a) Briefly discuss the risk factors for PET that you will obtain from her history. (8 marks) (b) How may you reduce the risk of her developing PET? (12 marks)

5. Mrs BOC is 36 years old, in her first pregnancy, at 38 weeks' gestation. She attended the antenatal clinic and was found to have blood pressure (BP) of 160/120 mmHg and two plusses of protein. She has had a headache associated with nausea and vomiting over the past 2 days. (a) Evaluate the options available to her. (6 marks) (b) Soon after an elective Caesarean section, she continues to bleed and investigations suggest that she has disseminated intravascular coagulation (DIC). Justify your management. (10 marks) What advice will you give her at her postnatal follow-up visit? (4 marks)

1. A primigravida presents with hypertension and proteinuria at 35 weeks' gestation. (a) Justify the investigations you will undertake on her. (8 marks) (b) How will you manage her pregnancy? (12 marks)

Common mistakes

- Discussing the diagnosis of PET
- Listing the complications of PET
- Manage in the community
- Refer to hypertensive team
- Deliver by Caesarean section
- Monitor fetus

A good answer will include some or all of these points

(a) Justify the investigations you will undertake on the patient. (8 marks)

- Maternal:
  - Full blood count (FBC) – checking for thrombocytopenia – gauge severity of disease
  - Urea and electrolytes (U&Es) – creatinine and urea
  - Serum urates – abnormally high values indicate severe disease
  - Clotting screen – fibrinogen and fibrinogen degradation products (FDPs)
  - Liver function test (LFT) – alanine aminotransferase (AST)/alkaline phosphatase
  - Quantification of proteinuria – 24-hour urine collection for protein – quantification is more reliable than dipstix
  - Urinary protein: creatinine ratio – a useful tool for assessing and provide baseline for monitoring of disease
  - 24-hour BP measurement (ambulatory BP measurement) – provides a more reliable assessment of severity of hypertension and the rhythm – any change in diurnal pattern?
- Fetal:
  - Ultrasound scan for growth – abdominal and head circumference and liquor volume
  - Doppler scan of the umbilical artery, middle cerebral artery and ductus venosus may be indicated where there is severe fetal growth restriction (FGR)
  - Cardiotocography (CTG)

(b) How will you manage her pregnancy? (12 marks)

- Admit and monitor:
  - Monitor:
    - Signs of severe disease, etc.

- 4-hourly BP
- Daily urinalysis
- Twice-weekly biochemistry and haematology tests or more frequent, depending on the severity and progression
- Fluid balance – intake and output
- BP – high – treat:
  - Intermediate: nifedipine oral (20 mg slow release (SR)) or intravenous labetalol or hydralazine
  - Control BP – methyldopa, nifedipine, labetalol
- Severe disease – indwelling catheter, intensive therapy unit charts, group and save, involve anaesthetist and paediatricians (severe disease, baby likely to be small), magnesium sulphate, etc.
- Deliver:
  - Severe disease – once stabilised deliver after assessment of cervix, unlikely to be favourable; therefore most likely a Caesarean section. If favourable, induce (prostaglandin or artificial rupture of fetal membranes and Syntocinon®)
  - When and how, Caesarean section, induce, etc.
- Other options – manage as outpatient once stabilised and mild disease?
- Monitor fetus – serial growth scan every 2 weeks and Doppler studies if indicated

Sample answer

(a) Justify the investigations you will undertake on the patient. (8 marks)

These will either be maternal or fetal. Maternal investigations would first confirm the diagnosis and then form the baseline on which subsequent monitoring for progression would be based. These include a FBC (specifically thrombocytopenia whose presence indicates disease severity), U&Es, which are indicators of renal impairment, serum uric acid (values above gestation-specific upper limits are useful in gauging disease severity), fibrinogen and FDPs (fibrinogen levels fall while FDPs rise with disease severity), LFT (AST and serum proteins – transaminases rise with hepatocellular damage while protein levels fall with severe disease) and quantification of proteinuria from a 24-hour urine collection (more reliable than random urinalysis). Additionally, the creatinine clearance rate and protein: creatinine ratio could be estimated from the urine collection. A 24-hour BP recording will provide a better assessment of the degree of hypertension. These investigations should be repeated with a frequency determined by the disease severity and perceived progression.

Fetal investigations include an ultrasound scan (head circumference, abdominal circumference, femur length and amniotic fluid index) to assess growth. FGR is an important complication of early onset and severe PET. When FGR is present, Doppler studies of the umbilical artery and other vessels such as the ductus venosus and middle cerebral artery become useful in monitoring and therefore the timing of delivery. If the woman is admitted for the disease, it would be reasonable to perform regular CTG although its value is questionable. In addition, how often this should be done remains controversial but at least once daily would be reasonable.

(b) How will you manage her pregnancy? (12 marks)

The patient should be admitted for further assessment. The severity of the disease, which depends on associated symptoms and signs, and the results of various investigations, will determine subsequent management. The symptoms are headaches, visual disturbances, right upper abdominal pain and altered sensorium while the signs include hyper-reflexia, ankle clonus and right hypochondrial tenderness.

Her initial inpatient monitoring should include a strict fluid input/output chart, 4-hourly BP measurements and observation for early signs of imminent eclampsia, such as nausea and vomiting, severe headaches, epigastric pain, altered sensorium and visual disturbances.

For mild disease (BP <150/95 mmHg and normal or slightly deranged biochemical and haematological indices), there may be a case for allowing the patient home with close monitoring by the community midwife. However, she must have ready access to the hospital and should not be on her own. Appropriate counselling about the signs of deterioration and imminent eclampsia should be offered before she is allowed home. In some units, this is not an option, the reasoning being that PET is known to progress very rapidly to eclampsia without any warning. If the patient's BP is high (consistently above 150/100 mmHg or mean arterial pressure (MAP) >110 mmHg) then treatment with an antihypertensive, such as methyldopa, labetalol or nifedipine, should be instituted. In addition to maternal monitoring, fetal monitoring in the form of regular CTGs, biophysical profilometry and Doppler velocimetry of the umbilical and middle cerebral arteries will be performed. Fetal kick charts, though often used, are not reliable and are of little objective benefit.

Pregnancy should be allowed to progress to term and labour induced if there are no contraindications to a vaginal delivery with mild disease. For severe disease, the patient should be delivered. How and where delivery occurs will depend on several factors including fetal presentation, the state of the cervix and the fetus, and the wishes of the patient. If the cervix is unfavourable and there is deterioration in the maternal condition, delivery by Caesarean section would be the best option. However, in the absence of any obvious deterioration in maternal condition or a contraindication, a vaginal delivery with epidural analgesia in labour should be the option of choice, provided the cervix is favourable and the platelet count is normal.

The management of this patient must be tailored to suit her needs. Inpatient management on an outpatient basis may be suitable but the danger of rapid progression to eclampsia and its attendant complications needs to be recognised before accepting such an approach.

2. A 32-year-old primigravida with PET at 39 weeks' gestation has just had a fit in labour. (a) What complications may ensue if she is poorly managed? (7 marks) (b) Justify the steps you will take in her management. (13 marks)

Common mistakes

- Take a history and do a physical examination
- Observe the fit and then exclude other causes of fits
- Deliver by Caesarean section
- Offer general anaesthesia
- Intravenous hydrazaline/labetalol
- Investigate and manage accordingly

A good answer will include some or all of these points

(a) What complications may ensue if she is poorly managed? (7 marks)

- Hypertensive stroke
- Cardiac failure
- Hepatic failure
- Maternal death
- DIC and postpartum haemorrhage
- Renal failure
- Cortical blindness
- Intrauterine fetal death
- Venous thromboembolism (VTE)
- Psychological sequelae

(b) Justify the steps you will take in her management. (13 marks)

- Ensure availability of senior obstetrician (consultant) and anaesthetist – obstetric emergency requiring multidisciplinary team working
- Stop the fits – magnesium sulphate ($MgSO_4$) intravenous 4 g stat, then maintenance with 2 g every 4 hours
- Control airway and ensure breathing
- Control BP – immediate and long term
- Intravenous line and take bloods for FBC, blood group and save, U&Es, LFTs, uric acid
- Indwelling catheter – fluid input/output
- Monitor fetus – is fetus alive and not in distress?
- Assess cervix – vaginal delivery?
- Caesarean section if unfavourable

- Epidural?
- Watch oxygen saturation levels and central venous pressure (CVP)
- High dependency unit (HDU)/intensive care unit (ICU) care
- Any clotting problems?
- Counselling after

Sample answer

(a) What complications may ensue if she is poorly managed? (7 marks)

The complications of poorly managed eclampsia can be categorised under various systems. Cardiovascular complications include hypertensive stroke (more commonly due to elevated systolic BP and cardiac failure. A constricted intravascular volume may result in renal failure and VTE; while hepatocellular damage may lead to hepatic failure. Other complications are DIC and HELLP syndrome (haemolysis, elevated liver enzymes, low platelet count), cortical blindness, intrauterine fetal death and maternal death. Following delivery, postpartum haemorrhage may result from DIC, placental abruption or severe hepatocellular damage. Maternal mortality may result from any of the complications above, although it may be iatrogenic (secondary to fluid overload caused during management). Most patients who have had an eclamptic fit suffer from psychological sequelae which may be non-specific.

(b) Justify the steps you will take in her management. (13 marks)

This is an obstetric emergency and its management should involve a consultant obstetrician, an anaesthetist and experienced midwives. Management should aim for maximum safety to the mother and the fetus. The airway must be secured to ensure that the patient is breathing. This could be achieved by turning the patient on to her left side and inserting a Guedel's mouthpiece, or another mouthpiece, which will prevent the tongue from falling back and blocking the airway or being bitten during another fit.

Any fits should be stopped by the administration of intravenous $MgSO_4$ 4 g slowly over a period of 10–15 minutes followed by 2 g every 2 hours for maintenance and suppression of further fits. Randomised controlled trials have shown conclusively that this regimen is not only more effective in stopping convulsions but is associated with fewer side-effects (both to the mother and fetus) than intravenous diazepam in the management of eclampsia. With the administration of this drug, an intravenous line should be secured and bloods collected for a FBC, U&Es, creatinine and uric acid levels, group and save, LFTs and fibrinogen and FDPs. An indwelling urethral catheter will facilitate the monitoring of urinary output, especially as eclampsia may be complicated by prerenal renal failure. A strict fluid input/output chart would identify any significant imbalance between input and output, which could precede overload and resulting pulmonary oedema.

The BP should be controlled, as failure to do so may result in cerebrovascular accidents. The first option to achieve this will be a fast-acting antihypertensive agent. The choice will be between hydralazine, nifedipine or labetalol. The best drug for this patient would be hydralazine; this is fast-acting and can be given intravenously. It may have to be repeated to lower the BP. The disadvantage of hydralazine administration this way is that the rapid drop in BP that it induces may cause significant fetal hypoxia. Maintenance doses may thereafter be administered intravenously using the MAP as a tool to titrate the dose of antihypertensive. Labetalol is equally effective and could therefore be given as an alternative. However, to use nifedipine the patient should ideally be able to swallow, although it may be administered sub-lingually.

The ultimate treatment for eclampsia is delivering the baby. However, before this is achieved, the mother must be stabilised, as contractions may provoke further fits. She should therefore be given a continuous infusion of $MgSO_4$ and monitored for toxicity by magnesium levels, knee reflexes, urinary output and respiratory rate. Once she is stable and her BP is controlled, the baby must be delivered. The best means of delivery is vaginal, unless there are contraindications. The cervix should first be assessed, and if it is favourable, the fetal membranes should be ruptured and Syntocinon® commenced to initiate contractions. Where the cervix is unfavourable, a Caesarean section is preferable to a difficult, and possibly failed, induction. It is important to keep stress to a minimum in this patient as this may precipitate further fits. Before embarking on the plan of delivery, fetal wellbeing should be assessed. CTG will confirm that the fetus is alive and also whether it is in distress. If in distress, delivery is best achieved quickly, usually by Caesarean section under general anaesthesia. If the fetal heart rate is normal and there is no coagulopathy, an epidural will be ideal for Caesarean section as it not only lowers the BP but minimises further stress, which could provoke further fits.

A central venous line will minimise the risk of circulatory overload. A pulmonary wedge pressure may be required in some cases. A HDU monitoring chart should be commenced and transfer to a HDU or ICU considered if there is deterioration or there are no facilities for optimum monitoring. Once the clinical symptoms have improved, time must be set aside to offer supportive counselling and a detailed explanation of the complication, the management and implications for any future pregnancies.

3. A 27-year-old known hypertensive, in her first pregnancy, books for antenatal care at 10 weeks' gestation. (a) Discuss the complications that she may have and how you will diagnose them. (6 marks) (b) What steps will you take to improve the outcome of pregnancy? (14 marks)

Common mistakes

- Refer her to a physician
- Routine screening for antenatal clinic
- Take a history and do a physical examination
- Treat cause of hypertension
- Offer dietary advice
- Refer patient to tertiary centre

A good answer will include some or all of these points

(a) Discuss the complications that she may have and how you will diagnose them. (6 marks)

Maternal:
- Superimposed PET – most common (complicates 5–50 per cent of chronic hypertensive pregnancies)
- Congestive heart failure
- Acute renal failure
- Placental abruption – most common
- DIC
- Maternal death
- Fetal:
  - FGR
  - Intrauterine fetal death
  - Iatrogenic preterm delivery

(b) What steps will you take to improve the outcome of pregnancy? (14 marks)

- Assess disease – any associated complications?
- Medication – switching to less teratogenic agents?
- Screening for indicators
- Complications of hypertension
- Severity of hypertension
- Pregnancy complications
- FGR

- PET
- Control of BP – medication
- Involvement of physicians
- Monitoring of fetal growth
- Monitor renal function
- Delivery
- Role of uterine artery Doppler scans plus aspirin?

Sample answer

(a) Discuss the complications that she may have and how you will diagnose them. (6 marks)

The maternal complications of hypertension in pregnancy include superimposed PET and eclampsia, congestive cardiac failure, acute renal failure, placental abruption, DIC and maternal death. Superimposed PET occurs in approximately 5–50 per cent of chronic hypertensive pregnancies. The diagnosis of most of these complications will be based on early warning signs such as an increase in BP and proteinuria. Close monitoring (clinical, biochemical and haematological) is therefore essential to ensure early diagnosis and timed interventions.

Fetal complications include intrauterine growth restriction, intrauterine fetal death and iatrogenic prematurity and its associated consequences. Regular ultrasound scans for fetal growth and associated fetal monitoring by means of biophysical profilometry and Doppler velocimetry of the umbilical artery and other fetal vessels will not only identify FGR but will enable timely interventions which will minimise the risk of intrauterine fetal death.

(b) What steps will you take to improve the outcome of pregnancy? (14 marks)

The first step must be one which excludes other risk factors, the presence of which will significantly increase the risk of complications. These risk factors include the cause of the hypertension (essential or secondary to renal/other diseases), a family history of hypertension and PET, obesity or associated medical conditions that are independent of the hypertension.

The next step would be to assess the severity of the hypertension. If the patient's BP is very high and she is not on regular medication, she needs to be placed on an antihypertensive agent. This must be after consultation with a physician. Drugs with known teratogenicity (e.g. angiotensin-converting enzyme (ACE) inhibitors) should be avoided. If she is already on medication, this must be reviewed and changed to a less teratogenic agent if necessary. Hypertension may be due to several causes. If the cause is known, appropriate screening must be offered to ensure that there is no deterioration in this cause. The renal and cardiovascular systems need to be examined and investigated thoroughly for evidence of involvement secondary to the hypertension. The fundi should also be examined, as they may indicate the severity of the disease.

Ultrasound scan of the fetus to exclude anomalies will be performed as routine, but if the patient's antihypertensive drugs were teratogenic, then she must be screened for the specific

49

anomalies that may result. In addition, a uterine artery Doppler scan at 20 and 24 weeks' gestation may indicate the risk of the patient developing PET. Later in pregnancy, serial growth scans and liquor volume estimation will identify abnormal fetal growth. Unfortunately, FGR cannot be prevented, but early identification and timely intervention will prevent the complications of intrauterine fetal death and severe intrauterine hypoxia.

During pregnancy, tight control of the patient's BP and regular screening for proteinuria will be necessary to reduce the risk of FGR and PET. It is essential to involve physicians in the care of the patient throughout the pregnancy, even more so if her BP is difficult to control. Renal function should be monitored regularly, and whenever necessary her drug requirements should be reviewed. This is especially important in view of altered physiology during pregnancy. In the first trimester, vomiting may require more frequent administration of antihypertensive drugs, whereas in the second trimester dosages may be reduced in view of the physiological drop in BP.

The timing of delivery will depend on the control of the patient's BP and associated complications. In the absence of any complications, pregnancy should be allowed to go to term. However, when complications occur, appropriate measures need to be taken, including delivery. The method of delivery will be determined by several predominantly obstetric factors.

The role of aspirin in the management of this patient is controversial. If uterine artery Doppler scans are abnormal, she is certainly at a greater risk of PET. However, by the time the uterine Doppler scans are undertaken it may be too late for aspirin to be of any benefit. It may, therefore, be advisable to start the patient on aspirin (75 mg daily) at 10 weeks' gestation and await the results of the uterine artery Doppler scans. If the Doppler scans are normal, the aspirin could be discontinued and if not, it should be continued to at least the end of 34 weeks, as this has been shown to reduce the incidence and severity of PET.

4. A 26-year-old books for antenatal care at 8 weeks' gestation. (a) Briefly discuss the risk factors for PET that you will obtain from her history. (8 marks) (b) How may you reduce the risk of her developing PET? (12 marks)

Common mistakes

- Assuming that the patient has severe PET
- Delivery by Caesarean section
- Discussing the complications of PET
- Assessing the state of the cervix and delivery at 30 weeks' gestation without justifying why
- Monitor mother and fetus – being non-specific

A good answer will contain some or all of these points

(a) Briefly discuss the risk factors for PET that you will obtain from her history. (8 marks)

- General:
  - Obesity – BMI 30 kg/m^2 is associated with an approximate doubling of the risk
- Genetic factors:
  - Mother with history of PET, risk of developing PET is 20–25 per cent
  - Sister with PET, risk may be as high as 30–40 per cent
- Past obstetric history:
  - Primiparity (risk 2–3-fold)
  - Multiple gestation (2-fold increase risk for twins)
  - Previous PET (7-fold increased risk)
  - Long birth interval (2–3-fold increased risk)
- Medical factors:
  - Pre-existing hypertension
  - Renal disease
  - Diabetes mellitus (pre-existing or gestational)
  - Antiphospholipid syndrome
  - Connective tissue disease
  - Inherited thrombophilia

(b) How may you reduce the risk of her developing PET? (12 marks)

- Identification of risk factors
- Aspirin in high risk (e.g. previous PET)
- Uterine artery Doppler at 20–24 weeks (presence of notching and high resistance index)
- Close monitoring of BP and urine after 24 weeks' gestation

- Treatment of risk factors and prophylaxis where appropriate (Fragmin® for antiphospholipid syndrome)
- Steroid for connective tissue disorders
- Early institution of treatment with safe and long-acting drugs
- Timely delivery based on clinical and obstetric factors

Sample answer

(a) Briefly discuss the risk factors for PET that you will obtain from her history. (8 marks)

Risk factors for PET can be grouped under general, genetic, medical and past obstetric. Obesity (BMI >30 kg/m²) is associated with a doubling of the risk of PET. Genetic factors include a history of PET in the mother or sister. A positive maternal history is associated with a 20–25 per cent increased risk while a history of PET in a sibling increases the risk by 30–40 per cent. Risk factors in the past medical history include pre-existing hypertension (5–10 per cent of these patients will develop PET), renal disease, diabetes mellitus (pregestational and gestational), antiphospholipid syndrome, connective tissue disorders and inherited thrombophilia. The precise rate by which these factors increase the risk is uncertain.

Being a primigravida increases the risk of PET 2–3-fold, while multiple pregnancies increase the risk by at least 2-fold (for twins). A history of PET increases the risk 7-fold while a long birth interval is reported to increase the risk by 2–3-fold. The timing of onset and severity of PET in previous pregnancies is important as the earlier the onset, the more likely it is to be severe and this is associated with a greater risk of recurrence.

(b) How may you reduce the risk of her developing PET? (12 marks)

The first step in reducing the risk of developing PET is identification of any risk factors. Those at risk should then be referred for further screening (by means of haematological or biochemical investigations) if appropriate. The administration of low-dose aspirin has been shown to reduce the chances of PET developing in the high-risk population. Where there is known thrombophilia, low-molecular-weight heparin (unfractionated heparin) initiated early not only reduces the risk of early pregnancy demise but that of PET. In those with connective tissue diseases, institution of steroids may be beneficial. Those with pre-existing hypertension should be treated with appropriate medication ensuring that those contraindicated in pregnancy, such as ACE inhibitors, are avoided.

The best screening tool for PET is uterine artery Doppler between 20 and 24 weeks' gestation. The presence of notches and or high resistance after 22 weeks is taken to represent incomplete physiological adaptation of the spiral arteries. Such patients are at a significant risk of developing PET and should be monitored closely preferably in a consultant-led unit. They may also be given aspirin (low dose).

Early identification of early-onset disease will ensure timely interventions to reduce consequences and progression to eclampsia. This is dependent entirely on monitoring of BP and regular urinalysis. When PET develops, timely delivery will minimise the risk of complications.

5. Mrs BOC is 36 years old, in her first pregnancy, at 38 weeks' gestation. She attended the antenatal clinic and was found to have a BP of 160/120 mmHg and two plusses of protein. She has had a headache associated with nausea and vomiting over the past 2 days. (a) Evaluate the options available to her. (6 marks) (b) Soon after an elective Caesarean section, she continues to bleed and investigations suggest that she has DIC. Justify your management. (10 marks) What advice will you give her at her postnatal follow-up visit? (4 marks)

Common mistakes

- Take a history and physical examination
- Treat with $MgSO_4$ – no details
- Antihypertensives – which ones?
- Refer to tertiary centre – no reason
- Uterine artery Doppler scan to monitor pregnancy
- Ultrasound scan for fetal growth and Dopper scans – why?

A good answer will include some or all of these points

(a) Evaluate the options available to her. (6 marks)

- Diagnosis – PET
- Options – admit to the ward? Or delivery suite? Why?
- Benefits of admission – investigate for severity – bloods, etc.
- Examine for sign of severity – why?
- Treat hypertension – which drug to administer and when to treat?
- Nifedipine? Hydrazaline? Labetalol? Methyldopa?
- $MgSo_4$ – why?
- Deliver – how?
- Examine/assess cervix?
- Caesarean section or vaginal delivery?
- Monitor fetus – how and benefits?
- Monitor mother – biochemistry, fluid balance, etc.

(b) Soon after an elective Caesarean section, she continues to bleed and investigations suggest that she has DIC. Justify your management. (10 marks)

- Intravenous cannulae – large bore (preferably at least size 16 but preferably size 12–14)
- Inform haematology laboratory
- Involve consultant obstetrician and obstetric anaesthetists
- Consider CVP or central line

- Group and cross-match 6 units of blood
- Cross-match platelets and frozen plasma
- Recombinant factor VII
- Surgery – brace suture, hysterectomy

(c) What advice will you give her at her postnatal follow-up visit? (4 marks)

- Recurrence risk – high
- Needs to be investigated if not already investigated – FBC, U&Es, LFTs, thrombophilia screen, antiphospholipid screen
- May benefit from acetylsalicylic acid in early pregnancy
- If positive for thrombophilia or antiphospholipid syndrome, will require Fragmin® throughout pregnancy and the puerperium
- Antenatal care and delivery should be in a consultant-based unit with ICU facilities for the neonates

Sample answer

(a) Evaluate the options available to her. (6 marks)

Mrs BOC has PET and requires admission and delivery. The options are admission onto the ward or the delivery suite and the timing of delivery. Admission will ensure close monitoring, early identification of deterioration and timely intervention. Admitting to the delivery suite has several advantages over admission onto the ward – there is likely to be more intense observation than on the ward. In addition, there is usually easy availability of medical and better skilled midwifery staff, should she develop eclampsia. She is 38 weeks and will require delivering, which would be achieved on the delivery suite. Admission also allows for investigations for severity of disease and the state of the fetus. Such investigations include biochemistry, haematological, frequent urinalysis and a strict input and output chart.

Examination of the patient will identify any signs of severe disease such as hyper-reflexia and ankle clonus. An automatic BP measurement will provide regular measurements although the values obtained may be lower than those with a traditional mercury sphygmomanometer.

The treatment options will depend on the severity of the PET. If there is need to control her BP quickly, and she is able to tolerate it orally, nifedipine SR is one of three options. The others are labetalol and hydrazaline. These other options are administered intravenously. Hydrazaline can cause a rapid fall in BP and associated fetal hypoxia; hence when administered, it should be given over a period of 5–10 minutes.

Whether she is given $MgSO_4$ will depend on the assessment of the severity of the PET. If it is considered severe, $MgSO_4$ has been shown to reduce progression to eclampsia.

Delivery will depend on the state of the cervix, and fetal health. An abdominal examination, fetal monitoring and a vaginal examination will be the appropriate options following admission. Where the cervix is unfavourable or the fetus is in distress, delivery would be advisably by Caesarean section. An epidural in the absence of thrombocytopenia is recommended, as it lowers BP and reduces the stimulation of pain which could provoke an eclamptic fit.

(b) Soon after an elective Caesarean section, she continues to bleed and investigations suggest that she has disseminated intravascular coagulation (DIC). Justify your management. (10 marks)

The first step is to ensure that there she has at least two large-bore cannulae. During the securing of an intravenous access, blood should be sent for an FBC and cross-match of at least 6 units of blood. In addition, platelets should be cross-matched and fresh frozen plasma requested. It may be necessary to get the anaesthetist to site the Venflon® if this is proving difficult, as is often the case in these patients because of oedema. The consultant obstetrician and haematologist (including the blood bank) should be informed. The anaesthetist should insert a CVP line. Her management will consist of blood transfusion – replacement of especially coagulation factors and for this, fresh frozen plasma will be ideal. Blood transfusion should be administered to ensure that the haemoglobin does not fall significantly. If the bleeding continues despite replacement therapy, recombinant factor VII may be considered.

Surgery should only be considered as a last option; even this is fraught with difficulties as bleeding tends to be generalised and difficult to control. The surgical options include the brace suture, a hysterectomy and, rarely, interventional radiology in the form of uterine artery embolisation. Prior to this a balloon (e.g. Bakri®) catheter may be applied into the uterus to establish whether this will stop the bleeding through a tamponade effect. Renal failure may result from hypovolaemia, hence an indwelling catheter is essential for strict monitoring of fluid intake and output. In addition, regular renal function tests should be performed.

(c) What advice will you give her at her postnatal follow-up visit? (4 marks)

At the postnatal visit, the advice she will be offered will contain the recurrence risk, which is higher than the background risk. In addition, she will need to be investigated if this had not been already undertaken. This is unlikely as transfusion or the administration of fresh frozen plasma is known to alter the profile of some of the indices being screened. Enough time must therefore be given for these to return to normal. The investigations to be instituted will include those for acquired and inherited thrombophilia, antiphospholipid syndrome, an LFT and renal function tests. If any of the thrombophilias are positive, she will benefit from unfractionated heparin throughout the next pregnancy and possibly the puerperium. Any subsequent pregnancies must be cared for in a consultant unit with facilities for intensive care.

4

Medical disorders in pregnancy

1. A 28-year-old known epileptic on sodium valproate presents at 10 weeks' gestation. (a) What complications may she have by virtue of this condition? (6 marks) (b) What steps will you take to minimise these complications? (10 marks) (c) If she had presented for pre-pregnancy counselling, what advice would you have given her? (4 marks)

2. A 33-year-old woman presented at 38 weeks' gestation with chronic cough, night sweats and right-sided chest pain. She is unemployed and has two other children at home. You suspect that she may have tuberculosis (TB). (a) What additional relevant information will you obtain from her? (4 marks) (b) How will you confirm the diagnosis? (4 marks) (c) Briefly outline your management of this patient if the diagnosis is confirmed. (12 marks)

3. Critically appraise the screening for diabetes mellitus in pregnancy. (20 marks)

4. An obese diabetic woman books for antenatal care at 6 weeks' gestation. (a) Enumerate the risks of this pregnancy. (8 marks) (b) What steps will you take to improve the pregnancy outcome? (8 marks) (c) What advice will you give her postnatally? (4 marks)

5. A 26-year-old woman with cardiac disease grade III is admitted in labour at 40 weeks' gestation. (a) What steps will you take to minimise the complications of her cardiac disease? (6 marks) (b) Briefly outline the steps you will take to minimise these complications. (14 marks)

1. A 28-year-old known epileptic on sodium valproate presents at 10 weeks' gestation. (a) What complications may arise because of her epilepsy? (6 marks) (b) What steps will you take to minimise these complications? (10 marks) (c) If she had presented for pre-pregnancy counselling, what advice would you have given her? (4 marks)

Common mistakes

- Take a history and do a physical examination
- Discussing different types of epilepsy and the risks associated with each type of epilepsy
- Elaborating on the past obstetric and medical histories
- Listing the complications of epilepsy in pregnancy
- Management to be transferred to physician
- Offer Caesarean section, irrespective of any other indication or reason
- Failure to distinguish between the different parts of the question
- Paediatrician to be present at the time of delivery

A good answer will include some or all of these points

(a) What complications may she have by virtue of this condition? (6 marks)

- Increased seizures – 33 per cent of women have an increased frequency of seizures during pregnancy
- Risk of status epilepticus – but this is not significantly higher than outwith pregnancy
- Complications related to antiepileptic drugs (AEDs). These depend on the type of AED:
  - Neural tube defects (NTDs)
  - Facial clefting
  - Fetal AED syndrome (a combination of malformations)
  - Coagulopathies in approximately 50 per cent of neonates whose mothers are on phenobarbitone, primidone or phenytoin (most women are on more modern AEDs)
- Increased risk of seizures in offspring
- Fetal asphyxia from repeated seizures

(b) What steps will you take to minimise these complications? (10 marks)

- Optimise antiepileptic therapy to ensure good seizure control – combined care with physician:
  - Assessed by physician (neurologist) – evaluation of patient for factors that will favour withdrawal of AEDs:
    - Seizure free for more than 2 years?
    - Age at onset of seizures
    - Seizure type
    - Number of seizures before control achieved

- Folic acid 5 mg to continue throughout pregnancy
- Control of seizures – should be determined clinically using drug levels to provide guidance only
- Screen for malformations – detailed ultrasound scan
- Serum screening – alpha-fetoprotein (AFP); part of aneuploidy testing but may be useful for NTDs (not as reliable as ultrasound scan)
- See regularly to ensure no need to increase dosage of AED
- Oral vitamin K 10 mg daily from 36 weeks' gestation
- Intrapartum management – similar to that of any obstetric patient but must avoid hyperventilation (potent analgesia recommended)
- Postpartum – monitor drug levels (physiological alterations cause an increase during pregnancy which must be reduced)
- Watch out for tonic–clonic convulsions, which occur in 1 per cent of patients during the first postnatal day
- Intramuscular vitamin K to the neonate
- Driving and bathing baby
- Contraception – less effective with AEDs

(c) If she had presented for pre-pregnancy counselling, what advice would you have given her? (4 marks)

- Should be seen by a physician or in a combined clinic (by an obstetrician and physician)
- Review medication with a view to:
  - Converting to monotherapy or less teratogenic drugs
  - Stopping, depending on various factors (e.g. time of last seizure)
- General advice about lifestyle factors (smoking, alcohol, drugs, etc.)
- Folic acid 5 mg pre-pregnancy and throughout pregnancy
- Counselling about the risk of malformations
- Early booking, combined care

Sample answer

(a) What complications may she have by virtue of this condition? (6 marks)

The complications may be maternal or fetal. Maternal complications are either related to the condition itself or to the AEDs. Those in the former category include an increased in seizure rate (reported in a third of women during pregnancy) and the risk of status epilepticus (this risk is not increased in pregnancy). Immediately after delivery, the risk of tonic–clonic seizures is increased. Complications related to AEDs depend on the type of drugs but in general are NTDs (1–3 per cent with sodium valproate (Epilim®)), facial clefting, fetal AED syndrome (a combination of malformations) and coagulopathies in the neonates (approximately 50 per cent of neonates whose mothers are on phenobarbitone, primidone or phenytoin). The fetuses are at an increased risk of asphyxia if fits are poorly controlled and their risk of developing seizures is also increased.

(b) What steps will you take to minimise these complications? (10 marks)

There are several steps that could be taken to minimise these complications. Antiepileptic treatment should be optimised to ensure good seizure control. This is best achieved in consultation with physicians (neurologists). The patient should be evaluated for factors that will favour withdrawal of treatment (e.g. being seizure free for 2 years, age at onset of seizures, type of seizure and the number of seizures before control was achieved). As she is already 10 weeks, attempts to switch therapy to more modern drugs should not be encouraged, especially if her fits are well controlled on Epilim®. The control of her seizures should be determined clinically and using drug levels to provide guidance only. Regular attendance at a joint neurologist/obstetrician clinic will ensure a tight control of her seizures by adjusting the AED dose when appropriate or indicated.

It is important that she is on folic acid 5 mg daily and should continue with this throughout pregnancy. Serum screening may provide a useful means of suspecting open NTDs (raised AFP) although ultrasound scanning would be a better tool for screening. Oral vitamin K (10–20 mg daily should be given to the mother from 36 weeks' gestation.

Her intrapartum care will not be different to that of any other obstetric patient but attempts must be made to avoid hyperventilation – hence a potent analgesic is advisable. Postpartum monitoring of drugs levels may be required, as altered physiology may mean an increase in drug availability. The first day postpartum may be complicated by a tonic–clonic seizure, hence it is advisable for the patient to be monitored in the hospital. The neonate should be given vitamin K to reduce the risk of vitamin-K-dependent coagulopathy. The mother should be counselled against driving and bathing the baby. Prior to discharge, counselling about contraception should include the reduced efficacy of hormonal contraception by AEDs.

(c) If she had presented for pre-pregnancy counselling, what advice would you have given her? (4 marks)

If she had presented pre-pregnancy, the advice would have been provided ideally by a joint obstetric and neurological team. This will include a review of her medication and converting her to monotherapy or less teratogenic drugs and stopping treatment if she fulfils the criteria for doing so. General advice will be provided on lifestyle factors such as smoking, alcohol and drugs, and folic acid 5 mg pre-pregnancy and throughout pregnancy. Counselling will be offered about the risk of malformations, the need to book early and drug compliance.

2. A 33-year-old woman presented at 38 weeks' gestation with chronic cough, night sweats and right-sided chest pain. She is unemployed and has two other children at home. You suspect that she may have TB. (a) What additional relevant information will you obtain from her? (4 marks) (b) How will you confirm the diagnosis? (4 marks) (c) Briefly outline the management of her pregnancy. (12 marks)

Common mistakes

- Not asked to discuss the differential diagnoses of TB (such as sarcoidosis)
- Diagnoses of the differentials
- History of chronic cough, pulmonary embolism, cystic fibrosis, chronic bronchitis
- Not asked to justify suspicion of diagnosis of TB
- Irrelevant investigations, such as blood cultures, infection screen, stool culture, etc.
- No need to dwell on history

A good answer will include some or all of these points

(a) What additional relevant information will you obtain from her? (4 marks)

- History of the following:
  - Symptoms – associated haemoptysis and weight loss
  - Travel outside the UK to an endemic or high-infection area
  - Contact with someone with chronic cough or known diagnosis
  - Associated pyrexia – timing (night, etc.)
  - Other factors – members of family with similar symptoms
  - Lifestyle factors – drugs, smoking, living conditions, etc.

(b) How will you confirm the diagnosis? (4 marks)

- Tuberculin skin test (TST) – Mantoux test – safe and reasonably sensitive in pregnancy
- Chest X-ray (CXR) with shielding of the abdomen (best in those TST positive) – presence of opacities in the upper lung zone
- Sputum – for acid fast bacillus stain (Ziehl–Neelsen stain), culture and sensitivity or polymerase chain reaction (PCR)
- Bronchoscopy for PCR

(c) Briefly outline your management of this patient if the diagnosis is confirmed. (12 marks)

- Baseline maternal investigations prior to commencement of treatment:
  - Full blood count (FBC)

- Liver function test (LFT), especially the transaminases
- Human immunodeficiency virus (HIV) testing – this should be offered to all patients with TB
- Treatment – should be joint management with chest physicians (pulmonologist):
  - World Health Organization (WHO) recommendation:
    - Initial phase treatment for 2 months with a combination of ethambutol, pyrazinamide, rifampicin and isoniazid (also called INH)
    - Subsequent 4 months' therapy with rifampicin and INH
    - Commence pyridoxine 25–50 mg daily to reduce the neuropathy associated with INH
  - Monitoring:
    - Regular LFTs
    - Recheck sputum after 2 weeks (should be negative after treatment)
- Fetal investigations and monitoring:
  - Ultrasound scan for growth and liquor volume
  - Doppler scans of umbilical artery and other vessels if indicated
- Intrapartum:
  - Sputum negative – manage as normal (interventions only for obstetric reasons)
  - Sputum positive – isolate and barrier nurse
- Postnatal:
  - Sputum negative, no specific measures other than administer INH-resistant bacille Calmette–Guérin (BCG) to neonate
  - Sputum positive – separate mother and baby until sputum becomes negative. Breastfeeding should not be discouraged – express and feed
  - Contraception – combined oral contraceptive pill not as effective (impaired by anti-TB drugs)
- Public health measures:
  - Notify public health department (notifiable disease in the UK)
  - Screen other members of the family (children, husband, etc.)
  - General advice on diet, environmental hygiene, smoking, alcohol and drugs

Sample answer

(a) What additional relevant information will you obtain from her? (4 marks)

It is important to establish whether the patient has recently travelled outside the UK to a country with a high prevalence of TB and whether she has been in contact with someone with chronic cough or a known diagnosis of pulmonary TB. Other features of TB that need to be excluded include associated haemoptysis and weight loss. Pyrexia, which is predominantly in the evenings, is also important. Are there any other members of the family with similar symptoms? Although not directly related to the diagnosis, lifestyle factors such as smoking and living conditions are useful during rehabilitation.

(b) How will you confirm the diagnosis? (4 marks)

The diagnosis can be achieved by a thorough clinical examination supported by ancillary investigations. General and chest examination may reveal signs of TB. Again, these may not be very specific as other differentials may present with similar features. Ancillary investigations that should be offered to confirm the diagnosis include a CXR (with the abdomen/fetus shielded) and a Mantoux test. This is safe in pregnancy and is the best means of detecting TB. The CXR may reveal opacities on the upper right lobe (the most common site of pulmonary TB) or other areas of opacities in the lungs. A Mantoux test will indicate the presence of TB antigens in the patient. This test may produce a false-positive result with some other tropical diseases, such as leprosy, and in malnourished or immuno-suppressed patients. Where the patient is producing sputum, this should be sent for acid-fast bacilli testing. A sputum for acid fast bacilli (Ziehl–Neelsen stain), culture and sensitivity or PCR will be diagnostic. Bronchoscopy and lavage for PCR offers the most accurate means of making a diagnosis.

(c) Briefly outline your management of this patient if the diagnosis is confirmed. (12 marks)

Once the disease has been confirmed, the public health department should be notified as this is a notifiable disease. Subsequent treatment should be by a team consisting of a pulmonary physician, a general practitioner (GP), a health worker, a midwife, a paediatrician and an obstetrician. A FBC, LFT and HIV testing should be offered before commencing treatment. An initial 2 months' treatment with a combination of rifampicin, INH, ethambutol and pyrazinamide is recommended by the WHO. This is followed by 4 months of rifampicin and INH. In addition, she should be commenced on pyridoxine 25–50 mg daily to reduce the neuropathy associated with INH. Monitoring should be in the form of regular LFTs.

Fetal investigations and monitoring include regular ultrasound scan for growth and liquor volume (since pulmonary TB may be complicated by fetal growth restriction (FGR)) and, where indicated (i.e. where FGR if confirmed), regular Doppler scans of the umbilical and middle cerebral arteries. The sputum should be rechecked 2 weeks after the commencement of treatment – it should be negative if it was originally positive. The initial treatment may require hospital admission if the symptoms are severe. If this is necessary, she should not be admitted to an open ward. She should either be barrier nursed or admitted to an isolation unit until she is rendered sputum negative. This will usually follow 2 weeks' treatment.

The patient may resist admission because of her children, in which case she may be managed at home. As part of her management, she must be educated on how the disease spreads, the need for better hygiene at home to minimise the risk of transmitting the infection to other members of the family (if they are not already affected) and advice on nutrition. Appropriate support must be offered and advice given if her living conditions are damp and dirty.

Provided she has been rendered sputum negative, the rest of the pregnancy should be monitored as routine and labour allowed to follow the normal course. However, if there is a suspicion of severe pulmonary compromise as a result of the infection, then second stage may be supported with an elective forceps delivery to avoid unnecessary pushing. If she has not been rendered sputum negative (and goes into labour within 2 weeks of therapy) she should be barrier nursed. The danger at this stage will be to members of staff.

However, after delivery, there is also the danger of transmitting the infection to the neonate. If the patient is to breastfeed, the baby must be given INH-resistant BCG and isolated for a week before the mother is allowed to breastfeed. During this time, expressed breast milk may be used to feed the baby. If she is not going to breastfeed, isolation is still required. The 7-day isolation period is to allow the vaccine to become effective. It is important that the paediatrician is notified when the patient is admitted in labour. Plans for the care of the baby should be documented in the notes in case the medical staff on-call (when the patient is in labour) are different to those involved in her antenatal care. An important part of the management of this patient must be to screen all contacts, including her children, for the disease. These contacts must be offered appropriate treatment. The role of the GP and health visitor in this regard is extremely important.

3. Critically appraise the screening for diabetes mellitus in pregnancy. (20 marks)

Common mistakes

- Complications of diabetes mellitus in pregnancy
- How to perform a glucose tolerance test (GTT)
- Management of diabetes in pregnancy
- Need for physician involvement
- Ultrasound scan for fetal abnormalities
- Management of neonatal complications

A good answer will include some or all of these points

- History – obstetric and family – reliability
- Maternal weight – obesity?
- Definition
- Race/age – reliability
- Obstetric risk factors/indications
- Fetal risk factors
- Other risk factors
- Methods
- Random blood glucose/fasting blood glucose
- GTT
- Glycosylated haemoglobin (HbA1c)
- ACHOIS Study (Growther *et al.*, 2005) and National Institute for Health and Clinical Excellence (NICE) guidelines

Sample answer

Diabetes is one of the most common medical disorders of pregnancy, associated with a high perinatal morbidity and mortality. Although the risks associated with gestational diabetes are well recognised, it remains uncertain whether screening and treatment to reduce maternal glucose levels reduces risk. NICE guidelines did not recommend screening but the recent ACHOIS study confirmed that screening and treatment significantly improved outcome. One of the difficulties with this complication is that not all patients present with pre-existing disease. Indeed, some are recognised for the first time in pregnancy and some develop the disorder in pregnancy as a consequence of the diabetogenic effects of pregnancy. Screening for diabetes in pregnancy therefore assumes enormous significance if all cases are to be identified and managed appropriately to improve outcome.

Unfortunately, screening still fails to identify all cases. Screening for diabetes in pregnancy starts with a detailed obstetric and family history. A previous macrosomic baby, unexplained stillbirth, congenital malformation (especially those common in diabetic pregnancies), poly-hydramnios and a family history in a first-degree relative is associated with an increased risk of diabetes mellitus. Unfortunately, some of these risk factors are poorly defined. For example, the definition of fetal macrosomia depends on the population and the racial group. The use of a cut-off point of 4000 g, for example, may include too many women, whereas increasing it to 4500 g may exclude some cases. It is also not uncommon to fail to identify close relatives affected with diabetes mellitus. Although a close relative is regarded as a first-degree relative, the exact role of second-degree relatives in increasing the risk of diabetes mellitus is unclear.

Maternal weight is another risk factor. Obesity is poorly defined. For example, in some units, this is regarded as weight over 90 kg at booking, whereas in others, a body mass index of over 30 is the cut-off point. Such wide variation in standards suggests too many divergences for the use of maternal weight as a screening tool. Race and age are also regarded as demographic risk factors. In some units, all those of Asian origin and women over the age of 35 years are considered at risk. It may be seen as discriminatory to label women from one particular ethnic group, or older women, as at risk. Such risk factors are not universally acceptable and it is, therefore, not uncommon to have units that offer screening to all women defined by the above criteria, and others that do not. The rate of diabetes detection will therefore depend on the screening tools used.

During pregnancy, various risk factors may be identified and indicate the need for screening. These include glycosuria, polyhydramnios, macrosomia and recurrent infections, especially in the vulva and vagina. Glycosuria occurs in about 4 per cent of pregnancies because of reduced renal threshold. Therefore, as a risk factor for diabetes, it is unreliable. A large number of women will therefore be offered further screening on account of this alone. Various attempts have been made to refine this indication, e.g. glycosuria on more than one occasion or in the early morning specimen of urine. Polyhydramnios is a late occurrence, as is fetal macrosomia. Congenital malformations, although occurring early, are often not identified until the second trimester. Although these may be identified in some patients with diabetes, identification is often late and the consequences would already have occurred. However, their presence must be regarded as an indication for second-stage screening.

Identification of at-risk groups is only the first step in the screening for diabetes mellitus. Following this, the definitive or second-stage screening must be offered. The most common form of screening is an oral GTT. In the UK and most of Europe, this is with a 75 g glucose load. In the USA 100 g is used. This is undertaken after an overnight fast. The disadvantage of this form of screening is nausea and vomiting, which may be induced by the glucose. In addition, there is some disagreement on the diagnostic criteria. Currently, the fasting and 120 minutes' glucose values are used for diagnosis. Whether venous or capillary blood is used for the test is another area of controversy.

Some attempts have been made to stratify this screening. Identifying patients based on the above risk factors has been shown to miss some cases of diabetes. To overcome this, it has been suggested that each patient be offered a random blood glucose test and the value related to the time of the last meal. Where the value is <5.4 mmol/L, and the last meal was more than 2 hours previously, or the levels are <6.4 mmol/L within 2 hours of the last meal, then a full glucose tolerance test is undertaken. However, this remains controversial. Some have advocated a 50 g glucose load followed by a 1-hour blood glucose test. This method will identify those who will further require a glucose tolerance test. Unfortunately, this regime is time consuming and expensive, and is unlikely to be adopted by all units.

Although HbA1c is used to monitor glycaemic control, it may be useful as a screening tool.

Reference

Growther CA, Hiller JE, Moss JR, McPhee AJ, Jeffries WS, Robinson JS *et al.* (2005) Effect of gestational diabetes mellitus on pregnancy outcomes (the Achois Trial). *NEJM* **352**: 2477–86.

4. An obese diabetic woman books for antenatal care at 6 weeks' gestation. (a) Enumerate the risks of this pregnancy. (8 marks) (b) What steps will you take to improve the pregnancy outcome? (8 marks) (c) What advice will you give her post-natally? (4 marks)

Common mistakes

- Discussing screening for diabetes mellitus
- Discussing the diagnosis of diabetes and the classification in pregnancy
- Discussing the management of diabetes in general
- Being very vague and not discussing what you will do
- Advising the patient to lose weight
- Detailing the intrapartum management of diabetes mellitus
- Involving the neonatologist in her intrapartum care

A good answer will include some or all of these points

(a) Enumerate the risks of this pregnancy. (8 marks)

- First trimester:
  - Miscarriage
  - Difficulties dating pregnancy
- Second trimester:
  - Unreliable biochemical screening
  - Unreliable ultrasound screening
  - Congenital malformations
  - Polyhydramnios
  - Preterm labour – spontaneous and iatrogenic
- Third trimester:
  - Fetal macrosomia
  - Polyhydramnios
  - Preterm labour – iatrogenic or spontaneous
  - Unexplained stillbirth
  - Difficulties assessing fetal growth and lie/presentation
- Labour:
  - Failure to progress
  - Shoulder dystocia
  - Trauma to the fetus – fractured clavicles, etc.
  - Difficult operative (abdominal and vaginal) deliveries
  - Venous thromboembolism (VTE)
- Neonatal:
  - Hypoglycaemia
  - Hypomagnesaemia

- Hypocalcaemia
- Tetany
- Neonatal jaundice
- Polycythaemia

(b) What steps will you take to improve the pregnancy outcome? (8 marks)

- Dating pregnancy – best with a transvaginal ultrasound scan (TVS)
- Good glycaemic control – using regular blood monitoring and HbA1c. Diabetic control: insulin (change oral hypogylycaemic agent to insulin); maintain BM stix® between 5.5 and 6.5; HbA1c <6.5 per cent; regular blood glucose monitoring – 4-hourly profiles; calorie restriction
- Folate at the higher dose – 5 mg during pregnancy
- Detailed ultrasound scan including a fetal echography
- Blood pressure check with large cuff and regular checking of urine for proteinuria and nitrites
- Assessment by anaesthetists and discussion that epidural is best and administered early in labour
- Maternal complications: urinary tract infections – midstream urine samples; hypertension/pre-eclampsia (PET) – checking blood pressure may be difficult, so use large cuffs; diabetic complications – hypoglycaemia, etc.
- Fetal growth – macrosomia more likely, although FGR may occur; serial growth scans; abdominal palpation difficult; polyhydramnios needs to be excluded
- Intrapartum – regular fire drills for shoulder dystocia, anticipatory intervention
- Ensure that appropriate manpower is present
- Labour: induced or spontaneous; cephalopelvic disproportion; shoulder dystocia – precautions; neonatal complications – hypoglycaemia, respiratory distress syndrome (RDS), tetany, etc.

(c) What advice will you give her postnatally? (4 marks)

- Breastfeeding – improves insulin sensitivity and therefore reduced insulin requirements
- Counsel to lose weight before another pregnancy
- Pre-pregnancy insulin requirements (if increased during pregnancy)
- Contraception

Sample answer

(a) Enumerate the risks of this pregnancy. (8 marks)

The risks of the pregnancy could be grouped as fetal and maternal. The maternal risks include poor diabetic control in the first trimester if there is hyperemesis gravidarum, PET, hypertension, recurrent vulvovaginal and urinary tract infections, and hypoglycaemic episodes.

Fetal risks can be divided into those in the first, second and third trimesters, intrapartum and neonatal. The first trimester risks are miscarriage and difficulties dating pregnancies (by clinical examination and ultrasound). Much later, there are the risks of unreliable biochemical screening for aneuploidy, difficulties performing invasive diagnostic procedures (such as amniocentesis and chorionic villus sampling), unreliable ultrasound anomaly scan and therefore reduced accuracy in diagnosing congenital malformations, which are more common in diabetics (especially cardiac and skeletal).There is an increased risk of polyhydramnios, fetal macrosomia, unexplained fetal death, iatrogenic and spontaneous preterm labour and abnormal fetal lie. Because of her obesity, assessing fetal growth, lie and presentation may be difficult and therefore there is an increased risk of misdiagnosing abnormalities in fetal growth (fetal macrosomia and growth restriction). Ultrasound estimation of fetal weight may also be unreliable.

During labour the risks include failure to progress, poor uterine contractions, shoulder dystocia, trauma from difficult vaginal instrumental deliveries and infections after Caesarean sections (wound infections). The neonatal risks include those of hypoglycaemia, hypomagnesaemia, hypocalcaemia, tetany, polycythaemia, neonatal jaundice, and thrombosis. Reduced maternal mobility and increased risk of operative deliveries increase the risk of VTE. Early identification and treatment of these complications will minimise their consequences.

The fetus is at an increased risk of congenital malformations, such as NTDs, cardiac, musculoskeletal and caudal regression syndrome. Early anomaly scans and the routine 20–22 weeks anomaly scans will identify some of these. It is essential that a cardiologist undertakes an echocardiography to exclude major and minor cardiac malformations. Fetal macrosomia is a common complication of diabetes mellitus, especially when poorly controlled and with maternal obesity. Therefore, during her antenatal care, she should have serial ultrasound scans for fetal growth. This is even more important in this obese patient in whom abdominal palpations will be difficult.

(b) What steps will you take to improve the pregnancy outcome? (8 marks)

The first step to improve outcome is to ensure that the pregnancy is accurately dated. This is best achieved by a TVS. Ensuring good glycaemic control will reduce the risk of malformations and perinatal morbidity and mortality. This can be achieved by ensuring that the HbA1c is kept below 6.5 per cent and regular blood glucose values are between 5.5 mmol/L and 6.5 mmol/L. This is best achieved by 4-hourly blood glucose profiles, restriction of caloric intake and 6–8-weekly HbA1c.

Folate supplementation should be with the higher dose of 5 mg daily and it is advisable for this to continue throughout gestation. In order to improve the outcome of her pregnancy, there must be meticulous control of her diabetes, early recognition of complications and treatment and skilled care during the pregnancy. The patient's diabetic control must be very tight. This is best achieved within a team of dedicated clinicians and midwives, including a physician with an interest in diabetes mellitus, an obstetrician and the GP.

Blood glucose should be maintained between 5.5 and 6.5 mmol/L. If the patient is not already on insulin, this must be instituted. Insulin offers the advantage of better diabetic control and, since it does not cross the placenta, is unlikely to have any teratogenic effects on the fetus. The patient's HbA1c should be less than 6.5 per cent. This tight control is monitored by frequent blood glucose estimations – usually every 4 hours using BM stix®. The patient must keep a personal chart of her insulin regimen and her BM stix® values. At this early gestation, dietary advice must be offered. Using a standard cuff to measure her blood pressure will produce erroneously high readings; a large cuff should therefore be used. Hypoglycaemia may be fatal to the fetus, so educating the mother and her partner about this complication and ensuring that glucagon is readily available for its treatment is absolutely necessary.

Where diabetes is well controlled, labour may be allowed to start spontaneously. However, in most units, it may be induced at 38 weeks' gestation. Because of fetal macrosomia, complications such as obstructed labour, failure to progress and shoulder dystocia should be identified early and managed accordingly. Once the baby is delivered, complications such as hypoglycaemia, hypothermia, RDS, tetany, polycythaemia and jaundice may occur. These should be identified early and treatment instituted. If there is a possibility that the fetus may be delivered early, steroids (in the form of two doses betamethasone 12 mg 12 hours apart) must be given. The involvement of the paediatrician is crucial and must be from the time of admission of the patient to the labour ward.

In this patient, if all the adequate precautions are undertaken, the outcome of her pregnancy is likely to improve significantly.

(c) What advice will you give her postnatally? (4 marks)

After delivery she should be advised that there are no contraindications to breastfeeding. In fact she should be encouraged to breastfeed. Breastfeeding improves insulin sensitivity and therefore reduces insulin requirements. Prior to being discharged from the hospital, she should be advised on weight loss before embarking on another pregnancy. Her insulin should be changed to her pre-pregnancy dose if this was increased during pregnancy. Finally an appropriate contraceptive should be provided. If she is breastfeeding, the combined oral contraceptive pill will be contraindicated.

5. A 26-year-old woman with cardiac disease grade III is admitted in labour at 40 weeks' gestation. (a) What intrapartum complications of her cardiac disease may she develop? (6 marks) (b) Briefly outline the steps you will take to minimise these complications. (14 marks)

Common mistakes

- Details of the American classification of cardiac disease
- Refer to physicians for management
- Central venous pressure and Sengstak tubes
- Management to be controlled by anaesthetist
- Antibiotics for second stage
- Manage patient on the high dependency unit/intensive care unit (HDU/ICU) only
- Causes of cardiac disease in pregnancy
- Investigate for the causes of cardiac disease in pregnancy

A good answer will include some or all of these points

(a) What intrapartum complications of her cardiac disease may she develop? (6 marks)

- Hypotension – especially secondary to aortocaval compression by the gravid uterus (cardiac patients are particularly sensitive to aortocaval compression by the gravid uterus):
  - Risk is greatest after an epidural
- Fetal and maternal distress from rapidly developing hypotension
- Cardiac failure – related to fluid overload and physiological changes associated with labour including the use of oxytocics
- Fluid overload and pulmonary oedema
- Endocarditis
- Venous thrombosis

(b) Briefly outline the steps you will take to minimise these complications. (14 marks)

- Management must be in a multidisciplinary team including an obstetric physician or cardiologist, an anaesthetist (experienced in the management of severe cardiac disease patients in labour) and an experienced midwife
- Definition of grade III cardiac disease – non-specific – pathology could be any
- Hypotension – manage labour in the left lateral position (to decrease aortocaval compression):
  - Where epidurals are to be administered, preload guided by monitoring of the circulatory volume is recommended

71

- Continuous electrocardiography (ECG) to detect arrhythmias – where the cardiac disorder is associated with arrhythmias
- Monitor oxygen saturation in labour
- Consider pulmonary artery catheter and arterial line if deteriorating cardiovascular status
- May consider shortening the second stage of labour by an operative vaginal delivery (avoids increasing the risk of cardiac failure)
- Prophylactic antibiotics if the type of cardiac condition exposes patient to the risk of bacterial endocarditis (e.g. mitral valve prolapse, complex cyanotic heart disease, previous bacterial endocarditis, hypertrophic cardiomyopathy)
- Avoid ergometrine
- Postnatal – monitor fluid balance carefully especially for the first 24–72 hours – fluid shifts from extravascular to intravascular space and may therefore result in overload
- Counsel about subsequent pregnancies
- Postpartum management – watch out for risk of pulmonary oedema and fluid overload; may require HDU/ICU care
- Prophylaxis against VTE

Sample answer

(a) What intrapartum complications of her cardiac disease may she develop? (6 marks)

Intrapartum complications that may occur include hypotension (especially secondary to aortocaval compression by the gravid uterus although could be related to an epidural anaesthesia), cardiac failure and death. Rapidly developing maternal hypotension could then result in fetal and maternal distress. Cardiac failure is more likely to be related to fluid overload and physiological changes associated with labour including the use of oxytocics. Fluid overload may cause pulmonary oedema. Other complications include endocarditis and VTE. These complications are more likely to occur in the second and third stages and during the early puerperium. Fluid overload is the most common predisposing factor for these complications.

The complications of cardiac disease grade III in labour could be minimised by highly skilled management of the patient. In this case, it has to be by a multidisciplinary team including an obstetric physician or cardiologist, an anaesthetist (experienced in the management of severe cardiac disease in labour) and an experienced midwife. It is important to remember that cardiac disease grade III is non-specific and therefore the precise type of cardiac disease may influence the management.

(b) Briefly outline you steps you will take to minimise these complications. (14 marks)

Hypotension should be avoided by managing the patient in the left lateral position (to decrease aortocaval compression) and where epidurals are to be administered, a preload guided by monitoring of the circulatory volume is recommended. Continuous ECG monitoring should be offered to detect arrhythmias, especially where the cardiac disorder is associated with arrhythmias. Oxygen saturations should be monitored regularly in labour and where indicated a pulmonary artery catheter and an arterial line should be inserted – these are indicated if there is deterioration in the cardiovascular status.

The second stage of labour may be shortened by an operative vaginal delivery to avoid increasing the risk of cardiac failure. Prophylactic antibiotics are necessary if the type of cardiac condition exposes the patient to the risk of bacterial endocarditis (examples include mitral valve prolapse, complex cyanotic heart disease, previous bacterial endocardiatis, hypertrophic cardiomyopathy).

The third stage must be managed carefully. The use of intravenous Syntometrine® should be avoided as this would result in rapid venous return to the heart and subsequent heart failure. The only oxytocic agent that could be used for the third stage of labour is intramuscular oxytocin. There may be a case for the physiological management of the third stage. However, this must not be at the risk of postpartum haemorrhage and worsening maternal morbidity. The placenta should then be delivered by controlled cord traction.

In the postnatal period, a careful fluid balance is essential especially within the first 24–72 hours when fluid shifts from the extravascular to the intravascular compartments with the potential of fluid overload and cardiac failure. During the postpartum period, there should be a high vigilance for pulmonary oedema and fluid overload which may require HDU/ICU management.

Appropriate counselling about subsequent pregnancies should be offered before discharge from the hospital. These should be avoided if possible and appropriate contraception considered. The risk of VTE is considered to be significant in this patient. This should be minimised by administering subcutaneous heparin/Fragmin® for approximately 5 days after delivery. Early mobilisation of the patient is essential in this regard. Close monitoring of the vital signs during the puerperium is essential because increased venous return to the heart may result in cardiac failure.

Further reading

Nelson-Piercy C (2006) Heart disease. In: Nelson-Piercy C (ed.) *Obstetrics Handbook*, 3rd edn. London: Informa Healthcare, pp. 23–43.

Tomlinson M (2006) Cardiac disease. In: James DK, Steer PJ, Weiner CP, Gonik B (eds) *High Risk Pregnancy: Management Options*. London: Saunders, pp. 798–827.

5

Prenatal diagnosis and congenital malformations

1. Prenatal screening is an important part of modern obstetric care. (a) Briefly outline the pros and cons of first trimester screening. (8 marks) (b) What methods of first trimester screening will you offer a 35-year-old primigravida? (12 marks)

2. Mrs BT attended for a detailed ultrasound scan and the baby was found to have an exomphalus. (a) Briefly outline the steps you will take when you first see her in the clinic. (8 marks) (b) Justify your subsequent management of the patient. (12 marks)

3. A 15-year-old girl attended for a detailed ultrasound scan and her baby has been found to have a congenital cardiac abnormality. (a) What factors will influence your counselling? (6 marks) (b) Critically appraise how she will be managed. (14 marks)

4. Critically appraise the role of ultrasound scan in the diagnosis of trisomy 21. (20 marks)

5. Debate the statement that amniocentesis is soon to supersede chorionic villus sampling (CVS) in prenatal diagnosis. (20 marks)

6. A couple have just been told after an ultrasound scan at 15 weeks' gestation that their baby has a diaphragmatic hernia. (a) Outline very briefly the prognostic factors of this condition. (6 marks) (b) How will you counsel the patient now and throughout her pregnancy? (10 marks) (c) Justify how you will manage the labour. (4 marks)

1. Prenatal screening is an important part of modern obstetric care. (a) Briefly outline the pros and cons of first trimester screening. (8 marks) (b) What methods of first trimester screening will you offer a 35-year-old primigravida? (12 marks)

Common mistakes

- Listing all the malformations that may be diagnosed in the first trimester
- Restricting yourself to chromosomal abnormalities
- Failing to mention biochemical screening
- Excluding history as a screening method
- Justifying screening in the first trimester
- Discussing the differences between amniocentesis and CVS
- Take a history and do a physical examination
- Discussing the details of nuchal translucency (NT) and biochemistry screening in the first trimester and how the various analytes change with gestation

A good answer will include some or all of these points

(a) Briefly outline the pros and cons of first trimester screening. (8 marks)

- Offers opportunity to make a diagnosis before pregnancy becomes obvious
- More applicable to pregnancies of higher order (twins, triplets, etc.)
- Identifies fetuses at risk of other problems for more targeted screening, e.g. cardiac malformations
- Termination if indicated can be offered surgically
- CVS possible
- Biochemical markers not as reliable (most still rising)
- Ultrasound markers – fetal development may affect reliability of markers
- Newer techniques – fetal cells and deoxyriboso nucleic acid (DNA) in maternal circulation evolving and not yet as reliable

(b) What methods of first trimester screening will you offer a 35-year-old primigravida? (12 marks)

- History – personal, family, social, past obstetric and medical:
  - Personal – known chromosomal or structural (e.g. cardiac) abnormality in either or both parents
  - Family history of chromosomal, metabolic or structural malformation
  - Social history – alcohol, drugs especially recreational, occupation
  - Obstetric history – past history of stillbirth (especially unexplained or where baby is described as 'funny looking', associated structural malformations, chromosomal abnormality)

- Medical history – conditions that may be associated with malformations (e.g. diabetes mellitus, epilepsy, connective tissue disorders) or drugs that may be teratogenic, e.g. antiepileptics, lithium for endogenous depression
- Ultrasound scan – dating of pregnancy, number of fetuses, NT and structural abnormalities:
  - Dating will provide accurate interpretation of results of biochemistry and morphology
  - Number of fetuses and chorionicity
  - NT – value above cut-off for gestation and population – reliability depends on the operator and the fetal position. Most fetuses with abnormal NTs are normal but require scanning later for cardiac abnormalities and other (especially) thoracic compression anomalies
  - Structural abnormalities and markers, e.g. holoprosencephaly, anencephaly, nasal bone hypoplasia (skeletal) renal, cystic hygromas, anterior abdominal and other central nervous system (CNS) manifestations. Detailed knowledge of developmental embryology is essential to interpret results
- Biochemistry – human chorionic gonadotropin (hCG), alpha-fetoprotein (AFP), inhibin and pregnancy-associated plasma protein-1 (PAPP1):
  - Most reliable is hCG and inhibin
  - Timing – 11–13 weeks
- Fetal blood in maternal serum:
  - Still being refined
- Fetal DNA in maternal blood:
  - Still being refined
- Others – cells in cervical secretions

Sample answer

(a) Briefly outline the pros and cons of first trimester screening. (8 marks)

First trimester screening is increasingly becoming available in most obstetric units in the UK. It offers an opportunity for screening and diagnosis before the pregnancy becomes obvious to others. Where there is the need to terminate the pregnancy, surgery is an option. For most women, it will enable the identification of those at risk for whom more targeted screening and diagnostic testing could then be offered. The other advantage of screening in the first trimester is its application in pregnancies of higher order where traditional biochemical screening is unreliable. Where invasive testing (such as CVS) is required, this can be easily undertaken.

The disadvantages of screening in the first trimester include the fact that some of the screening methods, such as history, may not always be easy to obtain and in some cases may be unreliable. In addition, the biochemical analytes that are used in the second trimester may be changing very rapidly and therefore not reliable for use in this trimester unless the pregnancy is accurately dated. Newer techniques which are becoming more available in the first trimester, such as fetal DNA and fetal cells in the maternal circulation, are still evolving and their reliability is still being refined. The use of ultrasound markers in the first trimester may be affected by developmental embryology which is essential for interpretation.

(b) What methods of first trimester screening will you offer a 35-year-old primigravida? (12 marks)

The methods of screening that could be offered in the first trimester include history, ultrasound scan, biochemistry, fetal cells in maternal blood, free fetal DNA in maternal blood and in cervical secretions. With regard to history, this could be personal, family, social, obstetric or medical. A personal history will include that of a known chromosomal or structural (e.g. cardiac) abnormality in either partner. In the family history, important factors include that of chromosomal, metabolic and structural abnormalities. Social factors that increase the risk of abnormalities include alcohol, drugs (e.g. recreational drugs) and occupations at risk of exposure to teratogens (e.g. radiation).

A past obstetric history of relevance will include that of a stillbirth (especially unexplained or where the baby is described as looking funny) and associated structural or chromosomal malformations. The risk factors for malformation in the medical history include diabetes mellitus (predating pregnancy), epilepsy or treatment, connective tissue disease and endogenous depression on treatment with lithium carbamate. Other factors to be considered in the medical history will include drug therapy for medical disorders such as hypertension. This is more so where the drugs are known to be teratogenic, e.g. angiotensin-converting enzyme inhibitors for hypertension or sodium valproate (Epilim®) for epilepsy.

Ultrasound scan in the first trimester is an important screening tool. It allows the dating of the pregnancy, which is crucial for interpretation of biochemical screening tests, identifies multiple pregnancies and chorionicity, and is able not only to diagnose structural abnormalities but also to identify soft markers for chromosomal abnormalities. Structural abnormalities that may be identified in the first trimester vary from those of the CNS and skeleton to the gastrointestinal tract. The use of transvaginal ultrasound scanning and machines with a better resolution, along with a greater understanding of the structural embryology of the fetus, has significantly improved the accuracy of the early identification of some of these anomalies. However, because several organs may be too small at these early gestations, difficulties may be encountered in clearly defining some important abnormalities. Abnormalities that can be confidently diagnosed in the first trimester include holoprosencephaly, anencephaly and cystic hygroma. A sound knowledge of developmental embryology is essential to provide such a screening.

The most commonly applied screening test for aneuploidy in the first trimester is NT. This is performed between 11 and 13 weeks' gestation. It is a marker for chromosomal abnormalities and structural malformations, especially cardiac. The accuracy of this screening tool depends on training. A large study in the south-east of England demonstrated that most radiographers can be trained to provide a reliable service. When combined with biochemistry, approximately 80 per cent of chromosomally abnormal fetuses can be identified.

Nasal bone hypoplasia at 11–13 weeks' gestation was thought to be a reliable soft marker but the FASTER trial (Malone et al., 2004) has dampened enthusiasm for this. Fetal cells or DNA in the maternal circulation are currently being investigated and are increasingly being used for first trimester screening. Several published studies confirm the potential of this non-invasive screening/diagnostic test, which is likely to become more widespread with improved sensitivity and specificity.

Biochemical screening is becoming a recognised tool in the first trimester. The analytes measured in maternal serum include inhibin, PAPP1, βhCG and AFP. Because these analytes rise at a very fast rate in the first trimester they require very accurate dating of the pregnancy for interpretation. An ideal screening with these analytes must, therefore, be combined with a dating ultrasound scan in the first trimester, otherwise margins of error will be too wide for accurate interpretation.

Reference

Malone FD, Ball RH, Nyberg DA *et al.* (2004) First trimester nasal bone evaluation for aneuploidy in the general population. *Obstet Gynaecol* **104**: 1222–8.

Further reading

Ndumbe FM, Navti OB, CHilaka VN, Konje JC (2008) Prenatal diagnosis in the first trimester of pregnancy. *Obstet Gynecol Surv* **63**: 317–28.

2. Mrs BT attended for a detailed ultrasound scan and the baby was found to have an exomphalus. (a) Briefly outline the steps you will take when you first see her in the clinic. (8 marks) (b) Justify your subsequent management of the patient. (12 marks)

Common mistakes

- Discussing how to diagnose exomphalus
- Involving surgeons to make the diagnosis
- Comparing the implications of exomphalus with gastroschisis
- Multidisciplinary care – no details of what this means
- Assuming the baby has a chromosomal abnormality
- Discussing termination of pregnancy as the only option
- Failure to justify the second part of the question
- Discussing the pros and cons of amniocentesis versus CVS
- Ensuring paediatric surgeon is present at delivery
- Timing of delivery to be determined by surgeon or neonatologist – this is the responsibility of the obstetrician (who may do so in consultation)

A good answer will contain some or all of these points

(a) Briefly outline the steps you will take when you first see her in the clinic. (8 marks)

- Inform patient of the findings and explain implications. Offer to contact partner or relative/friend if alone
- Implication(s) of finding
- May be isolated, or
- May be associated with other structural abnormalities yet to be identified
- Increased risk of aneuploidy – therefore offer karyotyping
- Arrange further scanning (another opinion) at tertiary level if at secondary level, or in the fetal medicine unit (with consultant or equivalent) if in a tertiary hospital. (Remember you will not be asked to see a patient who has already been seen by an expert!)

(b) Justify your subsequent management of the patient. (12 marks)

- Three possible scenarios:
  - Isolated
  - Associated structural anomalies
  - Associated chromosomal abnormality
- At the fetal medicine unit, ultrasound scan will be to exclude subtle anomalies, which may point to a particular syndrome

- Karyotyping to exclude aneuploidy – risk of miscarriage associated with this. Absence of abnormality does not guarantee that the fetus will be normal:
  - Options – amniocentesis for fluorescent *in situ* hybridisation (FISH)
  - CVS for FISH
- Scanning reveals multiple anomalies associated with poor prognosis or karyotype is abnormal – options are termination of pregnancy or continuation after appropriate counselling
- No abnormality seen – multidisciplinary care (neonatologist, paediatric surgeon, geneticists):
  - Neonatologist – see and counsel about neonatal care
  - Paediatric surgeon – counsel about postnatal treatment and complications
  - Geneticist – need to exclude syndrome after birth
- Follow-up management – looking for prognostic features

Sample answer

(a) Briefly outline the steps you will take when you first see her in the clinic. (8 marks)

The first step is to explain the diagnosis to the patient but prior to this, she should be given the option of having her partner or someone with her. She may initially refuse to accept the diagnosis and a skilled counsellor may be necessary. Alarming the patient of the risk of severe abnormality may be counterproductive, as some patients will automatically opt for a termination of pregnancy. It is important to approach it sensitively, emphasising that the diagnosis of such a problem does not necessarily mean that the baby will be severely handicapped. Exomphalus is associated with a chromosomal abnormality in up to 40 per cent of cases. In the other 60 per cent, with no karyotypic abnormality, the baby may be syndromic.

Whether the baby has or does not have a chromosomal abnormality, there may be associated structural abnormalities (e.g. cardiac). The patient should be offered a further, detailed ultrasound scan at a tertiary level. The presence of such abnormalities, however, may not be diagnostic of a chromosomal abnormality, but when combined with the exomphalus may fit into a syndrome the prognosis of which may be easy to assign (if a known syndrome).

(b) Justify your subsequent management of the patient. (12 marks)

There are three possible scenarios to her subsequent management. These would be divided into: (1) an isolated exomphalus, (2) an exomphalus with associated structural abnormalities and (3) exomphalus with associated chromosomal abnormalities. Scanning at the tertiary level will exclude associated anomalies including subtle ones. Their presence may point to a specific syndrome. It may be necessary to refer the patient to a clinical geneticist for a syndromic diagnosis to be made, followed by appropriate counselling.

In view of the high risk of chromosomal abnormalities with exomphalus, invasive testing for fetal karyotype should be offered in the form of amniocentesis or CVS. The choice for either will depend on the patient. However, it may be advisable to offer amniocentesis as the risk of mosaicism is lower than with CVS. With modern FISH techniques, results should be available within 1–2 days; however, where this is unavailable, traditional amniocentesis will take approximately 2–3 weeks. Even if she had FISH with either a CVS or amniocentesis, it would still be advisable to have the full karyotype from the traditional analysis.

If the chromosomes are abnormal (incompatible with life or associated with significant handicap), or there are severe malformations found on additional scanning, termination of pregnancy would be discussed and performed if opted for. If termination is after 21 weeks, then counselling about intracardiac potassium chloride (KCl) administered prior to mifepristone and prostaglandins should be offered.

If the chromosomes are normal, then prognostic factors should be assessed and appropriate counselling offered. If the hernia is large, and the liver and other viscera are outside the abdominal cavity, the prognosis is poor. In these circumstances, a termination may be offered. A paediatric surgeon and a neonatologist should be involved in the patient's care. The paediatric surgeon will explain the management after delivery, whereas the neonatologist will explain the neonatal care of the fetus. An important part of the management is to follow up the pregnancy with serial ultrasound scans to assess the exomphalus and prognostic factors such as polyhydramnios.

Where the defect is small and only small parts of the abdominal viscera are in the hernia sac, the prognosis is good. It may be advisable to introduce the patient and her partner to families that have had affected children and or to associations that provide support for such parents. The timing and method of delivery will depend on the presence of complications. In their absence, there is no reason to intervene prior to term. Delivery should be as gentle as possible to avoid rupturing the hernial sac. A thorough postnatal examination may reveal features of a syndrome. Whatever the management, appropriate postnatal follow-up and counselling is mandatory.

3. A 15-year-old girl attended for a detailed ultrasound scan and her baby has been found to have a congenital cardiac abnormality. (a) What factors will influence your counselling? (6 marks) (b) Critically appraise how she will be managed. (14 marks)

Common mistakes

- Terminate pregnancy
- Offer neonatal surgery
- Perform chromosome investigations
- Discussing the aetiology of cardiac malformations
- Discussing intracardiac surgery
- Involve social workers

A good answer will include some or all of these points

(a) What factors will influence your counselling? (6 marks)

- Her ability to understand – maturity
- The type of congenital malformation
- Associated structural abnormalities
- Other risk factors for aneuploidy
- Availability of facilities for invasive testing
- Expertise for further imaging
- Postnatal care facilities – further investigation and management
- Possible aetiological factors

(b) Critically appraise how she will be managed. (14 marks)

- Explanation of the diagnosis to the patient:
  - She is young – any effects on her understanding?
- Involve paediatric cardiologist
- Counselling about the diagnosis
- Further investigations – karyotyping – normal or abnormal? Normal does not exclude other problems
- Management – neonatal period
- Other undiagnosed abnormalities not diagnosed
- Problems of diagnosis

Sample answer

(a) What factors will influence your counselling? (6 marks)

The first factor will be her ability to understand the findings and their implications. She is only 15 years old and is yet to reach the age of consent. She may also struggle to come to terms with the diagnosis and explanations offered. Her ability to assimilate the information should therefore be assessed before proceeding to in-depth counselling. It may be necessary to involve her parents or partner at a later date if not available at the time of the diagnosis. Additionally, if consent is required for further testing, she must be of sufficient maturity to understand before giving consent.

Another important factor will be the type of malformation. Is it correctable, or associated with a poor prognosis? This may depend on the availability of facilities for expert echocardiography and counselling.

Any subsequent counselling will be influenced by the level of expertise of the person who made the diagnosis. Most likely this was made by a radiographer or at a secondary-level ultrasound scan. In these circumstances, counselling must be undertaken with extreme caution as, unless a fetal echocardiography has been undertaken, it may be misleading especially as to the outlook and the subsequent management options after delivery. It is important that the diagnosis and the severity of the abnormality are confirmed by a fetal cardiologist. Further counselling must be offered by the cardiologist and preferably a fetal medicine obstetrician. Other structural abnormalities should be excluded by further ultrasound scanning. The type of abnormality and the implications for the outcome of the baby will be a major factor for how the mother is counselled.

Finally, the postnatal facilities for managing the baby and the possible aetiological factors (if any) will be helpful, not only for tailoring her care but also for providing information on the recurrence risk and prevention.

(b) Critically appraise how she will be managed. (14 marks)

Her management must start with an explanation of the diagnosis, its implications and further management. Prior to this, attempts should be made to contact her partner or next of kin (e.g. parents). This may not delay the counselling and most patients would be too nervous waiting for the arrival of relatives. Whether she is of sufficient maturity and understanding to give consent to any required procedures should be ascertained prior to counselling. If she is not, it would be advisable to ensure that there is a next of kin present.

A cardiac echo should be offered as well as counselling by a paediatric cardiologist. This further scanning will determine whether the abnormality is correctable or not. If it is, the paediatrician will provide details of postnatal care, prognosis and arrange subsequent follow-up. It is important that she also has a tertiary-level ultrasound scan to exclude other coexisting abnormalities, which together may point to a specific syndrome. In the presence of other abnormalities, a clinical geneticist should be asked to see and counsel the patient.

Major structural cardiac abnormalities may be associated with chromosome abnormalities, such as deletion of the short arm of chromosome 22. The type of cardiac abnormality is therefore important. An isolated minor abnormality will not require karyotyping; however, for a major abnormality, karyotyping should be discussed and offered if acceptable. This is most likely to be by amniocentesis although a CVS is an alternative. FISH on the sample will only exclude specific chromosomal abnormalities but counselling should include the fact that a normal karyotype on FISH does not guarantee a normal karyotype. If the karyotype is abnormal or the prognosis is poor by virtue of associated malformations or the abnormality is incompatible with postnatal survival, then termination of pregnancy is an option. This is best undertaken after KCl injection and with mifepristone and prostaglandins.

Irrespective of the findings, counselling must emphasise that cardiac scanning is difficult and, although major abnormalities may be identified, subtle ones may not be excluded confidently. Therefore, subsequent monitoring and repeat detailed cardiac scans need to be performed during the pregnancy in those continuing with the pregnancy. These will increase the chances of identifying other abnormalities as the fetal heart gets bigger.

Unfortunately, antenatal exclusion of associated structural or chromosomal abnormalities does not completely guarantee their coexistence. Counselling should therefore emphasise that definitive answers will only be provided after delivery. In some cases, these may not even be obvious until after the neonatal period. The neonatal care of the baby and possible complications need to be discussed. Ample opportunity should be provided for repeated counselling to reinforce information offered. Delivery should be planned but it is best in a unit where there is a neonatal cardiologist and *in utero* transfer is better than *ex utero* transfer. In addition, the neonate should be examined thoroughly to ensure that other subtle malformations that could point to a specific prognosis are excluded.

The recurrence risk will depend on the type of malformation and its association with chromosomal abnormalities. However, the definitive counselling will only be offered after delivery and must involve a neonatologist.

4. Critically appraise the role of ultrasound scan in the diagnosis of trisomy 21. (20 marks)

Common mistakes

- Discussion of prenatal diagnosis of trisomy 21
- Ultrasound features of Down's syndrome
- Amniocentesis
- CVS
- Biochemical analytes for screening for trisomy 21
- Therefore no point discussing all the soft markers for Down's syndrome; amniocentesis versus CVS; biochemical analytes and Down's syndrome; advantages of first trimester versus second trimester scanning; accuracy of soft markers versus biochemical versus invasive procedures

A good answer should include some or all of these points

- Recognise that ultrasound is not a diagnostic tool for Down's syndrome
- Its role is mainly as an adjunct in: screening; diagnostic procedures
- Screening:
  - Dating of pregnancy – important as 40 per cent of women do not remember their last menstrual period (LMP) and therefore interpretation of NT and biochemical screening will be inaccurate
  - Soft markers – first trimester, second trimester
- Adjunct to diagnostic procedures: amniocentesis and CVS done under ultrasound guidance
- Disadvantages: operator dependent; machine quality important; not reliable in picking up cases of Down's syndrome; markers may generate unnecessary parental anxiety (false-negative results)
- Conclusion: key role in prenatal diagnosis of Down's syndrome but only in conjunction with invasive procedures of amniocentesis and CVS

Sample answer

Trisomy 21 is the most common chromosomal abnormality in the UK, with an incidence of one in 600 live births. Diagnosis is based on chromosome analysis and is not radiological; therefore ultrasound is not a diagnostic method for this abnormality. However, its role in its diagnosis is mainly as an adjunct to screening and in the performance of the invasive diagnostic procedures.

Although maternal age and family history are important risk factors for screening for Down's syndrome, biochemistry has become a common screening method. This depends on an accurately dated pregnancy. Since about 40 per cent of women are uncertain of their LMP, to be able to interpret the biochemical screening correctly, the pregnancy must be dated accurately. In the first trimester, ultrasound scan will date the pregnancy to within 4 days and to within 7–10 days in the second trimester. In the first trimester, ultrasound is also used to measure the NT, which is now a well-recognised marker for both chromosomal and structural or compression thoracic and cardiac abnormalities. Increasingly, sonoembryology is allowing early identification of soft markers for karyotypic abnormalities. In the second trimester ultrasound scan is useful in the identification of soft markers for trisomy 21. It is also an adjunct for diagnostic purposes as the procedures of amniocentesis, CVS and fetal blood sampling are all performed under ultrasound guidance.

Although ultrasound is important, there are disadvantages of using this tool in the antenatal diagnosis of trisomy 21. It is operator dependent and, therefore, soft markers may be missed. On the other hand, the quality of the machine is extremely important. With better machines, soft markers and other structural abnormalities of uncertain significance may become more evident and thus cause more uncertainty and anxiety to prospective parents. Ultrasound is not reliable in the diagnosis of Down's syndrome and some of the soft markers may be transient. The absence of these markers does not therefore imply the absence of trisomy 21. In fact, about 50 per cent of cases of trisomy 21 have no associated soft markers.

Ultrasound scan plays a key role in the prenatal diagnosis of trisomy 21, but only as a screening tool or when used to guide the operator in various invasive diagnostic procedures. Unfortunately, it generates significant anxiety in prospective parents when it identifies soft markers, especially as most of these fetuses are chromosomally normal.

5. Debate the statement that amniocentesis is soon to supersede CVS in prenatal diagnosis. (20 marks)

Common mistakes

- Describing the procedure of CVS
- Describing the complications of amniocentesis
- Complications of both procedures
- Early amniocentesis/CVS:
  - Limb defects? – aneuploidy?
  - Amniocentesis between 9 and 11 weeks and at 11–12 weeks?
  - Polymerase chain reaction for prenatal diagnosis

A good answer will include some of the following

- CVS: timing; skilled operator; results; mosaicism; complications
- Amniocentesis:
  - Timing results – role of FISH (limitations to specific probes), expensive, lower complication rate
- Termination of pregnancy – surgical or medical
- Unlikely to be superseded but will remain as an alternative under specific indications
- FISH

Sample answer

Amniocentesis and CVS are the two most common methods of prenatal karyotyping. Amniocentesis was the first of these procedures introduced into obstetrics. When CVS was introduced, it was generally believed that this procedure might supersede amniocentesis. However, both procedures continue to be offered to women throughout the world. Each has advantages and disadvantages. The concept that one will supersede the other is fuelled by these differences.

CVS offers prenatal diagnosis between 9 and 11 weeks' gestation. Although it was initially offered as early as 8 weeks' gestation, reports of association with terminal limb defects discouraged many perinatologists from offering it before 9 weeks' gestation. The advantages of CVS include early and quicker diagnosis – usually within 48 hours (from direct preparations), thereby allowing surgical terminations. In addition, these terminations may be performed without the patient feeling fetal movements or other signs of pregnancy becoming too obvious. The procedure is only available in a few centres where the expertise exists and enough procedures are undertaken to ensure that standards are maintained.

The complications of the procedure include miscarriages which may occur in about 1–2 per cent of all cases. Placental mosaicism occurs in about 1 per cent of CVS. Although the results may be available within 48 hours, this may fail. For quality assurance, cultures are necessary to confirm results. These tend to take about 10 days. The need for a skilled operator and facilities to process these samples means that this option is not readily available to all patients in some hospitals.

Amniocentesis, on the other hand, is recommended to be performed from 14 completed weeks of gestation upwards. The procedure is easy to perform and most units offer it. The main disadvantage is the time it takes for results to be available. In most units, this takes between 14 and 21 days, and in some, it may even take up to 4 weeks. By the time the results are known, it is often too late for a surgical termination and most units will therefore offer medical terminations. Some patients find this very distressing. With the advent of FISH, this may no longer be applicable. This technique can produce results from amniocentesis within 48 hours.

The main disadvantage is its restriction to specific chromosomes for which there are probes. Although it will identify most of the major chromosomal abnormalities and the sex chromosome disorders, the subtle or uncommon chromosomal abnormalities are unlikely to be diagnosed. The complications of amniocentesis are less frequent that those of CVS with a miscarriage risk of 0.5–1.0 per cent. The risk of mosaicism is also lower. Unlike CVS, this procedure can be performed by trained specialist registrars and in most units in the UK.

The two procedures may be interchangeable in some situations, but in some cases they serve different purposes. The concept of one superseding the other is therefore very unlikely. These two procedures complement each other and are offered for specific indications. It is therefore likely that they will remain available to couples.

6. A couple have just been told after an ultrasound scan at 15 weeks' gestation that their baby has a diaphragmatic hernia. (a) Outline very briefly the prognostic factors of this condition. (6 marks) (b) How will you counsel the patient now and throughout her pregnancy? (10 marks) (c) Justify how you will manage the labour. (4 marks)

Common mistakes

- Offer termination of pregnancy
- Refer patient to a fetomaternal specialist
- Diagnose chromosomal abnormalities
- Discussing the pros and cons of amniocentesis and CVS
- Complications of the prenatal diagnostic test
- Outlining the risk factors for congenital diaphragmatic hernia (CDH)
- Discussing the differential diagnoses of CDH

A good answer will include some or all of these points

(a) Outline very briefly the prognostic factors of this condition. (6 marks)

- The size of the hernia
- Timing of the diagnosis
- Presence of abdominal viscera in the chest
- Associated malformations – cardiac, etc.
- Associated karyotypic anomalies
- Associated polyhydramnios
- Quality and volume of lungs

(b) How will you counsel the patient now and throughout her pregnancy? (10 marks)

- Explain the diagnosis to the patient and partner (if not present, ask for permission to involve him)
- Outline difficulties predicting prognosis antenatally
- Early diagnosis indicates poorer prognosis compared to late diagnosis
- Referral for tertiary ultrasound scan (at same or different unit) to confirm diagnosis and exclude other anomalies, the presence of which may influence counselling and prognosis
- Isolated – offer karyotyping
- Isolated or part of a complex of malformations?– need for karyotype
- Exclude cardiac malformations
- Involvement of geneticist, neonatologist and paediatric surgeon
- Monitor for factors for adverse outcome: level in the chest; polyhydramnios; associated congenital malformations; need for long-term follow-up

(c) Justify how you will manage the labour. (4 marks)

- Await spontaneous onset – may need to be planned if from a unit without tertiary care facilities
- Intrapartum care – normal (labour and delivery)
- Inform paediatrician when admitted in labour and ensure present at the time of delivery
- Intubate and mechanically ventilate soon after delivery
- Once stabilised, transfer to neonatal intensive care unit (NICU) for planned surgery

Sample answer

(a) Outline very briefly the prognostic factors of this condition. (6 marks)

The prognosis of diaphragmatic hernia is difficult to predict antenatally; however, there are several factors that provide guidance. The timing of the diagnosis is one of the prognostic factors – the earlier the diagnosis, the more likely it is to be a larger defect, hence a poorer prognosis. The presence of abdominal viscera in the thorax suggests a large hernia, which is likely to be associated with a poorer prognosis. An isolated hernia has a better prognosis than one with associated malformations such as cardiac and chromosomal abnormalities. In later pregnancy, polyhydramnios is a poor prognostic sign. Although there are currently no reliable means of assessing lung volume, where the fetal lung volume is considered to be small, the prognosis is likely to be poor. Finally, the earlier the delivery, the poorer the prognosis.

(b) How will you counsel her now and throughout the pregnancy? (10 marks)

Counselling will start with an explanation of the diagnosis to the patient and her partner (if he is present). If he is not present, permission should be sought from the patient to contact him or another relative. The difficulties with providing a reliable assessment of prognosis antenatally should be discussed. It is important to be sure that the diagnosis is certain and, to this effect, a further ultrasound scan by a perinatologist (tertiary-level ultrasound scan) must be offered to the couple if one has not already been performed. During this ultrasound scan examination, not only must the diagnosis be confirmed but other structural abnormalities should be excluded, especially those of the cardiovascular system. Fetal echocardiography is therefore recommended. The presence of any associated abnormality will influence counselling (poor prognosis, need for karyotyping, etc.).

Where the abnormality is isolated, the prospective parents must be informed that the prognosis for the condition is difficult to predict. There are currently no predictive tests to gauge prognosis. However, monitoring during pregnancy may identify polyhydramnios, which is a poor prognostic factor. In addition, because the diagnosis has been made so early, this is likely to be associated with a large defect in the diaphragm and therefore a poor prognosis. Another factor that may predict prognosis is the presence of other abdominal viscera such as the liver and bowel in the thorax.

Although diaphragmatic hernias are not necessarily associated with a significantly higher incidence of chromosomal abnormalities, these need to be excluded as their coexistence is associated with a poor prognosis and termination will be an option. Therefore, on the basis of this, prenatal karotyping by amniocentesis or CVS should be discussed and offered. If the karyotype is normal, then subsequent management of the pregnancy must be multidisciplinary – involving a paediatrician, paediatric surgeon and a geneticist. The paediatrician will counsel the couple about neonatal management, whereas the paediatric surgeon will discuss the surgical correction of the defect. The geneticist will introduce the concept of syndromic babies.

Although there may be no other structural abnormality on ultrasound scan, or no chromosomal abnormality, there may be subtle abnormalities which, combined with the hernia, would be indicative of a syndrome. This possibility must be discussed and a priori recognition of some of these subtle abnormalities may make their identification after delivery easier.

(c) Justify how you will manage the labour. (4 marks)

Diaphragmatic hernia is not an indication for induction of labour or Caesarean section. However, if it is necessary to deliver the baby in a unit with appropriate facilities for neonatal care, then a planned delivery may be more suitable. Intrapartum monitoring should not be dissimilar to that for other pregnancies. However, the paediatrician must be notified when the patient is admitted in labour and be present at the time of delivery. Ideally, the delivery should be in a hospital with NICU facilities and those for paediatric surgery.

The best option is to deliver the baby by Caesarean section. This allows immediate intubation and ventilation rather than awaiting the onset of spontaneous breathing, which allows air into the stomach which may prevent the expansion of the lungs. The outcome for this baby must remain guarded until after delivery and surgery. In about 50 per cent of isolated cases, the outcome is good. In the others this will depend on various factors, some of which may be identified antenatally but most of which may not be obvious until delivery. Whatever the decision, there is a need to follow up the couple and the pregnancy long term to provide appropriate support and information about future pregnancies.

6

Isoimmunisation

1. Critically appraise prophylaxis against Rhesus (D) isoimmunisation. (20 marks)

2. A 26-year-old woman is in her first pregnancy with Rhesus (D) antibodies (32 IU/L) at 26 weeks' gestation. (a) Critically appraise how you will monitor the pregnancy. (14 marks) (b) What factors will determine any antenatal interventions and the timing of your delivery? (6 marks)

3. Anti-D prophylaxis has significantly reduced morbidity and mortality from Rhesus (D) isoimmunisation. However, there are still many cases of isoimmunisation occurring during pregnancy. How may this be remedied? (20 marks)

1. Critically appraise prophylaxis against Rhesus (D) isoimmunisation. (20 marks)

Common mistakes

- Forgetting the first trimester
- Ignoring the recommendations from the Royal College of Obstetricians and Gynaecologists (RCOG) about prophylaxis
- Detailing the management of a Rhesus-isoimmunised pregnancy
- Elaborating on other types of isoimmunisation
- Discussing the basis of anti-D prophylaxis
- Details of the pathogenesis of alloimmunisation

A good answer will include some or all of these points

- Anti-D has reduced the incidence of haemolytic disease of the newborn
- Recommendations
- Selective:
  - Rhesus-negative women – indications for prophylaxis
  - Bleeding >12 weeks, abdominal pain after delivery – difficulties with these recommendations:
    - Ideally, Kleihauer testing should be performed before administration of anti-D
  - Also recommended after amniocentesis, chorionic villus sampling, fetal blood sampling (FBS) and external cephalic version (ECV)
  - Problems with selective prophylaxis
  - Failed administration
  - Failure of sensitisation
  - Silent sensitisation
  - Inadequate doses
  - Strict adherence to 72 hours when it is relatively effective within 10 days
- Recent recommendation about routine prophylaxis
- 28 and 34 weeks – 500 IU:
  - Problems
  - Cost implications
  - Still miss out some silent sensitisations
- Reluctance by patients to accept because of the fear of new variant Creutzfeldt–Jakob disease (CJD), human immunodeficiency virus and hepatitis
- Monoclonal anti-D may overcome this

Sample answer

The advent of anti-D in the 1960s resulted in a significant reduction in perinatal morbidity and mortality from Rhesus isoimmunisation. Prophylaxis against isoimmunisation has been the key to this reduction. This prophylaxis has been to a large extent governed by standard recommendations. Very recently, these recommendations were modified by a Consensus Group consisting of obstetricians and haematologists.

The traditional recommendations were selective, anti-D given after a sensitising event. These events included miscarriages, invasive diagnostic procedures, antepartum haemorrhage, ECV, FBS and after delivery. The criteria for prophylaxis in the first trimester have been modified so that women with a slight bleed before 12 weeks' gestation are no longer required to have anti-D.

The difficulties with these modifications lie in their implementation. How is a mild bleed defined and what happens to patients who have repeated bleeds? The rationale for restricting this early group is the fact that significant fetomaternal haemorrhage is unlikely before 10 weeks' gestation. Ideally, these women should have a Kleihauer test and, where this is positive, anti-D should be given. Another consideration is that since anti-D is expensive, offering it at a time when it is least likely to be useful is not cost effective.

The consequences of this are that women who require anti-D by virtue of repeated bleeds and abdominal pain (but who have a high pain threshold) will be missed. In addition, those who are uncertain of their last menstrual period, whose pregnancies are therefore dated inappropriately, will not receive anti-D. An ideal situation would include scanning to date pregnancies accurately – but this is only possible when patients present to hospital. Since some of them do not and their general practitioners (GPs) are likely to follow recommendations, it is possible that sensitised women will appear as a result of this policy.

Since Kleihauer testing is not routinely performed on every patient, the dose of anti-D administered (especially in the latter stages of pregnancy) may not be enough and therefore sensitisation may still occur. Administration is often recommended within 72 hours of the sensitising event, yet it is recognised that some protection is available within 10 days of the event. The guidelines fail to address this enigma and therefore when patients present late, anti-D may not be offered.

The recommendation that all pregnant Rhesus-negative women be offered anti-D at 28 and 34 weeks' gestation, irrespective of a sensitising event, recognises the fact that failure to prevent isoimmunisation in some patients is related to silent fetomaternal haemorrhages. Since anti-D remains in the circulation for 6 weeks, administration of 500 IU at these gestations will cover the period where fetomaternal haemorrhages are likely to be significant. There are unfortunately some women who would not accept anti-D because it is a human product and also because of the risk of new variant CJD. These problems may be overcome with the advent of monoclonal anti-D.

Although prophylaxis has successfully reduced the incidence of sensitisation, failure to administer anti-D, or to administer the correct dose, and failure to protect despite administration, continue to result in affected pregnancies. Although more recent recommendations have attempted to address some of the reasons for these failures, there remain several obstacles to complete implementation and so isoimmunisation will persist.

2. A 26-year-old woman is in her first pregnancy with Rhesus (D) antibodies (32 IU/L) at 26 weeks' gestation. (a) Critically appraise how you will monitor the pregnancy. (14 marks) (b) What factors will determine any antenatal interventions and the timing of your delivery? (6 marks)

Common mistakes

- Take a history and physical examination
- Refer to high-risk unit for further management
- Discuss the pathogenesis of sensitisation
- Discussing the reasons for the sensitisation
- Deliver by Caesarean section

A good answer will include some or all of these points

(a) Critically appraise how you would monitor the pregnancy. (14 marks)

- Further investigations are required to ascertain the severity of the disease on the fetus:
  - Two approaches – invasive (FBS and amniocentesis) and non-invasive (Doppler ultrasound of the middle cerebral artery (MCA))
  - Invasive:
    - FBS – determines haemoglobin (Hb), blood group, presence of antibodies, bilirubin and reticulocytes, and blood gases
    - Highly skilled and associated with increased risk of preterm labour and rupture of fetal membranes
    - Amniotic fluid, optical densitometric analyses at wavelength of 450 nm (OD450) and safety lines
    - Risk of infections (chorioamnionitis), premature labour and rupture of fetal membranes
  - Doppler ultrasound scan of the MCA for peak systolic velocities:
    - No procedure-related risk
    - Not as precise as FBS or amniocentesis (i.e. will fail to identify all cases requiring intrauterine transfusion)
    - Result may be influenced by the skill of the operator and, for example, the angle of insonation or pressure of the fetal head
- Monitoring – options:
  - Maternal antibody levels (weekly or more frequently):
    - FBS – repeated FBS will significantly increase risks
    - Uncomfortable to patient and only provided in highly specialised centres – patient may have to travel (if no local facilities)
    - However, if transfusion required, can be given at the time of sampling
  - Amniocentesis – invasive and associated with risks

- MCA Doppler scan – non-invasive, reliable and can be offered by skilled ultrasonographers.
- No risk to pregnancy except may be a false result resulting in unnecessary intervention
- Ultrasound scan for growth:
  - Fetal biometry and features of hydrops or hepatomegaly

(b) What factors will determine any antenatal interventions and the timing of your delivery? (6 marks)

- Administration of steroids – anticipated gestational age at delivery. High antibody titre would suggest fetus is affected and would require early delivery
- Severity of disease in the fetus – if MCA Doppler scans are abnormal or either amniocentesis or FBS indicates severe disease at a stage when fetal maturity is assured (e.g. after 28 weeks) when the risk of intrauterine transfusion outweigh those of prematurity
- Critical points on the various investigations for which transfusion is required
- Availability of facilities for transfusion
- Availability of facilities for intensive neonatal care

Sample answer

(a) Critically appraise how you will monitor the pregnancy. (14 marks)

The antibody level in this primigravida is significantly high and most likely to be associated with, or result in, severe fetal disease. The first step is to ascertain whether the fetus has been affected. This can be achieved invasively or non-invasively. The invasive procedure of FBS has the benefit of enabling the determination of the fetal Hb, blood group, presence of antibodies, bilirubin, reticulocytes and blood gases (where there is severe anaemia). It requires skill and is performed mainly in tertiary centres to which this patient should be referred. Procedure-related risks at this gestation include preterm rupture of fetal membranes and/or labour, haemorrhage and haematoma (which, if from the cord, could result in tamponade). The other invasive option is amniocentesis; fluid obtained is subjected to OD450 and plotted on Liley's charts, from which action lines are established. This is fraught with complications such as premature rupture of membranes, preterm labour and chorioamnionitis.

Non-invasive assessment of the fetus is by means of Doppler velocimetry of the MCA for peak systolic velocities. These are then plotted on a normal chart (Mari and Hanif, 2008) and where the values are above the 95th centile, severe anaemia is suggested and thus the need for further intervention such as FBS and transfusion. This is not as precise as the invasive procedures but is associated with no risks to the fetus or mother. Prospective studies have demonstrated that this approach will identify all fetuses that are severely affected. The skill of the operator in obtaining the Doppler waveforms may influence the result and therefore the proportion of false-positive or -negative results.

Once it has been established that the baby is or is not affected by the antibodies, monitoring must target the antibody levels and the fetus. Maternal antibody levels should be measured at least weekly. There may be a need to monitor more frequently. With regards to fetal monitoring, this is best achieved by serial MCA Doppler velocimetry (e.g. twice weekly), serial FBS or amniocentesis, twice-weekly biophysical profilometry and fortnightly scans for fetal growth. Amniocentesis and FBS carry significant risk but if transfusion is required, this can be undertaken during the FBS. Doppler velocimetry on the other hand is free of risks. The growth scans will allow for the early identification of hydrops.

(b) What factors will determine any antenatal interventions and the timing of your delivery? (6 marks)

The first factor influencing antenatal intervention will be the anticipated timing of delivery. Two doses of 12 mg intramuscular betamethasone (or dexamethasone) should be administered, as this baby is likely to be delivered early. Another factor that will influence interventions is the severity of the alloimmunisation on the fetus. This will be determined by the MCA Doppler scans or amniocentesis or FBS, depending on which of these procedures is offered. Most units will use MCA Doppler scans to determine interventions. The type of intervention will depend on the gestational age. If the indication for intervention is after 32 weeks' gestation, it may be better to deliver and transfuse *ex utero* as the risks associated with intrauterine transfusion may outweigh the benefits. The critical points for which interventions are indicated will be crucial in the timing of interventions. Finally, the availability of facilities, and the expertise for any interventions will determine to a large extent where and who does the intervention.

References

Mari G, Hanif F (2008) Fetal Doppler: umbilical artery, middle cerebral artery, and venous system. *Semin Perinatol* **32**: 253–7.

3. Anti-D prophylaxis has significantly reduced morbidity and mortality from Rhesus (D) isoimmunisation. However, there are still many cases of isoimmunisation occurring during pregnancy. How may this be remedied? (20 marks)

Common mistakes

- Discussing anti-D prophylaxis – when and how it is administered
- Risk factors for sensitisation
- Screening for Rhesus D in pregnancy

A good answer will include some or all of these points

- Identify why there is failure of prophylaxis – failed administration; inadequate dose; silent fetomaternal haemorrhage
- Overcoming the reasons for failure:
  - Patient/GP/midwife education – communication of results and importance
  - Strict adherence to RCOG/National Institute for Health and Clinical Excellence guidelines
  - Administration even after 72 hours and up to 10 days – offers protection in up to 75 per cent of cases; larger doses (determined by Kleihauer test/flow cytometry)
- RCOG/Consensus Group recommendation – routine prophylaxis at 28 and 34 weeks (500 IU):
  - Poor implementation (not widely implemented yet) – expense – unavailable anti-D – new variant CJD – fear from patients (if human anti-D); monoclonal antibodies
- Recognition of the effects of other antibodies and effective screening

Sample answer

The persistence of sensitisation against Rhesus disease occurs for four main reasons. These are: (1) failure to administer anti-D, (2) administration of inadequate doses, (3) late administration and (4) silent fetomaternal haemorrhages. Until all these are remedied, Rhesus sensitisation will continue to occur.

There are several approaches to overcome persistent sensitisation. The first is the education of patients, midwives, GPs and all those involved in the care of pregnant women. Communication of blood group results to patients ought to be accompanied by leaflets explaining the implications of being Rhesus negative and imploring them to ensure that anti-D is given whenever there is a sensitising event in any pregnancy. Second, there must be mechanisms to guarantee strict adherence to guidelines on the administration of anti-D. Included in these guidelines should be an explanation of the rationale for this practice and that, where the 72-hour limit has been missed, prophylaxis should still be given as it offers some protection within 10 days of the sensitizing event.

Where possible, Kleihauer testing or flow cytometry should precede all anti-D administration and larger doses given if required. This may not be necessary in the first trimester since the 250 IU often administered is enough to neutralise 4 mL of fetal blood and the volume of fetal blood at this gestation is not significantly more than this.

The RCOG/Consensus Group recommendations about routine administration of anti-D at 28 and 34 weeks' gestation should be implemented. For effective implementation, adequate resources must be provided. Poor implementation has been blamed on inadequate finances to fund anti-D. For those objecting to human-derived anti-D, monoclonal anti-D should be made available. The risk of acquiring new variant CJD from anti-D is considered to be extremely small. Better education will therefore minimise the chances of rejection on this basis. Although Rhesus isoimmunisation may soon become uncommon, other rarer types of isoimmunisation are becoming more common. These must be recognised and efforts made to identify and prevent them in the same fashion as Rhesus isoimmunisation.

7

Abnormal fetal growth

1. A 26-year-old primigravida presents at 26 weeks' gestation with severe fetal growth restriction (FGR) confirmed on ultrasound scan. (a) What additional information will you require to help plan her management? (6 marks) (b) Evaluate the options available for monitoring the fetus. (7 marks) (c) What factors will influence when and how the fetus will be delivered? (7 marks)

2. What factors will determine the mode of delivery of a severely growth-restricted fetus in a primigravida? (20 marks)

3. A 30-year-old primigravida attended for her routine anomaly scan at 20 weeks' gestation. Ultrasound scan revealed a viable fetus of appropriate gestation with anhydramnios. She denies a history of spontaneous rupture of fetal membranes. (a) How will you exclude the causes of this complication? (8 marks) (b) Discuss the fetal consequences of anhydramnios. (4 marks) (c) Justify your management of the patient. (8 marks)

4. A 39-year-old woman attends for pre-pregnancy counselling having delivered a severely growth-restricted 1.6 kg male infant 6 months ago. (a) Justify the investigations you will undertake on her. (7 marks) (b) What counselling will you offer her with regards to recurrence? (6 marks) (c) How will you modify her care to reduce the risk of repeat FGR? (7 marks)

5. Fetal growth restriction is an important cause of perinatal morbidity and mortality. (a) Discuss the methods of screening women for this complication. (5 marks) (b) What are the risk factors for this complication? (5 marks) (c) How may the incidence be reduced? (3 marks) (d) Discuss briefly the complications of FGR. (7 marks)

1. A 26-year-old primigravida presents at 26 weeks' gestation with severe FGR confirmed on ultrasound scan. (a) What additional information will you require to help you plan her management? (6 marks) (b) Evaluate the options available for monitoring the fetus. (7 marks) (c) What factors will influence when and how the fetus is delivered? (7 marks)

Common mistakes

- Take a history and perform a physical examination
- Do an ultrasound scan to confirm gestational age
- Serum screening for Down's syndrome
- Deliver by Caesarean section
- Monitor fetus regularly (no details of monitoring)
- Refer to tertiary unit for management
- Fetal blood sampling (FBS) before deciding when to deliver
- Prognosis is too poor; therefore do nothing unless she goes into labour
- Discussing her past obstetric history and saying it is important (she is a primigravida!)

A good answer will contain some or all of the following

(a) What additional information will you require to help plan her management? (6 marks)

- Information related to the pregnancy:
  - Any history /diagnosis of viral infections earlier in pregnancy?
  - What was the serum alpha-fetoprotein (AFP) at the time of biochemical screening if done?
  - Any congenital malformations at the routine anomaly scan?
  - Fetal movements – normal or reduced?
  - History of antepartum haemorrhage or abdominal pain?
  - Details about ultrasound scan:
    - Type of FGR
    - Liquor volume
    - Doppler scans – done and if so what were the values (umbilical artery and middle cerebral artery (MCA))
- Information about facilities for neonatal care:
  - Neonatal intensive care facilities
  - Level of staff in the neonatal unit
  - Availability of space/cots

(b) Evaluate the options available for monitoring the fetus. (7 marks)

- Ultrasound scan:
  - Serial growth scans and liquor volume at least 10 days apart

- - Interval between scans may not allow for serial scans when fetus is severely growth restricted
- Doppler scans:
  - Umbilical and MCAs, ductus venosus
  - Frequency
- Biophysical profilometry (BPP):
  - Five parameters including cardiotocography (CTG)
  - Comprehensive but time consuming
- CTG:
  - Unreliable at this gestation
  - How frequently should this be done?
- Fetal kick chart:
  - Unreliable and very subjective

(c) What factors will influence when and how the fetus will be delivered? (7 marks)

- Fetal:
  - State of the fetus
  - Abnormal Doppler indices indicating immediate delivery
  - Abnormalities on CTG or monitoring parameters indicating immediate delivery
- Associated malformations:
  - Lethal malformations?
  - Correctable?
  - Infections
  - Karyotypic? Any need for karyotyping?
- Prognosis:
  - Depends on several factors including the gestational age at delivery
  - Facilities available and associated malformations of causative factor
- Gestational age:
  - Earlier gestation at delivery will imply delivery in a unit with neonatal intensive care unit facilities
  - Earlier delivery – most likely Caesarean section
- Steroids administration:
  - This may delay delivery to allow steroids to be effective
- Other causes, e.g. infections:
  - Maternal:
    - Associated complications
    - Pre-eclampsia (PET)
    - Thrombophilia
    - Others
- Wishes of the parents:
  - Parents' wishes will depend on prognosis and consequences on subsequent pregnancies

- Facilities for neonatal care:
  - Intensive care facilities and proximity
  - Staffing levels

Sample answer

(a) What additional information will you require to help plan her management? (6 marks)

The additional information required can be classified into that related to the pregnancy and that related to the facilities available for supporting the baby. With regards to information about the pregnancy, a history of, or suggestion of, viral infection earlier in this pregnancy may provide information about possible causes of the FGR. An unexplained raised AFP at the time of biochemical screening is associated with FGR. A normal anomaly scan would have excluded malformations associated with FGR; however, it should be recognised that some of these malformations could have been missed (especially cardiac malformations). Reduced or absent fetal movements, antepartum haemorrhage or abdominal pains will provide vital information for the assessment and monitoring of the pregnancy.

Any maternal history of diseases that may be associated with severe FGR should be excluded. These include hypertension, renal disease, connective tissue disorders and thrombophilias. Not only will this point to the potential cause of the FGR but it will also influence management.

Additional information about the ultrasound scan will include the type of FGR (symmetrical or asymmetrical), the liquor volume, Doppler velocimetry of fetal vessels (especially the umbilical artery and MCAs) and presence or absence of fetal breathing movements and tone.

(b) Evaluate the options available for monitoring the fetus. (7 marks)

This is aimed at assessing the fetal health and thereby establishing baseline indices for subsequent comparisons and also at determining whether to deliver or manage conservatively. Serial ultrasound scans (at least 10 days between scans) for growth and liquor volume provide a non-invasive tool for assessing growth and fetal health. Where the liquor is normal and there is reasonably satisfactory growth, this provides some reassurance. However, it requires manpower and frequent visits and does not provide a continuous means of assessing or monitoring fetal wellbeing. In a severely growth-restricted fetus, there may be no opportunity to perform more than one growth scan; however, liquor volume monitoring may be done more frequently and at shorter intervals than the 10 days required for growth scans.

Doppler velocimetry of the fetal arteries such as the umbilical and MCAs will provide a tool for assessing fetal wellbeing and help with the timing of delivery. The frequency of this monitoring will be determined by the state of the fetus. It requires expertise and machine but most units should be able to provide this nowadays. This test is sometimes dependent on the operator and therefore may result in unnecessary interventions.

Biophysical profilometry is another option but it requires ultrasound scan and is time consuming. It combines ultrasound scan and CTG. When applied properly, it is associated with an improved outcome but there is some suggestion now that not all the indices of this tool are essential for monitoring. Cardiotocography and fetal kick chats may be used but these have a limited application as they are either unreliable or only assess fetal health at the time of the test. In addition, just how frequently CTGs will be done will remain a problem.

(c) What factors will influence when and how the fetus will be delivered? (7 marks)

The factors that will influence when and how the fetus is delivered include the state of the fetus, associated malformations, the prognosis, gestational age at delivery and the facilities available in the unit. With regards to the state of the fetus, absent or reversed end diastolic flow on the umbilical artery Doppler scan or evidence of compensatory flow on the MCA Doppler scan or a BPP ≤6 will be considered an indication for delivery. Fetal kick charts and CTG are unreliable, especially at this early gestation.

Where there are associated malformations, their compatibility with life and association with karyotypic anomalies, congenital infections and whether these malformations are correctable will influence where and when this baby is delivered. For example, it may require delivering in a unit where appropriate corrective surgery, treatment of infections or supportive care can be provided.

Where the prognosis is poor, an option may be to wait for the demise of the baby *in utero* rather than delivery by Caesarean section. However, this must be determined taking into account the wishes of the parents. The gestational age will determine not only how soon the baby will be delivered, but how and where. The earlier the gestational age at delivery, the more severe the FGR and therefore the more likely delivery will be by Caesarean section and in a unit with neonatal intensive care facilities. If delivery is planned, the timing of steroid administration is important to ensure maximum benefit. Associated maternal complications, especially those that could compromise the mother's health such as PET, and their severity could lead to early delivery. Finally, the wishes of the parents and the facilities available should be taken into consideration when making the decision about delivery.

2. What factors will determine the mode of delivery of a severely growth-restricted fetus in a primigravida? (20 marks)

Common mistakes

- Take a history and do a physical examination
- Management will depend on past obstetric history – therefore obtain information about past obstetric history
- Discussing the details of monitoring of a fetus with FGR
- Screening and Doppler scanning in FGR
- Mode of delivery should be determined by the patient in conjuction with a neonatologist

A good answer should include some or all of these points

- FGR is a high-risk pregnancy and the outcome is influenced by the time of diagnosis and severity
- Late onset – better prognosis; milder forms – better prognosis
- FGR is due to several causes, some of which cannot be resolved with delivery
- The mode of delivery should offer the best outcome for the fetus and minimal risk to the mother
- Factors influencing mode of delivery:
    - Gestational age at diagnosis – very severe and early diagnosis – Caesarean section best option, likely classical
    - Presentation – breech/transverse lie – Caesarean section/cephalic vaginal delivery if safe for baby and mother
    - Severity – determined by size and/or monitoring indices – no intrauterine compromise and monitoring indices normal – vaginal delivery
    - Associated complications – PET/ruptured membranes and infections/ oligohydramnios, placental position
    - State of the cervix
    - Wishes of the patient

Sample answer

Severe FGR is associated with significant morbidity and mortality. The magnitude of these complications depends on the gestational age at which the diagnosis is made – the earlier the onset, the poorer the prognosis. The mode of delivery should offer the best outcome for the fetus and minimal risk to the mother.

Where the onset of FGR is early (e.g. occurring before the late second trimester) and the fetus is not significantly compromised (so as to have an extremely poor prognosis), the best option would be a Caesarean section. It is most likely that, at this early gestation, the lower segment will be poorly formed. This, compounded with oligohydramnios (a common association of severe FGR), will make a standard lower-segment Caesarean section difficult. A classical Caesarean section or a modified lower-segment Caesarean section (such as DeLee, U-shaped or a J-shaped incision on the lower uterine wall) would be more suitable. Although this is the best option at this early gestation, it must be remembered that maternal morbidity with this type of delivery is significant and that it also has a significant influence on subsequent pregnancies.

At a more advanced gestation, the lower segment may be formed, in which case the Caesarean section would be for a breech presentation, a significantly compromised fetus which cannot withstand the stress induced by labour, or associated complications such as PET, placental praevia or ruptured membranes with chorioamnionitis. If the fetus is not significantly compromised, there may be a place for a vaginal delivery. This will only be suitable if the cervix is ripe or ripening, labour will not be prolonged, the presentation is cephalic, and there are no associated complications. Although this may be the safest option for the mother, there is always the risk of progression to emergency abdominal delivery, which is associated with more morbidity than that following an elective Caesarean section. Therefore, the decision to allow a vaginal delivery in a severely growth-restricted pregnancy must be made bearing in mind that a larger proportion of cases will require an emergency abdominal delivery.

Although attempts to deliver a live fetus seem to be the best approach in the management of this primigravida, if the fetus is considered to be severely compromised and with a very poor prognosis, there may be a case to allow it to die *in utero* and opt for a vaginal delivery. The other option would be to induce a vaginal delivery knowing that the outcome will be uniformly poor. Such a decision has to be made with appropriate counselling from obstetricians and paediatricians. Whatever the case, the mode of delivery should be determined only after counselling the patient and taking her wishes into consideration alongside the state of the fetus and its long-term outcome.

3. A 30-year-old primigravida attended for her routine anomaly scan at 20 weeks' gestation. Ultrasound scan revealed a viable fetus of appropriate gestation with anhydramnios. She denies a history of spontaneous rupture of fetal membranes. (a) How will you exclude the causes of this complication? (8 marks) (b) Discuss the fetal consequences of anhydramnios. (4 marks) (c) Justify your management of the patient. (8 marks)

Common mistakes

- Take a history and do a physical examination to exclude 'causes' of spontaneous rupture of fetal membranes and oligohydramnios
- Listing all the causes of oligohydramnios/anhydramnios
- Management will depend on the degree of oligohydramnios
- Discussing the methods of diagnosing spontaneous rupture of fetal membranes
- Terminate the pregnancy
- Delivery should be by Caesarean section
- Screen for abnormal Doppler scans
- Failing to critically appraise your answer
- Induce labour at 28–34 weeks' gestation

A good answer will include some or all of these points

(a) How will you exclude the causes of this complication? (8 marks)

- Spontaneous rupture of fetal membranes
  - History and examination – sudden gush of liquor, feeling wet, continuous leakage? Speculum examination and demonstration of leakage of fluid. Others include fern test, nitrazine test
- Renal agenesis/obstruction to the outflow – posterior urethral valve – ultrasound at tertiary level. Limitations of ultrasound scan with anhydramnios
  - Doppler to identify renal arteries – beware adrenal arteries may mimic renal arteries
- Karyotyping for aneuploides – unlikely to be in isolation. Done by placental biopsy or FBS. Be aware of placental mosaicism

(b) Discuss the fetal consequences of anhydramnios. (4 marks)

- Pulmonary hypoplasia
- Compression deformities
- Intrauterine death

(c) Justify your management of the patient. (8 marks)

- Arrange an ultrasound scan to exclude renal agenesis – may be done at a tertiary centre with amnioinfusion
- Counsel about findings and prognosis – poor
- Offer termination of pregnancy
- Continue with pregnancy but fetus may die *in utero*
- Karyotyping
- Discuss post mortem to confirm diagnosis
- Counselling and follow-up visit with regards to recurrence

Sample answer

(a) How will you exclude the causes of this complication? (8 marks)

Anhydramnios is defined as complete absence of liquor amnii around the fetus. At this early gestation, the prognosis is poor unless it can be corrected. This will depend largely on the cause, which in most cases is not compatible with survival. The most likely causes are renal agenesis, obstruction to urine outflow and rupture of fetal membranes. In some cases it may be due to chromosomal abnormalities or other structural abnormalities.

The first step in the management of this patient is to attempt to establish the cause of the anhydramnios. Since she has denied the history of rupture of fetal membranes, her notes should first be reviewed to establish whether she has had previous ultrasound scans that revealed normal liquor. A booking ultrasound scan is the most likely one and this is unable to correctly predict anhydramnios, as during the early gestation there is no significant production of liquor amnii. However, it might have identified possible aetiological factors.

Although the history has been denied, it is essential to undertake a speculum examination and perform a test to exclude rupture of fetal membranes. With anhydramnios, this is likely to be negative. If it is positive, it will suggest a possible premature rupture of fetal membranes, although this is unlikely to influence the management. The tests used for this are recognised to have both false negatives and positives and may, therefore, not provide conclusive evidence for, or against, spontaneous rupture of fetal membranes.

The absence of liquor means that detailed ultrasound scanning will be difficult. The detailed scan should therefore be organised in a tertiary centre where level-three ultrasound is available. It may be necessary to undertake an amnioinfusion in order to facilitate this procedure. However, amnioinfusion is associated with the risks of chorioamnionitis and spontaneous miscarriages. Sometimes this procedure may rectify the anhydramnios and allow the pregnancy to progress to viability. It is, however, rare in cases of anhydramnios and more likely where there is oligohydramnios.

Since renal agenesis is a common cause of this complication, demonstrating the presence of kidneys may help in the management. The presence of kidneys may support repeated amnioinfusions, provided there are no other abnormalities that are incompatible with life. The use of colour Doppler scanning to delineate the renal arteries may be useful. It must be remembered that where there is renal agenesis, the adrenal arteries may be confused with renal arteries.

(b) Discuss the fetal consequences of anhydramnios. (4 marks)

The consequences of anhydramnios include pulmonary hypoplasia, which is incompatible with extrauterine survival, compression deformities and eventually fetal death. The severity of these complications will depend on the timing of the anhydramnios, especially if the cause is not congenital – the earlier the onset, the more severe the complications. Where the fetus does not die *in utero*, it is most likely to die in the neonatal period.

(c) Justify your management of the patient. (8 marks)

Since chromosomal and metabolic abnormalities may also be responsible for this complication, karyotyping should be discussed and offered. The best approach in this case is placental biopsy (chorionic villus sampling (CVS)). This is unlikely to alter the management. In some cases, where termination is offered CVS may be done before termination. The problem of placental mosaicism is a recognised drawback of this method of karyotyping.

In the absence of any karyotypic or structural abnormality, repeated amnioinfusions may be associated with a relatively good prognosis, provided the infused saline is retained. The neonatologist should be informed and involved in the care of the neonate from such management. However, at this very early gestation, pulmonary hypoplasia and pressure deformities are most likely, and after delivery the neonate would most probably succumb to hypoplasia of the lungs. Where the prognosis is considered to be poor, termination of pregnancy should be offered and following this, an autopsy to confirm the antenatal diagnosis and exclude the presence of other abnormalities that could be combined to constitute a syndrome with an obvious risk of recurrence.

4. A 39-year-old woman attends for pre-pregnancy counselling having delivered a severely growth-restricted 1.6 kg male infant 6 months ago. (a) Justify the investigations you will undertake on her. (7 marks) (b) What counselling will you offer her with regards to recurrence? (6 marks) (c) How will you modify her care to reduce the risk of repeat FGR? (7 marks)

Common mistakes

- Take a history and do a physical examination
- Assuming that she has PET and treating PET
- Managing her as a case of thrombophilia
- Failure to justify the investigations and treatment
- Assuming that the fetus is malformed or has aneuploidy
- Assuming that aneuploidy and malformations have been excluded
- The question is about management after delivery and there is no point in discussing management predelivery, including the administration of steroids

A good answer will include some or all of these points

(a) Justify the investigations you will undertake on her. (7 marks)

- Thrombophilia – proteins C and S, antithrombin III, factor V Leiden (activated protein C resistance)
- Antiphospholipid syndrome – lupus anticoagulant, anticardiolipin antibody
- Hyperhomocysteinaemia – fasting homocysteine
- Blood pressure check and investigate for hypertension if appropriate
- Infection screening
- Karyotyping if appropriate
- Thyroid function test
- Others

(b) What counselling will you offer her with regards to recurrence? (6 marks)

- Depends on the aetiology
- Idiopathic – recurrence risk is increased approximately 10-fold
- Cause – isolated or recurrent
- Chromosomal – risk is that of the chromosome abnormality
- Infections – minimal recurrence risk, etc.

(c) How will you modify her care to reduce the risk of FGR? (7 marks)

- Pre-pregnancy – lifestyle modification (smoking, alcohol, drugs, e.g. recreational)

- Folic acid
- Treat causes of FGR before embarking on pregnancy
- Book for antenatal care in consultant-led unit
- Aspirin in early pregnancy until 34 weeks
- Serial growth ultrasound scans
- Uterine artery Doppler velocimetry at 24 weeks
- Low-molecular-weight heparin if antiphospholipid syndrome, or treat other recognised causes as appropriate

Sample answer

(a) Justify the investigations you will undertake on her. (7 marks)

These will concentrate on identifying the possible cause of the FGR and include thrombophilia screening (including protein C and S, antithrombin III, activated protein C resistance and homocystein). Interpreting the results of these investigations must take into consideration the physiological changes that occur in pregnancy (especially protein S, which falls). Other investigations include screening for antiphospholipid syndrome (lupus anticoagulant and anticardiolipin antibody). Abnormal results will need to be repeated at least 4–6 weeks later. Other investigations will depend on symptoms and these include investigating for hypertension, hyperthyroidism, renal disease and other systemic diseases. The placenta should be sent for histological examination, and genetic testing, including karyotyping, should be undertaken on the parents if the baby has any dysmorphic features or has been demonstrated to be aneuploidic. Maternal infection screening should be undertaken if this is suspected to be a possible aetiological factor.

(b) What counselling will you offer her with regards to recurrence? (6 marks)

The risk of recurrence of FGR is significantly greater after delivering a severe FGR fetus. This risk will be influenced by the aetiological factors and whether any preventative measures are instituted. The risk of recurrence for idiopathic FGR is increased 10 times; for chromosomal abnormalities, this will be that of the abnormality. For example, any major aneuploidy has a recurrence risk of 1 per cent, unless there is parental chromosomal abnormality. Where infections are the cause, the risk of recurrence is minimal. Treatment of the aetiological factors and preventative measures such as the institution of thromboprophylaxis in those with antiphospholipid syndrome and thrombophilias will reduce the risk of recurrence. Treatment of other conditions such as hypertensive disorders and thyroid dysfunction will also affect the recurrence rate.

(c) How will you modify her care to reduce the risk of repeat FGR? (7 marks)

The first step to minimise the risk of recurrence is to counsel the patient about modification of lifestyle factors that affect fetal growth. These include smoking, alcohol and drugs, especially recreational drugs. Folic acid supplementation at the recommended dose will reduce the risk of malformations that may be associated with FGR.

She will be encouraged to book early and her care will be in a consultant-led unit. There may be a place for starting low-dose aspirin early, although the evidence for the benefit of this will depend on the cause.

In addition to the various routine ultrasound scans (booking and detailed), serial growth scans should be instituted from 24 weeks. A uterine artery Doppler scan at 22–24 weeks may identify those who are at a greater risk of recurrence. Where thrombophilia has been identified as an associated factor, thromboprophylaxis such as low-molecular-weight Fragmin® should be introduced early. Overall, the outcome of the pregnancy will depend to a large extent on the monitoring and treatment introduced.

5. Fetal growth restriction is an important cause of perinatal morbidity and mortality. (a) Discuss the methods of screening women for this complication. (5 marks) (b) What are the risk factors for this complication? (5 marks) (c) How may the incidence be reduced? (3 marks) (d) Discuss briefly the complications of FGR. (7 marks)

Common mistakes

- Discussing the causes of perinatal mortality and morbidity and relating them to FGR
- Take a history and make a diagnosis
- Listing the causes of FGR and discussing the pathogenesis of FGR
- Umbilical artery for diagnosis of FGR
- Discussing screening for PET and its management – although this is a cause of FGR, the question is about FGR and not PET, although there is inevitably some overlap
- Referring patient to tertiary unit for screening and management
- Discussing the pros and cons of either induction of labour for FGR or Caesarean section at particular gestations
- Criticising the various methods of monitoring

A good answer will include some or all of these points

(a) Discuss the methods of screening women for this complication (5 marks)

- History
- Demographics
- Clinical – abdominal palpation, symphysiofundal height measurement
- Customised against maternal weight, height, parity and ethnicity
- Uterine artery Doppler scan
- Ultrasound scan

(b) What are the risk factors for this complication? (5 marks)

- Previous FGR
- Recurrent miscarriage
- Unexplained raised AFP
- Hypertension/PET
- Systemic medical disorders
- Antepartum haemorrhage
- Social factors – smoking, alcohol, drugs

(c) How may the incidence be reduced? (3 marks)

- Early identification

- Prophylaxis
- Early diagnosis
- Monitoring
- Timely interventions

(d) Discuss briefly the complications of FGR. (7 marks)

- Intrauterine:
  - Intrauterine fetal death
  - Asphyxia
- Intrapartum:
  - Abnormal heart rate patterns
  - Fetal hypoxia (acidosis)
  - Meconium aspiration
  - Stillbirth
  - Increased risk of Caesarean section
- Neonatal:
  - Hypothermia
  - Hypoglycaemia
  - Mortality
  - Feeding difficulties
  - Anaemia
  - Necrotising enterocolitis
- Long-term:
  - Chronic lung disease
  - Increased childhood death
  - Neurodevelopmental disability
  - Hypertension and cardiovascular diseases
  - Metabolic syndrome – diabetes mellitus, etc.
  - Early death as adults

Sample answer

(a) Discuss the methods of screening women for this complication. (5 marks)

The diagnosis of FGR is poor and as many as 50 per cent of unexplained stillbirths are growth restricted. The methods of screening and diagnosis include clinical assessments and imaging. Abdominal inspection and palpation will identify only about a third of cases of FGR. This is not diagnostic, hence a large number will be mislabelled FGR and vice versa. This may be improved by symphysiofundal height measurement but a single measurement does not significantly improve the sensitivity of this screening tool. However, serial measurements that are plotted on customised charts are associated with a significantly better identification rate. These measurements are customised to the mother's height and weight.

Ultrasound examination of the fetus provides a more objective means of not only screening for, but also diagnosing, FGR. This will enable measurement of the growth velocity or the abdominal circumference (AC) plotted on a customised chart of AC and estimated fetal weight. The measurements plotted either on a customised chart or used to determine growth velocity are more sensitive at predicting and diagnosing FGR. There is no place for using amniotic fluid volume either as a screening or diagnostic tool. However, once a diagnosis has been made, this is useful in monitoring. Uterine artery Doppler velocimetry is a useful screening tool, with an abnormal value in a low-risk population reported to be associated with a 3.6 times increase in the likelihood ratio of developing FGR and a reduction in the likelihood ratio for a normal test by about 0.8.

(b) What counselling will you offer with regards to recurrence? (5 marks)

The risk factors for FGR include previous FGR, recurrent miscarriages, especially in the late first and second trimesters, unexplained raised AFP in the second trimester, maternal thrombophilia, antiphospholipid syndrome, systemic medical disorders such as hyperthyroidism, renal disease, hypertension, connective tissue disorders, antepartum haemorrhage and social factors such as smoking, drugs and alcohol. The risk of recurrence depends on the various factors and whether these can be modified or not. In unexplained FGR, the risk of recurrence is 10-fold greater. The fetal risk factors for FGR include congenital infections, especially the viral infections, congenital malformations and aneuploidy.

(c) How may the incidence be reduced? (3 marks)

The incidence of FGR can be reduced by identifying the high-risk population and risk factors, and combining prophylaxis and surveillance. A good history will identify most of the risk factors enumerated above under (b) and appropriate steps can then be taken to reduce these risks. Treatment of medical complications such as hypertension, and ensuring that maternal health is maximised prior to fertilisation, will be very useful in this regard. In addition, prophylaxis with low-molecular-weight heparin in those with positive screening result will significantly reduce the incidence. When the diagnosis is made, appropriate monitoring and timely interventions will reduce the complications and consequences. Where possible, all at-risk patients should have consultant-led antenatal care where surveillance is more likely to be comprehensive.

(d) Discuss briefly the complications of FGR. (7 marks)

The complications of FGR can be classified as those in the intrauterine and neonatal periods and long-term childhood and adult complications. The main intrauterine complications include asphyxia, oligohydramnios and intrauterine fetal death. During labour, the fetus is at risk of abnormal fetal heart rate patterns, stillbirth, meconium asphyxia and fetal acidosis. The Caesarean section rate for these babies is also higher. The complications in the neonatal period include hypoglycaemia, hypothermia, necrotising enterocolitis, anaemia and feeding difficulties. Children are prone to chronic respiratory disorders, failure to thrive and neurodevelopmental disabilities. In adulthood, FGR babies are at a greater risk of cardiovascular disorders, metabolic syndrome and early death.

8

Abnormal presentation

1. External cephalic version (ECV), performed at 36 weeks' gestation, is not justified. Debate this statement. (20 marks)

2. During a 38 weeks' antenatal assessment, you establish that the patient has an unstable lie. (a) Justify the investigations you will undertake on the patient. (6 marks) (b) Assuming that nothing abnormal is found, evaluate your management options of the pregnancy. (14 marks)

3. A 42-year-old primigravida is found to have a breech presentation at 38 weeks' gestation. (a) What factors will influence the advice you will offer the patient with regards to mode of delivery? (10 marks) (b) Briefly outline how you will manage the rest of the pregnancy if the baby is found to be transverse at 41 weeks' gestation. (10 marks)

1. External cephalic version, performed at 36 weeks' gestation, is not justified. Debate this statement. (20 marks)

Common mistakes

- Discussing the process of ECV
- Complications of ECV
- Differences between ECV at 36 and 37 weeks' gestation
- Failing to debate (debate means – advantages, disadvantages and conclusion)

A good answer will include some or all of these points

- Advantages:
  - Easier
  - Higher success rate at the time of ECV
  - More liquor and smaller baby
  - Bypass preterm breech delivery before 37 weeks' gestation
- Disadvantages:
  - Large number of pregnancies will be offered ECV
  - Some will undergo spontaneous version after ECV
  - Complications increased morbidity and neonatal complications
- Conclusions – on balance not advisable

Sample answer

Breech presentation at 36 weeks' gestation occurs in about 5–7 per cent of singleton pregnancies. ECV has been shown to reduce the prevalence of breech presentation at term and, therefore, the need for Caesarean section for breech presentation in labour or at term. The timing of this procedure has significant bearings on the numbers presenting at term.

Although most experts recommend that ECV be performed at 37–38 weeks' gestation, it is accepted that it can also be performed at 36 weeks. At this gestation, the procedure is easier because there is more liquor around the fetus and therefore the chances of success are higher. It is also considered to be easier as the fetus is smaller. For pregnancies that may go into spontaneous labour before 37 weeks' gestation (preterm), performing ECV at this early gestation ensures that such patients present in labour with cephalic presentation. This will inevitably reduce the complications associated with preterm breech delivery.

However, there are significant disadvantages to performing ECV at this gestation. Although it may be easier and more likely to succeed, it may be argued that approximately 20–25 per cent of breech presentations at 36 weeks' gestation will turn spontaneously into cephalic presentation at term. Therefore, these pregnancies do not require intervention. Performing the procedure at 36 weeks' gestation will involve a larger population of patients. ECV is associated with complications, such as preterm labour, placental abruption and cord entanglement, all of which may necessitate immediate delivery. At 36 weeks' gestation, the risks of prematurity are still significant and, therefore, undertaking this procedure just because of an increased success rate, but with an increased risk of prematurity and its complications, may not be the ideal trade-off.

The timing of ECV should be influenced by the chances of success, associated complications and the number of patients requiring this procedure. On balance, although 36 weeks may be associated with a higher success rate, it is not the ideal time for this procedure. It should be performed at a gestational age when most cases that would have undergone spontaneous version have done so. In addition, it should be undertaken when fetal maturity is considered to be sufficient in case emergency delivery is necessary. On this basis, therefore, 36 weeks does not appear to be the best time for ECV. The best time for this procedure should be at 37 or more weeks' gestation.

2. During a 38 weeks' antenatal assessment, you establish that the patient has an unstable lie. (a) Justify the investigations you will undertake on the patient. (6 marks) (b) Assuming that nothing abnormal is found, evaluate your management options of the pregnancy. (14 marks)

Common mistakes

- Offer elective lower-segment Caesarean section
- Offer a classical Caesarean section
- Discussing the complications of cord prolapse
- Advantages and disadvantages of ECV
- Different types of Caesarean section

A good answer will include some or all of these points

(a) Justify the investigations you will undertake on the patient. (6 marks)

- Ultrasound scan to exclude causes:
  - Localise the placenta
  - Pelvic tumours
  - Uterine malformation
  - Polyhydramnios
  - Oligohydramnios
  - Fetal macrosomia
  - Fetal anomalies
  - Most cases are idiopathic and related to high parity
- Full blood count (FBC), group and save serum

(b) Assuming that nothing abnormal is found, evaluate your management options of the pregnancy. (14 marks)

- Educate patient on complications
- May be complicated by ruptured membranes – cord or hand prolapse, difficult Caesarean section
- Admission into hospital?:
  - Advantages – monitored daily
  - Rupture – immediate access to surgery and possible risks
  - Disadvantage – patient away from family
  - Expensive to hospital
- Management at home?:
  - Alternative to inpatient management

- Easy access to hospital
- Education on the complications
- Timing delivery:
  - ECV
  - Stabilisation induction
  - Caesarean section if fails
  - Caesarean section – emergency or elective
  - Rupture membranes
  - During version

Sample answer

(a) Justify the investigations you will undertake on the patient. (6 marks)

The single most valuable investigation is ultrasound scan. This will exclude causes such as placenta praevia, pelvic tumours (such as ovarian cysts, uterine fibroids), fetal malformations, polyhydramnios, oligohydramnios, fetal macrosomia and congenital malformations of the uterus. Although ultrasound diagnosis of congenital malformations in pregnancy is unreliable because of the changes associated with pregnancy, this is still worth doing as the diagnosis of one (which will negate version) will be considered a contraindication to a vaginal delivery. In most cases, no cause is identified. Another important investigation is FBC and especially the haemoglobin estimation, since emergency surgery may be required at very short notice. It may also be advisable to group and save serum.

(b) Assuming that nothing abnormal is found, evaluate your management options of the pregnancy. (14 marks)

The patient should be admitted to hospital until fetal lie is stabilised or the baby is delivered. This is to minimise the complications of spontaneous rupture of fetal membranes with the consequence of cord or hand prolapse. A problem may arise if the patient has other children at home or refuses hospital admission. A detailed explanation of the reasons (education on the risks, especially spontaneous rupture of fetal membranes and cord prolapse) for offering hospital admission should be given to the patient.

Where she refuses admission, it is essential that her concerns are addressed. There is a place for managing the patient at home provided she is within easy reach of the hospital and has been counselled to report immediately there are contractions (irrespective of how mild they are), any vaginal bleeding or suspicion of ruptured membranes.

However, if she is not within easy reach of the hospital, admission is likely to be the only option. Her subsequent management will consist of daily palpation of the fetal lie. Once the lie has become longitudinal and remained so for at least 48 hours, and especially where the head is engaged, she should be allowed home and the spontaneous onset of labour awaited. However, if fetal lie remains unstable, ECV may be offered and, if this is successful and the lie remains stable, again she could be allowed home.

The other option is to offer the patient stabilisation induction at 41 weeks' gestation. This involves external version into a longitudinal position followed by Syntocinon®. Once adequate uterine contractions have been established, fetal membranes should be ruptured and labour allowed to progress as normal. In some cases, if the cervix is favourable, the membranes should be ruptured after version (with the fetus held in the longitudinal position) during the rupture. Once the liquor has drained, the likelihood of the fetus changing its lie becomes very small. Contractions could therefore be initiated with Syntocinon®.

In the event that the fetal membranes rupture with the fetus in the transverse or oblique position, the first step must be to exclude cord prolapse. Thereafter, the fetus must be delivered by Caesarean section. This is one of the few recognised indications for a classical Caesarean section. However, where the Caesarean section is performed soon after the membranes have ruptured (i.e. before all the liquor has drained), a lower-segment Caesarean section may be possible, especially if the back of the baby is posterior.

3. A 42-year-old primigravida is found to have a breech presentation at 38 weeks' gestation. (a) What factors will influence the advice you will offer the patient with regards to mode of delivery? (10 marks) (b) Briefly outline how you will manage the rest of the pregnancy if the baby is found to be transverse at 41 weeks' gestation. (10 marks)

Common mistakes

- History, examination and investigations!
- Details of the reasons why women have a breech presentation
- Discussing the breech term trial in detail
- Details of intrapartum management of breech presentation
- Complications of delivery
- How to perform an ECV and its complications
- Discussing the management of the causes of breech presentation, e.g. placenta praevia and pelvic tumours

A good answer will include some or all of these points

(a) What factors will influence the advice you will offer the patient with regards to mode of delivery? (10 marks)

- Evidence for breech vaginal versus Caesarean section (Term Breech Trial)
- Other contraindications to a vaginal delivery
- Fetal status
- Malformations
- Growth abnormalities
- Compromised, e.g. severely growth restricted?
- Type of breech
- Expertise for ECV
- Expertise for breech vaginal delivery
- Wishes of the patient
- Others

(b) Briefly outline how you will manage the rest of the pregnancy if the baby is found to be transverse at 41 weeks' gestation (10 marks).

- Exclude malformations
- Discuss options – vaginal versus Caesarean section
- ECV
- If Caesarean section – plan for 39 weeks

- If ECV, arrange and perform with counselling for emergency Caesarean section
- If breech vaginal delivery – allow spontaneous labour – no Syntocinon® or induction
- Appropriate analgesia
- Paediatrician and consultant to be available when in labour

Sample answer

(a) What factors will influence the advice you will offer the patient with regards to mode of delivery? (10 marks)

The most important factor is what the patient wants. The two options for her are attempting an ECV or planning an elective Caesarean section. She may also wish to have a trial of vaginal breech delivery. The most important evidence for mode of delivery is the Term Breech Trial (Hannah *et al.*, 2000). This clearly demonstrated that a vaginal breech delivery is associated with a significantly greater perinatal morbidity and mortality. On this basis, therefore the Royal College of Obstetricians and Gynaecologists recommends elective Caesarean section at term.

Other factors that will influence the advice she is given on mode of delivery will include the presence of contraindications to a vaginal delivery. If any of these are present, then an ECV will also be contraindicated. A macrosomic fetus or one compromised by fetal growth restriction or malformations will be considered a contraindication for ECV.

If the patient elects for a trial of vaginal breech delivery, the type of breech will be important. A footling breech will be unsuitable for a trial of vaginal delivery, while an extended breech is more likely to be successful.

Whether she is offered an ECV or not will depend on the expertise available and facilities to monitor the fetus, and embark on an emergency Caesarean section if required.

(b) Briefly outline how you will manage the rest of the pregnancy if the baby is found to be transverse at 41 weeks' gestation (10 marks).

The options at 41 weeks for this woman with a transverse lie are either an elective Caesarean section, an attempt at ECV and awaiting the spontaneous onset of labour, stabilisation induction or waiting for version until 42 weeks when either a Caesarean section or a stabilisation induction can be offered.

Assuming that malformations have been excluded, then these options will be discussed with the woman. If not, an ultrasound scan would be performed to exclude a low-lying placenta and exclude fetal malformations which may be causing the transverse lie. In the absence of any contraindication, an ECV would be the first option if the patient does not object. This is easier with a transverse lie than a breech longitudinal presentation. The main risk is rupture of membranes and either cord or hand prolapse. Although it may be successful, there is no guarantee that it will not revert to the transverse lie.

The other option will be performing a stabilisation induction. In this case, ECV is performed and the membranes ruptured while stabilising the lie of the baby. Where the cervix is unfavourable for an artificial rupture of fetal membranes, prostaglandin pessaries may be given to ripen the cervix before the ECV.

The last option will be to perform an elective Caesarean section. This will be when there are contraindications to version or vaginal delivery. Such contraindications include lower-segment fibroids and malformations of the uterus.

Reference

Hannah ME, Hannah WJ, Hewson SA, Hodnett ED, Saigal S, Willan AR (2000) Planned Caesarean section versus planned vaginal birth for breech presentation at term: a randomised multicentre trial. Term Breech Trial Collaborative Group. *Lancet* **356**: 1375–83.

9

Preterm labour/premature rupture of fetal membranes

1. A woman who has had two previous preterm deliveries, at 24 and 26 weeks' gestation respectively, presents for pre-pregnancy counselling. (a) Justify the investigations you will discuss with the patient. (6 marks) (b) How will you manage her in her next pregnancy? (14 marks)

2. Preterm delivery is one of the most important causes of perinatal mortality. Evaluate the methods available for the prevention of preterm labour. (20 marks)

3. A 37-year-old primigravida with a history of infertility presents at 23 weeks' gestation with premature rupture of fetal membranes. (a) Critically appraise the non-radiological investigations you will undertake on the patient. (4 marks) (b) Justify how you will monitor the patient after confirmation of the diagnosis. (4 marks) (c) How will you manage the patient prior to delivery? (6 marks) (d) What factors will influence your timing and method of delivery? (6 marks)

1. A woman who has had two previous preterm deliveries, at 24 and 26 weeks' gestation respectively, presents for pre-pregnancy counselling. (6 marks) (a) Justify the investigations you will discuss with the patient. (b) How will you manage her in her next pregnancy? (14 marks)

Common mistakes

- Take a history and perform a physical examination
- Assume that she is pregnant
- Refer to tertiary centre
- Offer a cervical cerclage
- Admit for bed rest until delivery
- Induce labour at 34 weeks' gestation
- Offer prophylactic antibiotics
- Screen for cervical infections

A good answer will include some or all of these points

(a) Justify the investigations you will discuss with the patient. (6 marks)

- Investigations outside pregnancy:
  - Vaginal swabs/endocervical swabs
  - Hysterosalpingography (HSG)
  - Retrograde cervical dilatation – historic
  - Ultrasound scan for fetal anomalies
- Investigations during pregnancy:
  - Cervical ultrasound assessment – length and dilatation
  - High vaginal swabs (HVSs)
  - Asymptomatic bacteriuria

(b) How will you manage her in her next pregnancy? (14 marks)

- Lifestyle modification:
  - Alcohol
  - Smoking
  - Drugs – recreational
- Education about recurrence risk (approx. 30 per cent)
- Consultant-based antenatal care supported by appropriate neonatal care facilities
- Serial ultrasound scans from 14 weeks and interventions such as cerclage if appropriate
- Role of steroid and when?
- Tocolysis – role and when

- Antibiotics – role (Kenyon *et al.*, 2001) – no obvious benefit unless rupture of membranes
- Place of confinement

Sample answer

(a) Justify the investigations you will discuss with the patient. (6 marks)

The investigations must aim to exclude possible causes such as genital tract infections, anomalies and cervical weakness (incompetence). Specific investigations will depend on whether she is pregnant or not, and if pregnant the gestational age.

These investigations include high vaginal and endocervical swabs for bacteria vaginosis and group beta-haemolytic streptococcus and an ultrasound scan to exclude uterine anomalies that may be associated with preterm labour.

Although investigating for cervical weakness outside pregnancy is rarely performed, the two traditional methods are HSG and retrograde cervical dilatation. The former is painful and uncomfortable, and there is the added risk of ascending infections. Similarly, retrograde dilatation may introduce infections. The two methods are intrusive and unreliable. For the diagnosis of cervical weakness (incompetence) to be made, the cervix should be able to take a size 7 mm Hegar dilator without analgesia. The appearance of coning on HSG will also be diagnostic.

(b) How will you manage her in her next pregnancy? (14 marks)

The recurrence risk in this patient is considered to be approximately 30 per cent. An important part of her management is education, which will hopefully result in a change in lifestyle factors such as smoking, stress, alcohol, recreational drugs and poor diet – all of which increase the risk of preterm labour. It may be necessary to involve other disciplines in this regard. Ensuring that lifestyle changes introduced during pre-pregnancy are maintained is essential in pregnancy.

Screening for infections such as bacterial vaginosis in pregnancy is useful, although it does not imply that this was the cause of her preterm labours. Similarly, infections of the urinary tract must be excluded. During pregnancy, every effort must be made to identify asymptomatic bacteriuria and bacterial vaginosis – all of which are treatable and recognised causes of preterm labour. The presence of beta-haemolytic streptococcus will influence her management in labour but will not necessarily influence the prevention of preterm labour.

During the early second trimester, the patient will be offered serial cervical length and internal cervical os diameter assessment by transvaginal ultrasound scan. If the cervix becomes shorter, or is dilating, cervical cerclage will be inserted. However, on the basis of her previous history, some authorities may insert cervical cerclage at 14–16 weeks. The advantage of this is that it ensures that the cervix is not changing significantly prior to the stitch. If the cervix becomes too short or is dilated, the insertion may be difficult and accompanied by complications which may precipitate preterm labour.

Admission for bed rest could be offered from 24 weeks. There is no scientific evidence that this is effective but it has a psychological effect on the patient. Steroids should be considered in view of her past history. She should be offered two doses of betamethasone (or dexamethasone) (12 mg intramuscularly (i.m.) 12 hours apart) at 24 weeks. In the absence of any risk factors, adequate rest must be ensured, especially around 24 weeks. Tocolytic agents have almost no role in the management of this patient.

If she presented in preterm labour, the use of tocolytic agents may prolong the pregnancy and therefore outcome. There is some evidence to suggest that various biochemical markers, such as fibronectin, salivary oestriol and tenascin, and urocortin, may be used to predict which pregnancies will go into preterm labour. However, these are not very predictive and therefore are only available as research tools. Preterm labour is likely to recur in this patient. Her management should therefore aim to minimise the risk of recurrence by identifying the cause and also instituting treatment that is effective and acceptable.

Reference

Kenyon SL, Taylor DJ, Tarnow-Mordi W (2001) Broad-spectrum antibiotics for preterm, prelabour rupture of fetal membranes: the ORACLE I randomised trial. ORACLE Collaborative Group. *Lancet* **357**: 979–88.

2. Preterm delivery is one of the most important causes of perinatal mortality. Evaluate the methods available for the prevention of preterm labour. (20 marks)

Common mistakes

- Description of the procedures of cervical cerclage
- Stating that cervical cerclage is not of any proven benefit
- Inaccurate facts
- Detailed discussion on the causes of preterm labour
- Listing the causes of perinatal mortality
- Discussing the management of preterm labour

A good answer will include some or all of these points

- Identification of at-risk group
- Previous preterm labour – recurrent risk:
    - 1 = 15 per cent
    - 2 = 20–30 per cent
- Lifestyle factors – low socioeconomic group, smoking, drugs
- Vaginal infections – bacterial vaginosis
- Education to minimise the risk factors, e.g. smoking, etc.
- Treatment of conditions that may lead to iatrogenic preterm labour
- Early identification of such conditions and preventing progression which may lead to preterm labour, e.g. pre-eclampsia (PET)
- Other systemic diseases, e.g. diabetes mellitus, etc. – good control?
- Infection screen – urine for asymptomatic bacteriuria, HVS, endocervical swab for bacterial vaginosis, beta-haemolytic streptococcus
- Prelabour premature rupture of fetal membranes – antibiotics? (Kenyon *et al.*, 2001b)
- Cervical weakness (incompetence) – ultrasound scanning and cerclage. Diagnosis outside pregnancy – HSG and cervical retrograde dilatation with Hegar's dilators
- Biochemical – fibronectin, oestriol, tenascin and prophylactic tocolytic agents?
- Multiple pregnancy – selective feticide/fetal reduction
- Polyhydramnios – amnioreduction

Sample answer

Preterm labour accounts for about 33 per cent of all perinatal deaths. It occurs in about 5–10 per cent of all pregnancies. The aetiology is unknown in a large number of cases. However, in some this is iatrogenic, commonly secondary to other maternal complications of pregnancy such as PET. Prevention of preterm labour is therefore an important part of perinatal medicine if its impact on morbidity and mortality is to be reduced.

Prevention of any condition must start with the identification of the at-risk group. Previous preterm labour is the single most predictive risk factor for recurrence. The risk of recurrence is 15 per cent after one preterm labour, rising to 30 per cent after two and to 45 per cent after three. Other risk factors include lifestyle factors such as smoking, recreational drugs, alcohol and low socioeconomic class. Maternal systemic diseases, such as diabetes mellitus, and cardiorespiratory conditions increase the risk of preterm labour. Some of these risk factors can be identified from a detailed history from the patient. Although a physical examination may identify some risk factors, this is unlikely to be effective.

A cheap and effective means of preventing preterm labour must be to educate patients to change their lifestyles, e.g. stopping smoking and using recreational drugs. In addition, improvement in nutritional status and treatment of infections and systemic disease will significantly minimise the risk of preterm labour.

Identification of infections is easy and effective. Routine urinalysis of samples from all pregnant women will identify those with asymptomatic bacteriuria. Screening for diabetes mellitus and bacterial vaginosis will also identify others at risk. Once those at risk have been identified, appropriate treatment would significantly reduce the risk. Conditions amenable to treatment include urinary tract infections (symptomatic and asymptomatic) and genital tract infections (especially bacterial vaginosis).

The use of uterine artery Doppler scanning in patients at risk of PET may identify a subgroup of patients who may benefit from prophylactic aspirin and, in some cases, anticoagulants to reduce the risk of PET. In addition, close monitoring of these patients will identify this complication early and afford an opportunity for treatment to reduce its severity and therefore the need for early delivery. Serial ultrasound scanning of the cervical length and canal in the at-risk group will identify those at risk of preterm labour. Such an investigation should be offered to all those with mid-trimester miscarriages, previous surgery on the cervix, multiple pregnancies and premature rupture of fetal membranes. The use of antibiotics in those with preterm rupture of fetal membranes has been shown to prolong pregnancy by a few days in patients with intact membranes presenting with preterm labour (Kenyon *et al.*, 2001); however, this has not been shown to be beneficial.

The use of biochemical markers, such as fetal fibronectin, salivary oestriol and tenascin, and urocortin, for the prediction of preterm labour is associated with poor positive predictive values. However, these may be used in conjunction with other tests, such as cervical scanning. Fetal fibronectin, for example, may be able to identify a subgroup of patients likely to go into preterm labour and better monitoring of these patients may prolong pregnancy. However, these methods are expensive and require complex calculations of ratios. Therefore, most are not available as a clinical aid to predict preterm labour.

Although polyhydramnios and multiple pregnancy are not common causes of preterm labour, these are well recognised, and selective feticide and amnioreduction have been shown to reduce the risk of preterm labour. The latter is more common in pregnancies of higher order – usually above two.

Although preterm labour is predictable in some groups of patients, it is often unpredictable in a large majority. It is therefore not possible to offer some of these screening tools to the general population because of logistical and manpower limitations. Screening and targeted treatment, therefore, can only be to a selected group of patients.

Reference

Kenyon SL, Taylor DJ, Tarnow-Mordi W (2001) Broad-spectrum antibiotics for spontaneous preterm labour: the ORACLE II randomised trial. ORACLE Collaborative Group. *Lancet* **357**: 989–94.

3. A 37-year-old primigravida with a history of infertility, presents at 23 weeks' gestation with premature rupture of fetal membranes. (a) Critically appraise the non-radiological investigations you will undertake on the patient. (4 marks) (b) Justify how you will monitor the patient after confirmation of the diagnosis. (4 marks) (c) How will you manage the patient prior to delivery? (6 marks) (d) What factors will influence your timing and method of delivery? (6 marks)

Common mistakes

- Repeating the question
- Being very pedantic in your answer
- Performing repeated high vaginal and endocervical swabs
- Terminating the pregnancy because viability has not been achieved – the only option!

A good answer will include some or all of these points

(a) Critically appraise the non-radiological investigations you will undertake on the patient. (4 marks)

- Baseline full blood count (FBC)
  - Raised white cell count (WCC). Serial counts better at identify infections than a single test
- C-reactive protein
  - Single reading unreliable but serial measurements are reliable
- HVS/low vaginal swab (LVS)
  - Pros and cons of repeated tests

(b) Justify how you will monitor the patient after confirmation of the diagnosis. (4 marks)

- Admit for the following:
  - 4-hourly temperature, pulse and respiratory rate (TPR)
  - HVS – daily, or LVSs
  - C-reactive protein
  - Serial fetal blood sampling (2–3 daily)
  - Cardiotocography (CTG) – how frequent and how reliable?
- Ultrasound scan – volume and lung volume including fetal breathing movements

(c) How will you manage the patient prior to delivery? (6 marks)

- Admit or manage as outpatient?
- Antibiotics – erythromycin for 5 days

- Counselling by neonatologist – prognosis, facilities, etc.
- Steroids for 24 hours – 12 mg betamethasone 12 hours apart (× 2 doses)
- Tocolysis – any role
- Amnioinfusion – any role

(d) What factors will influence your timing and method of delivery? (6 marks)

- Gestational age at delivery
- Superimposed complications – infections (chorioamnionitis), fetal distress, intrauterine fetal death
- CTG
- Wishes of the parents
- Prognosis
- Facilities available for neonatal care
- Maternal condition
- Fetal conditions

Sample answer

(a) Critically appraise the non-radiological investigations you will undertake on the patient. (4 marks)

Initial investigations to be performed to establish a baseline for subsequent monitoring include a FBC (specifically the WCC and differentials), a C-reactive protein and a HVS (obtained during a confirmatory diagnostic speculum examination) for microscopy, culture and sensitivity. Unfortunately, these parameters are not very sensitive in predicting chorioamnionitis. For example, C-reactive protein is unreliable, although serial levels showing a consistent rise will be suggestive of infection but not necessarily from the uterus. Similarly, a rise in WCC, which is not uncommon in pregnancy, may also be indicative of infection elsewhere in the body. However, serial values showing significant changes will raise suspicions of chorioamnionitis unless other sources of infection can be identified. The FBC and C-reactive proteins need to be repeated at least twice weekly.

(b) Justify how you will monitor the patient after confirmation of the diagnosis. (4 marks)

Early maternal manifestations of chorioamnionitis are pyrexia, tachycardia and tachypnoea. These may be identified by 4-hourly TPR recordings. These should be performed on this patient, even if she is to be managed on an outpatient basis. In addition to these, daily palpation of the lower abdomen for tenderness and examination of a pad for the colour of liquor and its smell will help in identifying early chorioamnionitis. Unfortunately, these signs may not always be present with infections. The value of serial HVSs is limited, as frequent introduction of the swabs in the vagina may increase the risk of ascending chorioamnionitis. Some argue that LVSs may be useful but these may only yield normal lower genital tract flora of no clinical significance. However, the diagnosis of beta-haemolytic streptococcus will influence management.

An ultrasound scan in this patient will quantify liquor volume, assess fetal growth and afford an opportunity for Doppler studies of the umbilical and other fetal vessels. Serial ultrasound scans will allow for estimation of the liquor volume but, more importantly, will enable a visual subjective assessment of the lung volume and fetal breathing, which is associated with a better prognosis. Where there is anhydramnios the prognosis is poor and under these circumstances amnioinfusion may be considered. Problems with this procedure include infections and failure to achieve any satisfactory residual volume as it may leak out as soon as it is infused. This is not only a tedious process for the clinician but is uncomfortable for the patient, may not be successful and there is no strong evidence to support it.

(c) How will you manage the patient prior to delivery? (6 marks)

Neonatologists must be involved in the management of this patient. They will provide information about the chances of survival at different gestational ages, the neonatal course and management, and possible complications. Timing delivery should be decided in close liaison with the neonatologists.

Steroids should be administered (betamethasone or dexamethasone given in two doses of 12 mg i.m. 12 hours apart) to help accelerate fetal lung maturity. Although mostly given after 24 weeks' gestation, there is a case for offering them to this patient. Tocolytic agents may be used if the patient starts having contractions, but these have not been shown to significantly prolong pregnancy. Kenyon et al. (2001b) concluded that prophylactic antibiotics in these patients not only prolong pregnancy, but also reduce perinatal morbidity. Erythromycin will therefore be offered to the patient after admission.

Various experiments suggest that the treatment of amniorrhexis by use of a blood patch or fetoscopic insertion of a mesh over the rupture site may improve outcome. In this patient, if this expertise is available, these options must be considered. A controversial issue is whether to manage the patient as an inpatient or as an outpatient. The advantages of inpatient care are close monitoring and early intervention when necessary. In addition, bed rest can be enforced. Nowadays, some sensible and well-motivated patients may be able to monitor themselves at home and, with the help of midwives, undertake all the serial monitoring offered in the hospital. In this patient, in view of the very high risk, on balance it may be advisable to monitor her as an inpatient.

Cardiotocography is an important part of fetal monitoring, especially as cord compression may occur with oligohydramnios. At this very early gestation this will not be instituted as an abnormal trace is difficult to interpret and, in addition, adopting a more proactive approach may not be the best option. The timing of this monitoring will therefore remain controversial. However, it may be started between 25 and 26 weeks' gestation, when a Caesarean section may be considered if there is need to do one.

(d) What factors will influence your timing and method of delivery? (6 marks)

The timing and mode of delivery will depend on several factors. These include gestational age, the availability of neonatal intensive care (NICU) facilities and the perceived chances of survival. If there are no NICU facilities, *in utero* transfer is the best option. At the lower end of the gestational age spectrum delivery is difficult and Caesarean section may be the only option if the baby is to be given the best chances of survival. However, if survival is not possible, after appropriate counselling, a vaginal delivery may be allowed. The management of this patient therefore poses several problems which must be addressed together or individually.

The most common complications that may occur in this patient are preterm labour, chorioamnionitis and significant oligohydramnios, leading to pulmonary hypoplasia. This fetus is 1 week from viability and, taking into account her reproductive history, it would be unreasonable to offer her a termination at this gestation on account of the potential risks. This is unlikely to be acceptable and may arouse antagonism from the patient and her partner.

Even when the pregnancy progresses beyond viability, pulmonary hypoplasia should be considered an indication for termination of the pregnancy.

Reference

Kenyon SL, Taylor DJ, Tarnow-Mordi W (2001b) Broad-spectrum antibiotics for spontaneous preterm labour: the ORACLE II randomised trial. ORACLE Collaborative Group. *Lancet* **357**: 989–94.

10

Intrauterine and intrapartum stillbirth

1. A 25-year-old schoolteacher attended at 41 weeks' gestation with absent fetal movements for 24 hours and an ultrasound scan confirmed the diagnosis of an intrauterine fetal death (IUFD). (a) Briefly outline your initial management. (4 marks) (b) What investigations will you undertake and why? (12 marks) (c) What factors will influence your subsequent management of this patient's next pregnancy? (4 marks)

2. A patient is scheduled for a postnatal follow-up visit following the delivery of an IUFD at 34 weeks' gestation. The post-mortem examination showed that the fetus died from multiple severe congenital malformations. (a) What must you do in preparation for her follow-up visit? (6 marks) (b) How will you counsel her at this visit? (14 marks)

3. How will you counsel a couple whose baby died in the neonatal period from an autosomal recessive condition? (20 marks)

4. A 32-year-old patient who had a neonatal death 2 years ago is now 20 weeks into her second pregnancy. Her previous pregnancy had been uncomplicated but at 37 weeks' gestation, she had a prolonged labour which was followed by a failed ventouse and forceps and then an emergency Caesarean section under general anaesthesia of a very asphyxiated baby who died 1 week after delivery, from intracranial haemorrhage. She wishes to be delivered by an elective Caesarean section at 36 weeks' gestation. (a) What are the pros and cons of an elective Caesarean section in this case? (10 marks) (b) What are the pros and cons of offering her a vaginal delivery at 36 weeks' gestation? (5 marks) (c) How will you manage her? (5 marks)

1. A 25-year-old schoolteacher attended at 41 weeks' gestation with absent fetal movements for 24 hours and an ultrasound scan confirmed the diagnosis of an IUFD. (a) Briefly outline your initial management. (4 marks) (b) What investigations will you undertake and why? (12 marks) (c) What factors will influence your management of this patient's next pregnancy? (4 marks)

Common mistakes

- Refer to perinatologist
- Take a history and offer investigations (which and why?)
- Offer chorionic villus sampling (CVS)/amniocentesis in next pregnancy – for what?
- Discuss pre-pregnancy counselling and dietary control (about what)
- Refer to geneticist

A good answer will include some or all of these points

(a) Briefly outline your initial management (4 marks)

- Inform woman of diagnosis with empathy
- Give time to react to bad news and time together with family – if not present ask permission to call partner or member of family to be with her
- Discuss management plans – need for investigations, delivery (vaginal) and postnatal care and investigations
- Inform consultant and/or senior on duty
- Inform her general practitioner (GP) and midwife

(b) What investigations will you undertake and why? (12 marks)

- Immediate:
  - Full blood count (FBC), group and save – may require blood transfusion
  - Kleihauer–Betke test – to exclude fetomaternal haemorrhage as a cause of the IUFD
  - Glycosylated haemoglobin (HbA1c) – to screen for diabetes mellitus
  - Thyroid function test (free thyroxine (FT4) and thyroid-stimulating hormone (TSH)) to exclude thyroid dysfunction
  - Infection screen – antibodies for toxoplasmosis, rubella, cytomegalovirus (CMV), human papillomavirus, herpes virus, syphilis) – TORCHES screen (toxoplasmosis, rubella, CMV, herpes simplex)
- Late:
  - Thrombophilia – protein C, antithrombin III and factor V Leiden – may be associated with thrombophilia
  - Antiphospholipid antibodies – anticardiolipin antibodies, lupus anticoagulant, B2 glycoprotein

- Placenta:
  - Histology
  - Swabs for microscopy, culture and sensitivity (M/C/S)
- Fetal:
  - Autopsy
  - Swabs for M/C/S
  - Karyotype – blood (taken antenatally, amniotic fluid) and solid tissues

(c) What factors will influence your management of this patient's next pregnancy? (4 marks)

- Cause of IUFD
- Associated maternal condition – identified from investigations
- Facility for monitoring available

Sample answer

(a) Briefly outline your initial management. (4 marks)

The patient will have to be informed of the diagnosis. An attempt should be made to contact her partner or close relative if she is alone. Although she should be given this option, this should not delay the counselling. Following this, she needs time to react to the bad news. The family should therefore be given some time on their own. The initial reaction will be denial but eventually the response will turn to anger and frustration. The counselling and support must therefore be with sensitivity and demonstrate empathy and understanding. The next step will be to discuss the available options, which will include undertaking investigations before and after delivery to help identify a possible cause of the IUFD, delivery and postnatal care. It is important that the consultant on call, her GP and midwife should be informed.

(b) What investigations will you undertake and why? (12 marks)

The investigations will be classified as fetal and maternal. Some of these will be immediate and others will be later (i.e. after delivery). The immediate maternal investigations include: (1) a FBC to check her haemoglobin and white cell count as there could be an infection, (2) group and save serum (she may require transfusion after delivery), (3) Kleihauer–Betke test to exclude fetomaternal haemorrhage as a cause of the IUFD, (4) HbA1c and random blood glucose to screen for diabetes mellitus, (5) thyroid function test – thyroid dysfunction is a recognised cause of IUFD and (6) an infection screen for antibodies for various organisms such as CMV, toxoplasmosa, parvovirus, herpes and syphilis. A thrombophilia screen consisting of antithrombin III and activated protein C resistance is essential but this may be delayed until much later – at least 6–8 weeks after delivery to include protein S. Other investigations include anticardiolipin antibodies, lupus anticoagulant, homocysteine and an autoimmune profile.

At the time of delivery, swabs should be taken from the fetus and placenta for microscopy and culture and the latter sent for histology. With regards to the fetus, the immediate investigation prior to delivery will be karyotyping by amniocentesis, if the parents accept this. This provides the best chance of getting a result, since karyotyping from solid tissue is associated with failure in over 50 per cent of cases (Khare *et al.*, 2005). Permission must be obtained from the parents for an autopsy. However, a thorough external examination of the baby should be undertaken and where permission for autopsy is denied consideration should be given to magnetic resonance imaging and X-rays. An important part of the examination is weighing and measuring various neonatal indices that will help in determining whether the baby was growth restricted or not.

(c) What factors will influence your subsequent management of this patient's next pregnancy? (4 marks)

The identifiable cause of the IUFD will be the most important factor influencing her subsequent management, for example, is the factor recurrent and can it be prevented? If it is preventable, then appropriate steps would be taken to minimise its recurrence. This may be in the form of instituting treatment or prophylaxis. Additionally, the time of the IUFD will be an important factor and for this woman, the next pregnancy will not be allowed to go beyond 40 weeks' gestation. Finally, the facilities available for monitoring will, to a large extent, determine how the next pregnancy is monitored.

Reference

Khare M, Howarth E, Sadler J, Healey K, Konje JC (2005) A comparison of prenatal versus postnatal karyotyping for the investigation of intrauterine fetal death after the first trimester of pregnancy. *Prenat Diagn* **25**: 1192–5.

2. A patient is scheduled for a postnatal follow-up visit following the delivery of an IUFD at 34 weeks' gestation. The post-mortem examination showed that the fetus died from multiple severe congenital malformations. (a) What must you do in preparation for her follow-up visit? (6 marks) (b) How will you counsel her at this visit? (14 marks)

Common mistakes

- Discussing CVS or amniocentesis
- Discussing how to manage a woman whose baby has been diagnosed as having congenital abnormalities
- You have not been told that the congenital malformations are recurrent or are chromosomal – hence do not say so
- Need to start trying immediately, as Down's syndrome risk increases with age
- No one has said the baby had Down's syndrome

A good answer will include some or all of these points

(a) What must you do in preparation for her follow-up visit? (6 marks)

- Ensure that all the results of the investigations undertaken are available
- Discuss the investigation results and the multiple malformations with a geneticist and other experts that may provide answers
- Research into the possible causes, nature of abnormalities and associated problems, including the recurrence risk
- Book a room or place for the postnatal visit
- Ensure that the couple have been sent the letter confirming the appointment and directions to the venue
- Invite others with expertise to discuss the malformations if considered appropriate

(b) How will you counsel her at this visit? (14 marks)

- Take the patient through antenatal events
- Explain and relate antenatal findings, if any, and autopsy findings and differences, if any
- Other investigation results – discuss normal and abnormal
- Discuss any other obvious explanation for the malformations, such as epilepsy, diabetes mellitus, drugs, etc.
- Do the patient and her partner need to see a geneticist?
- Help with grieving process – Stillbirth and Neonatal Deaths Society (SANDS), etc.
- Recurrence risk – if known
- Pre-pregnancy advice – diet, folic acid supplementation, etc.

- Plan for next pregnancy
- Detailed scan – at tertiary level
- Karyotyping in pregnancy
- Neonatologist/geneticist involvement

Sample answer

(a) What must you do in preparation for her follow-up visit? (6 marks)

A thorough preparation for the counselling will ensure maximum benefit from the visit. It is important that all the results of the investigations performed at the time of delivery and after are available and are reviewed and filed in the notes. If there is uncertainty about any of the results, either they are repeated or the various experts contacted for clarification. It would be useful to discuss the results of the investigations and the various malformations (which would have been confirmed and/or identified at autopsy) with a clinical geneticist to ensure that a possible diagnosis is identified. Occasionally, this may require seeking expert opinion either on some of the samples/tissue being investigated or on the information available. This should not be delayed until after the patient has been seen as it would only prolong the grief and anxiety of the couple.

If necessary, some investigations should be undertaken about the possible causes of the malformations, associated problems and their recurrence risks. In most units, a perinatal mortality multidisciplinary meeting would have taken place and a summary of the discussions will be available. These should also be consulted for plans for the next pregnancy. A venue for the consultation should be arranged and the patient notified of the venue and time of the consultation. If possible, the patient should be contacted again close to the time of the appointment to ensure that she is coming. Finally, enough time must be allowed for the consultation, which should be not interrupted.

(b) How will you counsel her at this visit? (14 marks)

The first step is to express sympathy and then take the patient through any antenatal events that you feel are essential. An explanation of the results of investigations and their implications should then be offered. It is not necessary to offer details of how the autopsy was conducted. There may be other explanations for the stillbirth. Conditions such as diabetes, epilepsy and its drug treatment, and other teratogenic drugs, which might be implicated, should be identified and discussed in detail.

Information should then be provided about support groups if necessary. Groups such as SANDS would provide telephone counselling and information leaflets about how to cope with a stillbirth. Occasionally, the patient and her partner may have to be referred to another expert (e.g. a geneticist) for counselling about recurrence risks and the possibility of prenatal diagnosis. If the risk of recurrence is known, it should be discussed.

After counselling about the stillbirth, details about the next pregnancy should be discussed and documented. A plan for the identification of these abnormalities must be clearly documented and explained to the patient. If these are associated with a chromosomal abnormality, prenatal karyotyping should be discussed. The options of amniocentesis and CVS would be discussed, but details would be unnecessary at this stage. Where necessary, a neonatologist should be involved to discuss the potential problems of babies with such malformations when they are born alive. If necessary, pre-pregnancy dietary advice should be offered. Counselling of patients like this is easier where the cause of the stillbirth is known. Where it is unknown, it is more difficult to come to terms with it.

Counselling is incomplete without communication with the patient's GP, who will offer support in the community. Good practice will expect a copy of the communication with the GP to be sent to the patient. The midwife ought to be involved in this process and all information relevant to the diagnosis of the cause should be passed on to the midwife and the GP.

3. How will you counsel a couple whose baby died in the neonatal period from an auto-somal recessive condition? (20 marks)

Common mistakes

- Enquire about any previous normal child – this history should be obtained from the couple – what is the relevance of this?
- The recessive condition must be identified – is this not obvious?
- Offer termination in the next pregnancy and discuss surrogacy or adoption as their only option
- Quoting/regurgitating what the general approach is from textbooks
- Failing to focus your answer on this couple

A good answer will include some or all of these points

- Recessive condition – both parents are carriers and are unaffected
- Risks for any child:
  - Being affected – 25 per cent (one in four)
  - Being a carrier child – 50 per cent (one in two)
  - Being normal child – 25 per cent (one in four)
- The condition is likely to be a lethal one (unless there was a mutation):
  - Was it therefore lethal or was it a mutation? Is that information available?
- Is the condition known (is it defined?) – test both parents to confirm that it is not a mutation
- If prenatal diagnosis is possible, discuss options – CVS/amniocentesis, etc.
- If prenatal diagnosis not possible:
  - Any obvious markers on ultrasound that may help identify condition?
  - If none, parents must understand risks involved
- Prenatal diagnosis available – affected – termination of pregnancy
- Pre-implantation diagnosis – available?
- Other option – egg donation, artificial insemination with donor sperm and adoption

Sample answer

An autosomal recessive condition is one that will only manifest if homozygously present in the offspring. This couple must each carry the recessive trait, although it is possible that a muta-tion could result in the expression of a recessive condition.

When counselling this couple, the first step will be to discuss the inheritance pattern of the condition. The risk of having a normal child if both parents are carriers is 25 per cent (one in four), having an affected child is 25 per cent (one in four) and having a carrier child is 50 per cent (one in two). The condition is likely to be lethal since the baby died from it. There may, of course, be mutations which may reduce the severity of the disease but this cannot be predicted.

It is important to ascertain that the condition has been defined and that both parents have been tested to confirm that they are carriers. An important aspect of counselling is to discuss prenatal diagnosis. The options will include CVS and amniocentesis. If prenatal diagnosis is not possible, are there any possible soft markers on ultrasound and how soon can they be identified? It may be possible to diagnose this condition with ultrasound (if there are obvious markers). If it is not possible to diagnose the condition, from either amniocentesis or CVS or from ultrasound scan, the parents must be informed of the chances of having an affected baby. If this is possible then termination may be offered for an affected fetus. It may also be necessary to refer the couple to a unit where there are facilities for making a diagnosis. The recent advances in molecular biology techniques have increased the number of conditions that can be diagnosed preimplantation. If this option is available, the couple should be counselled appropriately and referred to the most relevant unit.

The last options for them will include artificial insemination with donor sperms or *in vitro* fertilisation with donor eggs or adoption where the couple are unwilling to take any chances or cannot afford other options. The counselling should ideally involve clinical geneticists.

4. A 32-year-old patient who had a neonatal death 2 years ago is now 20 weeks into her second pregnancy. Her previous pregnancy had been uncomplicated but at 37 weeks' gestation, she had a prolonged labour which was followed by a failed ventouse and forceps and then an emergency Caesarean section under general anaesthesia of a very asphyxiated baby who died 1 week after delivery, from intracranial haemorrhage. She wishes to be delivered by an elective Caesarean section at 36 weeks' gestation. (a) What are the pros and cons of an elective Caesarean section in this case? (10 marks) (b) What are the pros and cons of offering her a vaginal delivery at 36 weeks' gestation? (5 marks) (c) How will you manage her? (5 marks)

Common mistakes

- Discussing how to monitor the pregnancy – advantages and disadvantages of consultant-led care versus midwifery care, hospital versus community care
- Refer patient to a specialist unit
- Failing to debate (pros and cons)
- Simply outlining how you will manage her
- Involving a psychiatrist

A good answer will include some or all of these points

(a) What are the pros and cons of an elective Caesarean section in this case? (10 marks)

- Pros of elective delivery by Caesarean section at 36 weeks' gestation:
  - Memories of traumatic experience avoided – psychological benefit to the patient (37 weeks, when last complication occurred, not reached)
  - Planned procedure and unlikely to go into spontaneous labour (as most occur after 37 weeks)
  - Paediatrician present
  - Procedure done during day time and by the most experienced person, or supervised by the most experienced obstetrician available
  - Surgery most likely to be performed under regional analgesia
  - Complications of elective Caesarean section less than those of an emergency Caesarean section – maternal mortality, venous thromboembolism (VTE), risk of general anaesthesia and failed intubation, Mendelson's syndrome
- Cons of an elective Caesarean section at 36 weeks' gestation:
  - Increased risk of respiratory distress syndrome (RDS) and transient tachypnoea of the newborn (TTN) – associated with complications of neonatal intensive care unit (NICU) admission, e.g. iatrogenic infection and chronic lung disease
  - Risks of repeat Caesarean section – bladder and bowel injury, adhesion formation, VTE

(b) What are the pros and cons of offering her a vaginal delivery at 36 weeks' gestation? (5 marks)

- Avoids repeat Caesarean section and its complications
- Same advantage of delivery prior to 36 weeks
- Fear of reoccurrence
- May still require an emergency Caesarean section
- Induction at 36 weeks may be difficult as cervix may be unripe

(c) How will you manage her? (5 marks)

- Counselling, demonstrating empathy and understanding of her anxiety
- Reassurance that a planned delivery and close monitoring may minimise the psychological trauma of her last experience
- Aim for pregnancy to progress beyond 36 weeks
- Consider an elective Caesarean section at 38 weeks
- But if presents in labour before, an emergency Caesarean section should be considered
- A vaginal delivery is a possibility but this will depend on her attitude and support
- May be necessary to involve clinical psychologist in counselling

Sample answer

(a) What are the pros and cons of an elective Caesarean section in this case? (10 marks)

Her demand for elective delivery by Caesarean section at 36 weeks is a sensible and logical one. This will obviously be of an important psychological benefit to the patient. However, while it will reduce her anxiety and fear of reaching 37 weeks' gestation, delivering at this gestation is associated with possible neonatal complications. These include TTN and RDS, all of which are likely to require admission into the NICU. Such an admission may be associated with nosocomial infections acquired on the unit. The proportion of babies with long-term chronic lung disease delivered at 36 weeks' gestation is higher that that at 37–38 weeks.

Delivering by Caesarean section is also associated with maternal morbidity and possibly an effect on subsequent pregnancies and general health in later years. The advantages of delivery by Caesarean section at this gestation include the avoidance of uncertainty about the timing and the how of delivery and complete prevention of the psychological fear that will certainly grip her around the time of her last experience, and more so when she goes into labour. Although planning to deliver at this early gestation may seem logical, there is also the possibility that she may go into spontaneous labour before this time. If that were to happen, the fear and anxiety related to her last experience would become evident.

(b) What are the pros and cons of offering her a vaginal delivery at 36 weeks' gestation? (5 marks)

A vaginal delivery at 36 weeks will avoid a repeat Caesarean section and its complications such as visceral injury (bladder and bowel). Postdelivery hospital stay will be shorter and there will be less need for postdelivery analgesia. Bonding with the baby and breastfeeding will be better following a vaginal delivery. A successful vaginal delivery will ensure that the experience of the last pregnancy is not repeated.

However, at this gestation, a planned vaginal delivery is associated with several disadvantages. The cervix is unlikely to be ripe, an early induction is therefore more likely to be protracted and the longer the interval between induction and delivery, the more anxious the patient will be. An induction does not guarantee a vaginal delivery as she may end up with an emergency Caesarean section, which may cause more anxiety and distress to the patient.

(c) How will you manage her? (5 marks)

In the management of this patient, although the decision to deliver early is a reasonable request, appropriate counselling, empathy and support, coupled with reassurance that a planned delivery and closer monitoring may minimise the psychological trauma of her last experience may allow the pregnancy to progress beyond 36 weeks' gestation. An elective Caesarean section is not unreasonable, but this could be planned for 38 weeks or later, with the proviso that if the patient went into labour before then, an emergency Caesarean section could be performed.

A vaginal delivery is not unrealistic, but the stress associated with this may be difficult for the patient to cope with. This patient has been through a very traumatic experience, which should be avoided in the current pregnancy. She needs to be reassured that everything will be done to avoid a repetition of the previous pregnancy, although a cast-iron guarantee cannot be given. It may even be necessary to offer counselling by a clinical psychologist.

11

Labour, including induction – normal/abnormal

1. Induction of post-term pregnancies at or before 42 weeks is associated with a significant reduction in perinatal mortality. (a) What are the risks of prolonged pregnancy? (7 marks) (b) What are the risks of induction of labour? (5 marks) (c) What factors will influence how you induce labour in a 36-year-old woman at 41 weeks + 5 days? (4 marks) (d) Evaluate the methods of induction at 42 weeks' gestation. (4 marks)

2. Shoulder dystocia is an important cause of perinatal morbidity and mortality. (a) Evaluate the different manoeuvres you will apply to the management of shoulder dystocia. (14 marks) (b) What are the complications of shoulder dystocia? (6 marks)

3. A 29-year-old G2P1 (previous Caesarean section) is being induced at 41 weeks' gestation following an uncomplicated pregnancy. (a) What measures will you take to minimise the risk of uterine rupture? (14 marks) (b) How will you recognise this complication? (6 marks)

4. Critically appraise the methods of induction of labour of an uncomplicated pregnancy at 41 weeks' gestation in a grand multipara. (20 marks)

5. A primigravida was admitted in spontaneous labour at 40 weeks' gestation 14 hours ago. Fetal membranes had ruptured spontaneously 12 hours before admission. Her cervix was 3 cm on admission. The cervix has remained at 8 cm for the last 4 hours and, in addition, she now has a pyrexia of 37.8°C. However, the fetal heart rate is normal. (a) Under what conditions will you do a Caesarean section in this patient?) (6 marks) (b) What complications may affect this mother and fetus? (6 marks) (c) She is eventually delivered by Caesarean section because of obstructed labour after 20 hours. How will you minimise any maternal and fetal complications? (8 marks)

1. Induction of post-term pregnancies at or before 42 weeks is associated with a significant reduction in perinatal mortality. (a) What are the risks of prolonged pregnancy? (7 marks) (b) What are the risks of induction of labour? (5 marks) (c) What factors will influence how you induce labour in a 36-year-old woman at 41 weeks + 5 days? (4 marks) (d) Evaluate the methods of induction at 42 weeks' gestation. (4 marks)

Common mistakes

- Listing the indications for induction
- Details of the different methods of induction – oral prostaglandins, vaginal PGE$_2$, Foley's catheters, etc.
- How to date pregnancies to reduce the number of inductions at 42 weeks' gestation
- Failure to evaluate
- Stating that inductions should only be done at 41 weeks

A good answer will include some or all of these points

(a) What are the risks of prolonged pregnancy? (7 marks)

- Maternal – main risks are not from the pregnancy itself but from the consequences of induction of labour:
  - Psychological stress caused by the prolonged pregnancy
- Fetal:
  - Increased risk of stillbirth from approximately 1:3000 pregnancies >37 weeks to 1:1000 at 42 weeks and 1:500 from 43 weeks
  - To save one death, need to induce 500 pregnancies
  - Induction at around 42 weeks reduces this risk
  - Increased risk of meconium-stained labour
  - Increased risk of emergency Caesarean section
  - Neonatal encephalopathy decreased after 41–42 weeks' gestation
  - Cerebral palsy increased especially in primigravidas (if induced after 41 weeks)
  - Meconium staining associated with decreased cord arterial pH. Meconium aspiration syndrome increased after 42 weeks
  - Dystocia increased with delivery after 42 weeks' gestation

(b) What are the risks of induction of labour? (5 marks)

- Prolonged hospitalisation and stay on the delivery suite
- Increased risk of Syntocinon® augmentation
- Postpartum haemorrhage from prolonged and dysfunctional labour
- Fluid retention and neonatal jaundice
- Increased risk of VTE from prolonged hospitalisation

- Increased need for analgesia
- Psychological effect of interfering with a natural process
- Demand on resources, especially during day time

(c) What factors will influence how you induce labour in a 36-year-old woman at 41 weeks + 5 days? (4 marks)

- Parity and type of previous deliveries, if any
- State of the cervix
- Presentation
- Associated complications – fetal or maternal
- Need for monitoring
- Availability of facilities for induction (including drugs)
- Patient's choice

(d) Evaluate the methods of induction at 42 weeks' gestation. (4 marks)

- Vaginal prostaglandins
- Amniotomy
- Syntocinon® alone or in combination
- Other methods

Sample answer

(a) What are the risks of prolonged pregnancy? (7 marks)

The rationale for induction at or before 42 weeks' gestation is the increased risk of stillbirth and complications that may result in perinatal death, including a failing placenta. Perinatal mortality falls to a trough between 38 and 40 weeks' gestation and then starts to rise after 41 weeks' gestation. The risk of stillbirth is approximately 1:3000 at 37 weeks and falls to 1:1000 at 42 weeks and then to 1:500 at 43 weeks. Induction at or before 42 weeks' gestation is therefore said to be at the time when the perinatal mortality is beginning to rise, but is not high enough to warrant immediate delivery. A randomised trial by Cardozo *et al.* (1986) demonstrated that, in order to reduce one perinatal death at or before 42 weeks' gestation, at least 500 inductions have to be performed.

Postdate pregnancies are associated with an increased risk of meconium-stained liquor, decreased arterial cord pH, an increased in cerebral palsy rate, especially in primigravidas after 41 weeks, and neonatal encephalopathy. Shoulder dystocia is also increased after 42 weeks' gestation. With regards to the mother, a prolonged pregnancy has a psychological effect, often in the form of depression, frustration and difficulties coping.

(b) What are the risks of induction of labour? (5 marks)

Inductions are associated with prolonged hospitalisation, a higher postpartum haemorrhage rate and dysfunctional labour. A large proportion of patients end up having their labours augmented. Induction is associated with a high risk of postpartum haemorrhage and neonatal jaundice. In the past it had been argued that Caesarean section rates were higher in those who had inductions, but modern approaches to induction of labour have significantly reduced the Caesarean section rate. However, the consequences of hospitalisation (increased risk of VTE) remain higher in this group. For some patients, interference with the natural process is often unacceptable and considered unnecessarily intrusive. Although induction of labour at, or just before, 42 weeks is associated with a lower perinatal mortality and morbidity, the consequences on resources are tremendous.

(c) What factors will influence how you induce labour in a 36-year-old woman at 41 weeks + 5 days? (4 marks)

These include parity and type of previous delivery. In a multiparous woman, the cervix is likely to be more favourable and therefore induction may simply be via artificial rupture of fetal membranes (ARM), while in a primigravida there is more likely to be a need for prostaglandins. Previous Caesarean section will be considered a relative contraindication to the use of prostaglandins as this increases the risk of uterine rupture considerably. The presentation of the fetus is another factor. Breech presentation will be considered a contraindication while stabilisation induction will be offered to a patient with an oblique, transverse or unstable lie. The presence of maternal or fetal complications such as pre-eclampsia, cardiac disorders, fetal growth restriction or macrosomia, will influence how the patient is induced. In the presence of a compromised fetus or maternal complications, attempts will be made to shorten the induction–delivery interval.

The other factors to be considered include the facilities for monitoring the mother and fetus, the availability of the induction agents (e.g. prostaglandins, misoprostol, etc.) and the patient's choice.

(d) Evaluate the methods of induction at 42 weeks' gestation. (4 marks)

The options for induction in this patient include vaginal prostaglandins alone or in combination with ARM with or without Syntocinon®, Syntocinon® on its own or with ARM, ARM alone, or other methods such as the use of oestrogen, and laminaria tents. Prostaglandins have the advantage of helping ripen the cervix and making ARM possible; they are cheap and effective. However, they increase the risk of uterine rupture and may cause hyperstimulation. Patients are free to be mobile while being induced. In most cases, it must be combined with ARM and/or Syntocinon®.

Artificial rupture of fetal membranes on the other hand is cheap and mimics natural labour. It can be combined with other methods without any difficulties. However, following ARM, it may take too long for labour to be established. Consequently, there may be an increased risk of ascending infection. Also, ARM is only possible in those with a favourable cervix.

Syntocinon® on its own is effective in those with a favourable cervix. In others, it may take a considerable length of time before labour is established. It can be combined with the other methods. Another drawback is its association with neonatal jaundice.

Mechanical devices are not commonly used in the UK but may be useful where other induction agents are unavailable. They are cheap and often effective.

Reference

Cardozo L, Fysh J, Pearce JM (1986) Prolonged pregnancy: the management debate. *BMJ* **293**: 1059–63.

2. Shoulder dystocia is an important cause of perinatal morbidity and mortality. (a) Evaluate the different manoeuvres you will apply to the management of shoulder dystocia. (14 marks) (b) What are the complications of shoulder dystocia? (6 marks)

Common mistakes

- Causes of shoulder dystocia
- Prevention of shoulder dystocia
- Risk factors for shoulder dystocia
- Refer to senior colleague
- Take a history
- Review notes for risk factors for shoulder dystocia
- Discussing risk management
- Developing guidelines

A good answer will include some or all of these points

(a) Evaluate the different manoeuvres you will apply to the management of shoulder dystocia. (14 marks)

- McRobert's technique
- All fours
- Corkscrew
- Suprapubic pressure
- Symphysiotomy
- Zavanelli
- Manual rotation

(b) What are the complications of shoulder dystocia? (6 marks)

- Maternal:
  - Emergency Caesarean section
  - Perineal trauma
  - Postpartum haemorrhage
  - Psychological distress
- Fetal:
  - Stillbirth
  - Birth asphyxia
  - Fracture of clavicle and humerus
  - Trauma to internal organs
  - Erb's or Klumpke's palsy

Sample answer

(a) Evaluate the different manoeuvres you will apply to the management of shoulder dystocia. (14 marks)

The most commonly used manoeuvre is McRobert's technique. This involves hyperflexion and abduction at the hip joints. Ideally, this should be undertaken by two operators. This enlarges all the pelvic dimensions through straightening of the lumbosacral angle and superior rotation of the symphysis pubis, and with suprapubic pressure, allows delivery of the shoulders. It is thought to be successful in over 80 per cent of cases. This manoeuvre is easy to apply and is successful in most cases.

Another manoeuvre involves turning the patient to the lateral position or on to all fours. This allows for easy manipulation and effective delivery. By adopting these positions, the pelvic dimensions are increased slightly and allow mild dystocias to be overcome. However, in severe cases, this is unlikely to be successful. Although effective in some cases, it may be difficult turning a labouring patient to these positions.

Where these fail, other manoeuvres have to be applied. The first of these is the lateral suprapubic pressure with the patient in the lithotomy position and maximum abduction at the hip joints. Here, an assistant applies lateral suprapubic pressure behind the anterior shoulder and the accoucher simultaneously applies backward traction on the fetal neck. The aim is to push the anterior shoulder into the pelvis in an oblique fashion. It results in the adduction of the shoulders and the bisacromial diameter. The pressure should be continuous for about 30 seconds and, if this is unsuccessful, it should be abandoned and the next manoeuvre embarked upon.

The next option is the corkscrew manoeuvre, which involves internal rotation of the shoulders away from the anterior posterior position. The operator inserts a hand into the vagina posteriorly and moves it up to the posterior aspect of the anterior shoulder. This is then pushed from behind into an oblique position. This may not succeed, in which case the posterior shoulder should be rotated through 180°. This allows it to be disimpacted whilst permitting the trapped anterior shoulder to enter the pelvis. Further rotation will then bring down the other shoulder and the delivery will be effective. These manoeuvres require confidence and skill, especially during the insertion of the hand and undertaking the rotation. Often, they are undertaken after others have failed and the concerns of delay in delivering make them more complicated.

Another option is to deliver the posterior shoulder, which is already in the pelvis, and then rotate the fetus and deliver the other shoulder. Here, the operator inserts a hand vaginally, flexes the elbow and shoulder and brings the forearm across the chest of the baby to deliver. If the anterior shoulder does not follow, the baby is rotated to allow it to be delivered.

Where all the above methods fail, more uncommon methods may be used. These are the Zavanelli's replacement of the head or symphysiotomy. The former involves the risk of annular detachment of the uterus. In good hands, the latter is associated with a good outcome, provided care is taken to avoid damaging the urethra and the hip joints.

(b) What are the complications of shoulder dystocia? (6 marks)

The complications of shoulder dystocia can be fetal or maternal. The immediate fetal complications include intrapartum death, fracture of the clavicle and humerus, birth asphyxia, trauma to internal organs and injury to the cervical nerve plexus resulting in either Erb's or Klumpke's palsy. The long-term complications include cerebral palsy and prolonged consequences of the injuries outlined earlier, especially where some of these have not healed properly.

The maternal complications include trauma to the genital tract, PPH and the psychological stress of the experience. Where the manoeuvres have failed to deliver a live baby, the additional procedures such a Zavanelli's, Caesarean section and symphysiotomy are associated with specific maternal injuries. The risk of recurrence is relatively high.

3. A 29-year-old G2P1 (previous Caesarean section) is being induced at 41 weeks' gestation following an uncomplicated pregnancy. (a) What measures will you take to minimise the risk of uterine rupture? (14 marks) (b) How will you recognise this complication? (6 marks)

Common mistakes

- Discussing methods you will undertake preinduction (decision has already been made about induction)
- Avoid adding too many variables, e.g. breech presentation, previous classical Caesarean section – you ought to know that these will be classified as contraindications for induction
- Do you cross-match blood, or group and save?
- Classical Caesarean section – will not be induced (this is considered by some as criminal or gross negligent practice) – therefore do not discuss induction in such a patient
- Do not mention anything no longer regarded as contemporaneous practice
- No need to go into the details of the induction process, e.g. delay Syntocinon® for 22 hours, etc.

A good answer will include some or all of these points

(a) What measures will you take to minimise the risk of uterine rupture? (14 marks).

- Prior to starting induction:
    - Exclude contraindications (assume they have been excluded)
    - Ruptured uterus is more commonly caused by hypertonic contractions, malpresentation or fetopelvic disproportion
    - Only induce for correct reason – ensure that there is a just reason for the induction
- During induction:
    - With Prostin® alone or in combination – extreme caution needed:
        - Caution with number of Prostin® tablets per day – may need to limit them
        - When in established labour
        - Must avoid hyperstimulation
        - Palpation? Cardiotocography (CTG) – not reliable
        - Intrauterine pressure tip catheter best – but why not commonly used?
    - With Syntocinon®:
        - Syntocinon® – non-judicious use must be avoided
        - Progress in labour
        - Good contractions, cervical dilatation and exclusion of fetopelvic disproportion.
    - ARM with or without any of the other methods above:
        - Avoid hyperstimulation when combining with oxytocics
    - Hyperstimulation – intravenous (i.v.) ritodrine

(b) How will you recognise this complication? (6 marks)

- Recognition:
  - Sudden and persistent bradycardia
  - Persistent abdominal pain/shoulder-tip pain
  - Maternal hypotension and tachycardia
  - Vaginal bleeding
  - Fetal parts easily felt per abdomen or presenting part receding into the abdomen

Sample answer

(a) What measures will you take to minimise the risk of uterine rupture? (14 marks)

The first step to minimise the risk of rupture is to recognise the risk factors for its occurrence and, if possible, to avoid them. These include hypertonicity/hypertonic contractions, malpresentations, fetopelvic disproportion and the type of scar on the uterus. In general, a classical Caesarean section will be considered a contraindication, whereas a complicated previous Caesarean section, especially one where there was postoperative infection, may be a relative contraindication.

Multiple prostaglandins are more likely to result in hypertonia and therefore a limit should be put on the number of prostaglandins to be used. Once labour is established, contractions should be monitored closely and the use of Syntocinon® should be with extreme caution. The use of Syntocinon® and prostaglandin for induction in women with a previous Caesarean section is reported to be associated with a 16-fold increase in risk of uterine rupture (Lyndon-Rochelle et al., 2001). It is also important to exclude contraindications to induction, such as fetopelvic disproportion, and only offer induction for genuine obstetric reasons.

Once the patient is in labour, avoiding injudicious use of Syntocinon® will minimise the risk of overstimulation. This can only be achieved by titrating the dose of Syntocinon® against carefully monitored uterine contractions. Where hyperstimulation occurs, i.v. ritodrine or subcutaneous terbutaline may be given to counteract it. Uterine contractions should be monitored objectively to ensure that their strength and frequency are within normal limits. The ideal method is by means of an intrauterine pressure tip catheter, but these are rarely used.

Continuous fetal monitoring will offer a better objective estimation of the frequency and duration of contractions. Palpation of contractions may complement this method of monitoring, but this should not be the only method of monitoring contractions in this high-risk group.

An important aspect of any labour is progress. This should be monitored and charted carefully and any early signs of obstruction or disproportion recognised, and the induction abandoned for an abdominal delivery. Similarly, if progress is poor, induction should be discontinued in favour of a Caesarean section.

(b) How will you recognise this complication? (6 marks)

The early signs of rupture must be recognised. These include a sudden bradycardia, abdominal pain breaking through an epidural, vaginal bleeding, maternal hypotension, tachycardia, receding fetal head, easily palpable fetal parts and shoulder-tip pains. In most cases, the sudden and non-recovering bradycardia is the first sign, especially in those with epidural anaesthesia.

Reference

Lyndon-Rochelle M, Holt VL, Easterling TR, Martin DP (2001) Risk of uterine rupture during labour among women with a prior caesarean delivery. *N Engl J Med* **345**: 3–8.

4. Critically appraise the methods of induction of labour of an uncomplicated preg-nancy at 41 weeks' gestation in a grand multipara. (20 marks)

Common mistakes

- Take a history and do a physical examination to determine
- Complications of previous labour
- Methods of delivery in previous pregnancies
- Birth weights of babies
- Contraindications to a vaginal delivery
- Discussing the benefits of awaiting spontaneous labour and suggesting inductions should be delayed
- In view of the parity, precautions must be undertaken
- Listing the complications of induction of labour in this woman

A good answer all include some or all of these points

- A grand multipara is at a greater risk of uterine rupture and precipitate labour
- Assumption made – no contraindications for a vaginal delivery
- Options
- ARM alone – if cervix is favourable (may not be). Onset of uterine contractions may be delayed with the risk of chorioamnionitis
- Least likely to be associated with increased risk of hypertonia and therefore rupture
- ARM + Syntocinon® – only if favourable. Syntocinon®, if used injudiciously, may result in rupture. Syntocinon® infusion can be stopped if hyperstimulation
- Prostaglandins – unripe cervix. Initiate contractions, mobilise. Risk of hypertonia and rupture. Unable to control once administered. Ritodrine (i.v.) may counteract hyper-tonia
- Laminaria tents – mechanical, dilatation of the cervix. Insertion may be uncomfortable
- Foley's catheter – balloon to dilate cervix and release endogenous prostaglandins. Same as for the laminaria tents
- Oestrogens – outdated

Sample answer

A grand multiparous woman is one who has had at least five (although there appears to be a move to reducing this to four by some experts) deliveries after 24 weeks' gestation. By virtue of this high parity, this patient is at an increased risk of uterine rupture, precipitate labour and postpartum haemorrhage during labour, especially one that is either induced or augmented. Postdates is one of the common indications for induction of labour. Various methods are available for induction of labour, ranging from simple ARM to the use of a combination of surgical and medical methods. It has to be assumed in this patient that there are no contraindications to a vaginal delivery, otherwise she would not be undergoing an induction.

Where the cervix is unfavourable for ARM, a membrane sweep may be followed by spontaneous onset of labour. Randomised trials have shown that sweeping the membranes and even massaging the cervix results in the onset of labour in a large proportion of patients, especially multiparous women. In this grand multipara, this may be an effective option. Its main advantage is that is allows labour to start spontaneously and this may be at the expense of waiting for a few days. Since the patient is at only 41 weeks' gestation, this method provides significant advantages as she could wait for a few days before further intervention.

The second option is ARM where the cervix is ripe. A ripe cervix is one with a Bishop's score of at least six. If the membranes are ruptured, the patient may go into spontaneous labour. However, she may require Syntocinon® to initiate contractions or augment labour. Artificial rupture of fetal membranes alone is less likely to be associated with hypertonic contractions and therefore is associated with no increased risk of uterine rupture. However, because it may require Syntocinon®, the risk remains high with this combination. In addition, waiting for contractions to start spontaneously may increase the risk of ascending infections, although this is rare.

Prostaglandins (PGE$_2$) and misoprostol are the most effective agents for the induction of labour in this patient. This is especially where the cervix is not favourable for ARM. One of the advantages of prostaglandins is that the patient is not confined to bed during the early phase of induction. Apart from ripening the cervix, the patient is more likely to go into spontaneous labour with prostaglandins. However, these may induce hypertonic contractions, which may result in uterine rupture in this grand multiparous woman. Once administered, it is difficult to control the absorption rate. Therefore the only means to overcome hyperstimulation is by the administration of i.v. or subcutaneous sympathomimetic agents. The prostaglandins, whether given orally or vaginally, are associated with systemic side-effects, such as vomiting and diarrhoea.

Mechanical methods of induction that could be used in this patient include Foley's catheter – usually with a 30 mL balloon. The catheter is inserted into the cervical canal and the balloon inflated and left *in situ* until it falls out. This will happen when the cervix is sufficiently dilated, and at this stage, the patient either goes into spontaneous labour or the membranes are ruptured and Syntocinon® initiated if necessary. This method is cheap, available to all units and effective. It may be difficult to insert the catheter and some patients may find this extremely uncomfortable. Other hygroscopic devices, such as laminaria tents, offer the same advantages as the Foley's catheter, except that they may be more expensive. Although 17-beta-oestradiol has been used in the past, this is rarely used nowadays.

5. A primigravida was admitted in spontaneous labour at 40 weeks' gestation 14 hours ago. Fetal membranes had ruptured spontaneously 12 hours before admission. Her cervix was 3 cm on admission. The cervix has remained at 8 cm for the last 4 hours and, in addition, she now has a pyrexia of 37.8°C. However, the fetal heart rate is normal. (a) Under what conditions will you do a Caesarean section in this patient? (6 marks) (b) What complications may affect this mother and fetus? (6 marks) (c) She is eventually delivered by Caesarean section because of obstructed labour after 20 hours. How will you minimise any maternal and fetal complications? (8 marks)

Common mistakes

- Do a physical examination to identify the cause of the pyrexia
- She has an obstructed labour and should be delivered by Caesarean section (you cannot make this diagnosis without justifying it)
- Criticising the management of patient so far – not really asked to do this
- Involve anaesthetist and paediatrician in the decision to deliver
- Discussing the methods of delivery with the patient and giving her the options so she can make a decision on how to be delivered

A good answer will include some or all of these points

(a) Under what conditions will you do a Caesarean section in this patient? (6 marks)

- Maternal:
  - Exhaustion
  - Failure to progress despite maximum Syntocinon®
  - Other risk factors in pregnancy
- Fetal:
  - Abnormal CTG
  - Abnormal pH and blood gases
  - Evidence of obstruction or disproportion
  - Abnormal presentation – brow or face mentoposterior

(b) What complications may affect this mother and fetus? (6 marks)

- Mother:
  - Obstructed labour
  - Complications of Caesarean section – increased risk of VTE, infections, etc.
  - Uterine rupture
  - Vesicovaginal or rectovaginal fistula

- Obstetric neuropraxia
- Chorioamnionitis
- Asherman's syndrome
- Psychological trauma
- Fetus:
  - Asphyxia
  - Stillbirth
  - Neonatal infections
  - Trauma to the fetus from difficult vaginal or abdominal delivery

(c) How will you minimise any maternal and fetal complications? (8 marks)

- Rest the bladder for 6–10 days with an indwelling catheter
- Broad-spectrum antibiotics
- Thromboprophylaxis for at least 5 days
- Neonate to be admitted onto the neonatal unit for observation and antibiotics
- Postpartum haemorrhage – best prevented by a Syntocinon® drip

Sample answer

(a) Under what conditions will you do a Caesarean section in this patient? (6 marks)

The maternal reasons for performing a Caesarean section include exhaustion and unwillingness to continue with labour, failure to progress, or other complications that may considerably jeopardise the life of the mother. The fetal indications include fetal distress (abnormal CTG alone or better still, an abnormal CTG and scalp pH), evidence of fetopelvic disproportion (significant moulding and caput formation) and abnormal presentation (e.g. brow or face in the mentoposterior position). In this pyrexial patient, if there is evidence of chorioamnionitis (e.g. foul-smelling liquor) and there is fetal tachycardia and delivery is not considered to be imminent, then a Caesarean section may be better, as it will allow timely institution of antibiotics to the baby and also reduce the risk of significant peritonitis after delivery.

(b) What complications may affect this mother and fetus? (6 marks)

The maternal complications include obstruction, which may result in uterine rupture, compression necrosis of the bladder and vagina resulting in a vesicovaginal fistula or compression necrosis of the vagina and rectum resulting in a rectovaginal fistula, obstetric neuropraxia, chorioamnionitis, Asherman's syndrome and psychological trauma from the difficult labour. The fetal complications include asphyxia, stillbirth, neonatal septicaemia, trauma due to a difficult delivery and cerebral palsy. Neonatal septicaemia may result in jaundice, renal failure, meningitis and other complications with resultant significant morbidity.

(c) How will you minimise any maternal and fetal complications? (8 marks)

The most severe immediate complication that the mother is likely to have is PPH (prolonged labour and chorioamnionitis) and the risk of this can be minimised by starting a Syntocinon® drip (40 IU/500 mL saline) and running it for 4 hours. Vesicovaginal fistula is a complication related to obstructed labour and this can be minimised by resting the bladder for about 6–10 days and giving broad-spectrum antibiotics. Where neuropraxia is suspected, resting the foot and physiotherapy are essential. The risk of VTE in this woman is considerably high; she should therefore be placed on thromboprophylaxis for at least 5 days. This could be in the form of low-molecular-weight heparin (e.g. Fragmin® 5000 mg daily) combined with early mobilisation and thromboembolic deterrent stockings.

The main complication that the neonate may suffer from is sepsis and for this the baby should be admitted into the neonatal intensive care unit for observation for at least 3–4 days, during which broad-spectrum antibiotics covering Gram-negative and -positive organisms and anaerobes would be instituted.

12

Intrapartum care and complications of labour

1. (a) Comment critically on the manoeuvres used in the management of the after-coming head in a breech delivery. (14 marks) (b) How may the complications of a planned vaginal delivery be avoided? (6 marks)

2. Mrs BB is 27 years old. She is mentally subnormal. In her first pregnancy, she refused intervention but fortunately had a normal delivery, which was complicated by a retained placenta that was delivered spontaneously with a postpartum haemorrhage of 800 mL. She presented in labour at 41 weeks' gestation with spontaneous rupture of fetal membranes and regular uterine contractions and, again, refused a vaginal examination and any form of intervention. (a) Identify the potential problems with the management of this woman. (6 marks) (b) Outline how you will deal with them. (14 marks)

3. You suspect that a primigravida induced by oxytocic agents and prostaglandins at 41 weeks' gestation has a ruptured uterus. (a) What clinical features will support your diagnosis? (8 marks) (b) Justify your subsequent management of the patient. (12 marks)

4. The morbidity and mortality associated with cord prolapse is high. (a) What steps will you take to reduce the risk of this complication? (10 marks) (b) How will you manage it when it occurs? (10 marks)

5. A 27-year-old teacher, in her second pregnancy, wishes to deliver at home. Her first pregnancy was uncomplicated and she had a 4-hour normal delivery of a 3.5 kg male infant. (a) What are the advantages and disadvantages of home delivery? (12 marks) (b) What factors will influence your decision to support her choice? (8 marks)

1. (a) Comment critically on the manoeuvres used in the management of the after-coming head in a breech delivery. (14 marks) (b) How may the complications of a planned vaginal delivery be avoided? (6 marks)

Common mistakes

- Take a history and do a physical examination
- Establish the indications for breech delivery
- Extolling the virtues of delivering all breeches by Caesarean section (Canadian trial)
- Ultrasound scan to estimate the diameter of the fetal head
- Ensure that the pelvis is adequate
- Pelvimetry – radiological/clinical
- Examine the patient to ensure that she is fully dilated

A good answer will include some or all of these points

(a) Comment critically on the manoeuvres used in the management of the after-coming head in a breech delivery. (14 marks)

- Three common approaches to management:
  - Burns–Marshall technique – pros and cons
  - Mauriceau–Smellie–Veit manoeuvre – pros and cons
  - Forceps to after-coming head – pros and cons
- Uncommon methods:
  - Symphysiotomy – pros and cons
  - Zavanelli technique; destructive operation – pros and cons
  - Caesarean section – pros and cons
- Conclusion

(b) How may the complications of a planned vaginal delivery be avoided? (6 marks)

- Selection of cases
- Ensuring that the most appropriate expertise is available
- Anaesthetist available
- Assessment of progress and aborting the process early
- Timing of manoeuvres, ensuring that there is no undue delay
- Training and education of medical and midwifery staff in breech vaginal delivery (using models, etc.)

Sample answer

(a) *Comment critically on the manoeuvres used in the management of the after-coming head in a breech delivery. (14 marks)*

The management of the after-coming head requires a good understanding of the mechanisms and processes of labour and the pelvic anatomy. There are traditionally three classical approaches. These include the Burns–Marshall technique, the Mauriceau–Smellie–Veit manoeuvre and the application of forceps. However, in some circumstances these may not be successful and other options must therefore be considered.

The Burns–Marshall technique allows the breech to hang until the nape of the neck is visible. This allows the fetal head to descend into the pelvis. Either the operator or an assistant then grasps the fetal ankles and feet and raises the body/trunk above the mother's abdomen. A hand is placed over the perineum to prevent precipitate delivery. The head is then delivered either with maternal effort or with some pressure from the suprapubic region. This technique is simple to apply; however, it may be associated with precipitate delivery of the head and intracranial haemorrhage, secondary to tentorial tears. By raising the trunk above the abdomen, hyperextension may result and make delivery complicated.

Application of forceps to the head after raising the trunk above the mother's abdomen allows gentle and better-controlled delivery of the head and therefore minimises the risk of intracranial haemorrhage. However, during the application of the forceps, failure to recognise that the lowest part of the fetal head is, indeed, the smallest, and therefore prematurely straightening the forceps may cause undue pressure on the fetal head and may result in fractures. This complication is more common if forceps with short shanks are used. Prolonged interval between application and delivery may also result in unnecessary compression of the fetal head.

The third technique is the Mauriceau–Smellie–Veit manoeuvre. The operator places the fetus over one forearm and then inserts the middle finger of that hand into the baby's mouth and the index and ring fingers on the malar eminences. The second hand applies pressure downwards on the occiput of the fetus. Combining this pressure with downwards traction to the mandible allows delivery. Occasionally, an assistant may apply suprapubic pressure to assist the delivery. Exerting too much force on the mandible may result in dislocation or fracture of the mandible. Inserting the finger too far into the throat and exerting pressure may also result in the creation of a pseudo-diverticulum.

Although these techniques are effective in most cases, occasionally delivery is impossible. A symphysiotomy may therefore be performed. This is an uncommon procedure in developed countries and is associated with damage to the urethra and instability at the pelvic joints. It may also be complicated by symphysitis. Another manoeuvre that is uncommon is pushing the baby back into the abdomen and performing a Caesarean section. The difficulty is in pushing the fetus into the abdomen, as usually the uterus is contracting on the fetus. The risk of annular detachment of the uterus is quite high in this procedure.

Craniotomy is an uncommon procedure but may be performed in cases where the fetus is dead and delivery is impossible, or if there is hydrocephalus. This operation is only performed as a last resort and parts of the bone may cause maternal injuries such as vesicovaginal fistula.

(b) How may the complications of a planned vaginal delivery be avoided? (6 marks)

The best way to avoid complications is case selection. Very strict criteria should be used to select those cases suitable for vaginal breech delivery. In addition, such deliveries must be conducted by trained and experienced staff with appropriate and timely supervision by senior staff including anaesthetists. Adequate analgesia will reduce the need for premature interventions or premature bearing down, especially when the breech has not descended into and out of the pelvis. Regular and competent assessment of progress will ensure that labour is interrupted by timely Caesarean sections. During the vaginal breech delivery the various stages and manoeuvres should be timed to prevent undue delay whenever one is not being effective. Finally training and education of junior medical and midwifery staff on breech deliveries, with regular fire drills, will ensure competency levels are maintained.

2. Mrs BB is 27 years old. She is mentally subnormal. In her first pregnancy, she refused intervention but fortunately had a normal delivery, which was complicated by a retained placenta that was delivered spontaneously with a postpartum haemorrhage of 800 mL. She presented in labour at 41 weeks' gestation with spontaneous rupture of fetal membranes and regular uterine contractions and, again, refused a vaginal examination and any form of intervention. (a) Identify the potential problems with the management of this woman. (6 marks) (b) Outline how you will deal with them. (14 marks)

Common mistakes

- Outline details of the diagnosis and management of labour
- Complications of spontaneous rupture of fetal membranes
- Management of postpartum haemorrhage
- Refer patient to psychiatrist
- Ought to have made a plan before delivery, therefore substandard care
- Care of patient should be in specialised unit

A good answer will include some or all of these points

(a) Identify the potential problems with the management of this woman. (6 marks)

- Mentally subnormal, therefore potential issues of:
  - Consent
  - Communication and understanding
- In established labour (rupture of fetal membranes and contractions) – need to exclude cord prolapse
- Monitoring of labour and fetal heart rate
- Increased risk of retained placenta and postpartum haemorrhage
- Care of the baby
- Where an emergency arises – how to proceed

(b) Outline how you will deal with them. (14 marks)

- Examine the notes for any antenatal documentation of discussions and plan of care in labour (if any)
- Involve senior member of obstetric, midwifery, anaesthetic and management team on duty
- Ensure relative and woman's midwife present if possible
- Vaginal examination to exclude cord prolapse
- Precautions against retained placenta

- Would the courts be involved? Seek advice from administration and Trust solicitors
- Planned postnatal care and involve social workers in the community

Sample answer

(a) Identify the potential problems with the management of this woman. (6 marks)

This patient poses several problems with her management. The first is to do with consent to the various procedures to be undertaken during labour. If she is so subnormal that she cannot understand and has no insight into implications of any interventions, she cannot provide consent. The second is communication and understanding. It will be difficult to explain with some clarity the various steps in the management of her labour and to be certain that these have been understood.

As she has presented with suspected rupture of fetal membranes, this has to be confirmed and a cord prolapse excluded. In addition, consent will be needed for monitoring the labour and the fetal heart rate. She has an increased risk of retaining the placenta and therefore of postpartum haemorrhage. An important issue is the potential of an emergency Caesarean section and how to proceed, since she is refusing any form of intervention.

(b) Outline how you will deal with them. (14 marks)

The antenatal notes should be examined for any documentation of discussions and plan of care in labour, if any. It is expected that this would have been identified antenatally and necessary precautions taken to address this problem. If there is no such documentation, appropriate steps need to be taken.

The patient's management should involve the most senior member of the obstetric, midwifery, anaesthetic and management team on duty. A relative who would have been with her throughout pregnancy, and her midwife, have to be present as they may provide support in a strange and perhaps frightening environment. Issues relating to consent about her care include assessment of progress of labour, monitoring of the fetus (first, to exclude cord prolapse), prophylaxis against retained placenta and primary postpartum haemorrhage (which are more likely to occur) and the necessary steps to take in the case of an emergency.

A close relative and the patient's midwife may be able to persuade her to allow the fetus to be monitored. In fact, they could encourage her to place the cardiotocograph (CTG) on her abdomen herself. Provided the fetal heart is normal and the patient is not in distress, labour can be allowed to continue without the need for vaginal examinations (provided cord compression has been excluded) and when there is anal dilatation she will start to push by reflex. This is more likely since she has had a normal delivery before.

Administrators may have to seek permission from the courts to treat in her best interest if necessary. Such authority may allow for the forced administration of oxytocic agents and transfusion, if required in cases of life-threatening massive postpartum haemorrhage. Such permission should also make provisions for an emergency Caesarean section if it is thought necessary (in the best interest of the patient).

The postnatal care of the baby must be reviewed and confirmed if there are any instructions documented in the patient's notes. If there are none, clues could be gleaned from the care of her previous baby. If the baby was fostered or has been adopted, a similar approach must be followed unless there are relatives who can guarantee looking after the child. The baby may, therefore, be made a ward of court and cared for in the hospital until appropriate steps have been taken to ensure its care in the community. The care of the mother after delivery must also be planned. In this case, the midwife and social workers involved will offer the necessary support and provide the required care in the community. Although contraception may not be offered at this stage, it must be discussed and a plan made on how to prevent further pregnancies.

In the care of this patient, there should be adequate communication between social workers, psychiatrists, senior obstetricians and anaesthetists, paediatricians and midwives, and all the necessary decisions must be agreed upon. Discussions at all levels will ensure that all aspects are considered as deemed necessary.

3. You suspect that a primigravida induced by oxytocic agents and prostaglandins at 41 weeks' gestation has a ruptured uterus. (a) What clinical features will support your diagnosis? (8 marks) (b) Justify your subsequent management of the patient. (12 marks)

Common mistakes

- Take a history and do a physical examination
- Discussing the risk factors for ruptured uterus
- Review notes to determine whether she has had any surgery
- Do a 30-minute CTG to monitor the fetus
- Only the consultant should manage such a patient as she is very high risk
- Anaesthetist must insert a central venous pressure monitor
- Input/output

A good answer will include some or all of these points

(a) What clinical features will support your diagnosis? (8 marks)

- Maternal:
  - Abdominal and/or shoulder-tip pain – pain breaking through epidural (if any sited)
  - Vaginal bleeding
  - Shock – hypotension and tachycardia
  - Fullness of the abdomen in the flanks (irregular in shape)
  - Weak pulse
- Fetal:
  - Bradycardia – sudden and persistent (i.e. non-recovering)
  - Fetal parts easily palpable per abdomen
  - Presenting part receding

(b) Justify your subsequent management of the patient. (12 marks)

- Fetus still alive or not – laparotomy and deliver fetus
- Repair if rupture is clean (i.e. not ragged)
- Repair and tubal ligation
- Hysterectomy
- Most important step – resuscitation: intravenous (i.v.) access; anaesthetist; involve haematologist
- Risk management – complete incident form, investigation, multidisciplinary meeting and education (steps to prevent recurrence)

Sample answer

(a) What clinical features will support your diagnosis? (8 marks)

The maternal features suggestive of a ruptured uterus include abdominal and/or shoulder-tip pain. The pain may have broken through an epidural if any had been sited. This pain is constant compared to the intermittent pain of labour. There may be associated vaginal bleeding, the volume of which varies greatly. The patient may be in shock as evidenced by hypotension and tachycardia. In addition, she may appear pale, sweaty and have cold and clammy extremities. The abdomen will appear irregular in contour with fullness at the flanks. Fetal parts will be palpated easily and no contractions will be palpable.

The fetal features are typically a sudden and persistent bradycardia that fails to respond to any resuscitative measures and is often accompanied by disappearance of the fetal heart when demise has set it. As described above the fetal parts become easily palpable per abdomen and the lie more difficult to define. The presenting part is seen to recede on pelvic examination.

(b) Justify your subsequent management of the patient. (12 marks)

An immediate laparotomy must be performed, preferably under general anaesthesia, to save the baby. This should be performed through the quickest means; therefore, a midline subumbilical skin incision may be preferred to a Pfannenstiel incision. Where possible, this procedure should be performed by a skilled obstetrician; however, in the absence of one, delivery cannot be delayed but a senior obstetrician should be involved in the patient's management.

Haemorrhage from an unscarred uterus is more likely to be life threatening. A second i.v. access should therefore be secured immediately the diagnosis is suspected. This could be shortly after the patient is under general anaesthesia. Blood should also be cross-matched, and it may be necessary to have uncross-matched blood available. The involvement of an experienced anaesthetist, haematologist and obstetrician is an important part of the management of this patient. This would ensure that complications of the rupture, such as haemorrhage and the need for massive transfusion, are properly managed.

Once the baby has been delivered, options are repairing the rupture alone, repairing and ligating the tubes, or a hysterectomy. The decision has to be made based on the nature of the rupture. If it is a linear rupture, a simple repair is all that is necessary. In this primigravida, this must be the preferred option, but it must not be at the risk of losing her life. Confidential enquiries into maternal mortality state that delay in offering hysterectomy to patients was partly responsible for some mortalities from haemorrhage.

Where there is very extensive damage to the uterus and it is perceived that it will not be able to carry another pregnancy after it has been repaired, tubal ligation will be necessary. Again, this decision must be made against the background of the patient's parity. In cases where the uterus has been extensively damaged and repair is not possible, a hysterectomy will have to be performed.

One of the most important aspects of this patient's management is postnatal counselling. Details of the events leading to the rupture must be discussed, as well as the type of treatment offered and its implications for subsequent pregnancies. If the rupture is linear and in the lower segment (and therefore mimics a Caesarean section scar) there is a place for allowing a trial vaginal delivery in subsequent pregnancies, but the use of oxytocic agents must be avoided. However, in some cases, the rupture will be in the upper segment and this must be considered as a classical Caesarean section scar and subsequent pregnancies managed appropriately. It may be necessary to involve a psychologist in the counselling of this patient.

4. The morbidity and mortality associated with cord prolapse is high. (a) What steps will you take to reduce the risk of this complication? (10 marks) (b) How will you manage it when it occurs? (10 marks)

Common mistakes

- Forgetting that there are two parts to the question
- Listing all the causes of cord prolapse and not discussing prevention
- Assuming that the prolapse has occurred in labour or only in a singleton pregnancy
- Delivery by Caesarean section – the only option

A good answer will include some or all of these points

(a) What steps will you take to reduce the risk of this complication? (10 marks)

- Cord prolapse is an obstetric emergency – results in hypoxia and intrauterine fetal death if no immediate intervention
- Risk factors: polyhydramnios; preterm labour; abnormal presentation (breech, transverse lie); unengaged head; second twin – intrapartum
- Minimising risk factors: polyhydramnios – defining causes, treating polyhydramnios and therapeutic reduction; unengaged head – avoid rupturing membranes unless necessary; prematurity – be aware of risk, especially when membranes rupture prematurely; management of second twin – avoid early intervention

(b) How will you manage it when it occurs? (10 marks)

- Management:
  - Early recognition on delivery suite – push presenting part away from the cord with hand in the vagina and retain it in place until delivery, or fill bladder
  - Rupture of fetal membranes – cord prolapse
  - Is the fetus alive?
  - Cervix fully dilated – fetus alive:
    - Vaginal delivery possible – ventouse
  - Cervix not fully dilated or cervix dilated and vaginal delivery not possible – Caesarean section; twins – high head – membranes just ruptured – internal podalic version and breech extraction

Sample answer

(a) What steps will you take to reduce the risk of this complication? (10 marks)

Cord prolapse is an obstetric emergency that requires immediate delivery, otherwise the fetus will die from severe asphyxia. It occurs after spontaneous rupture of fetal membranes (prelabour, intrapartum or after delivery of a first twin). To reduce the risk of this complication, those at risk must be identified and appropriate steps taken to minimise the risk.

Risk factors for cord prolapse include polyhydramnios, preterm labour, premature rupture of fetal membranes, abnormal lie (oblique and transverse) and presentation (breech and shoulder), a high head (especially at term) and multiple pregnancies, especially in those undergoing a vaginal delivery. The risk of cord prolapse may be minimised in some of the high-risk groups listed above, but in some it cannot. Where there is polyhydramnios, the cause should be found and, if possible, attempts made to reduce the liquor volume, especially where the patient is uncomfortable (in cases of acute polyhydramnios). The problem with this risk factor is that, in many cases, treatment is unable to reduce the liquor volume significantly and, therefore, the risk of cord prolapse. Other means of minimising the risk factors include counselling high-risk patients on when to present (especially when they are contracting, bleeding or suspect rupture of fetal membranes). Rupture of membranes when the head is unengaged should be avoided if possible and induction of labour undertaken only when it is appropriate, especially where the head of the fetus is high.

(b) How will you manage it when it occurs? (10 marks)

Once the diagnosis has been made, the fetus must be delivered as soon as possible. For all scenarios other than twin delivery, a hand must be maintained in the vagina, or alternatively the bladder is filled, to push the presenting part away from the cord until the baby is delivered. The quickest method of delivery is Caesarean section. Asphyxia in these cases is often secondary to spasm of the vessels in the cord, and compression. By minimising compression, most cases where the diagnosis is made early are not compromised. Where the diagnosis is made in a twin delivery, and the cervix is fully dilated, the cord can be pushed to one side and the baby delivered with a ventouse if the presenting part is cephalic. If it is breech and the membranes have only ruptured, it may be possible to do a breech extraction. Occasionally, the head may be too high to apply a ventouse. If this is the case a Caesarean section should be performed, but where the membranes have just ruptured it may be possible to undertake an internal podalic version and a breech extraction. Where the cervix is not fully dilated, the same principles should apply as when managing cord prolapse in a singleton pregnancy. However, it is possible to undertake a ventouse delivery when the cervix has reformed after the delivery of a first twin. The main problem is the delivery may be delayed and the fetus may be compromised.

5. A 27-year-old teacher, in her second pregnancy, wishes to deliver at home. Her first pregnancy was uncomplicated and she had a 4-hour normal delivery of a 3.5 kg male infant. (a) What are the advantages and disadvantages of home delivery? (12 marks) (b) What factors will influence your decision to support her choice? (8 marks)

Common mistakes

- Discussing the details of how to conduct a home delivery
- Discourage her from a home delivery
- Details of the conduct of a normal delivery
- Complications of labour
- Failure to give the advantages and disadvantages
- Decision depends on past obstetric history

A good answer will include some or all of these points

(a) What are the advantages and disadvantages of home delivery? (12 marks)

- Advantages of a home delivery:
  - Home environment
  - No high-technology monitoring of fetus
  - One-to-one midwife care
- Disadvantages:
  - No doctors available at short notice
  - If need for urgent intervention, may not have enough time – average transfer to hospital is more than 30 minutes
  - Psychological/guilt feelings if outcome is poor
  - Neonatologist unavailable
  - No facilities for epidural
- Overall – perinatal mortality high

(b) What factors will influence your decision to support her choice? (8 marks)

- Recognise that is an option in the UK
- Criteria for this option – uncomplicated pregnancy:
  - Fetal growth restriction (FGR)
  - Abnormal presentation and lie
  - Polyhydramnios
  - Antepartum haemorrhage
  - Fetal macrosomia
  - Complications such as pre-eclampsia (PET), diabetes, etc.

- Past obstetric history:
  - Shoulder dystocia
  - Postpartum haemorrhage
  - Retained placenta
  - Previous Caesarean section
- Easy access to the hospital
- Skilled midwife to conduct labour
- No contraindications to a vaginal delivery
- If happy to take the risks

Sample answer

(a) What are the advantages and disadvantages of home delivery? (12 marks)

Home delivery is an option that should be open for all uncomplicated pregnancies in the UK. In fact, the Government White Paper on changing childbirth supports this option. Despite this, it is still only taken up by a minority of women. Counselling of the patient should be objective and based on evidence rather on personal beliefs. Home births are supervised by either an independent midwife practitioner or hospital staff. The option will only be available to this patient if there are midwives who are prepared to supervise the delivery.

The advantages and disadvantages of home births need to be discussed. The main advantage of home confinement is that of 'demedicalisation' of the birth process. In addition, the patient and her family are in their own environment where high technology is unavailable. Care is provided either by a named midwife whom she is likely to have seen throughout the pregnancy or by someone with whom she has built a rapport. This makes the experience more fulfilling. In hospital delivery, although there is a real desire to have a named midwife this is difficult to implement in practice. It is therefore common for patients to have several midwives supervising their labour in hospital and it is not unusual for some of them to be meeting the patient for the first time. Home births are also associated with less analgesia intrapartum and postdelivery and better mother and baby bonding. The availability of family support is another benefit. The risk of acquired hospital infections is reduced.

The disadvantages of home confinement include the absence of facilities for more intensive surveillance of the fetus. That said, the Dublin trial did not show any benefits from continuous fetal monitoring. If anything, there was an increase in the operative delivery rate. Since there are no high-technology facilities for monitoring, it may be difficult to recognise fetal distress early and to intervene. In this situation, intervention may be delayed whilst the patient is transferred to hospital. This disadvantage has been supported by evidence indicating that perinatal morbidity and mortality in those who are transferred to hospital from a planned home birth is significantly higher than that from planned hospital confinement. The absence of a neonatologist and facilities for ventilation is another disadvantage. This means that even if the baby were delivered normally, but started grunting or required immediate intubation and ventilation, this would be impossible.

Although adverse events are rare, the patient should be informed that statistics may be acceptable when they do not apply to oneself, whereas, if there are complications, she must live with her decision. If she is fully aware of this, and is prepared to have the delivery at home, this option should be made available. The alternative is for her to have a hospital delivery (in a home-from-home unit, if available) with her named midwife and to be discharged home 4–6 hours after delivery.

(b) What factors will influence your decision to support her choice? (8 marks)

The factors that will influence the decision will include the availability of midwives to attend the delivery, whether the pregnancy is uncomplicated (complications such as PET, FGR, fetal macrosomia, polyhydramnios, abnormal presentation, antepartum haemorrhage, diabetes mellitus, etc. are contraindications) and her previous obstetric history (e.g. previous shoulder dystocia, previous Caesarean section, previous postpartum haemorrhage, third-degree perineal tears, etc. would be against a home confinement).

Easy access to hospital and facilities available for transporting the patient to the hospital are crucial. Another factor is the availability of facilities in the community for resuscitating the baby and mother, should the need arise. If there are no contraindications to a vaginal delivery, manpower is not an issue and there is ready access to the hospital, the decision would be supported. However, this must be viewed together with her understanding of the risks involved and willingness to accept these risks.

13

Operative obstetrics

1. A 34-year-old teacher, in her third pregnancy, the previous two having been delivered by Caesarean section, presents at 37 weeks' gestation requesting for a trial of vaginal delivery. (a) How will you counsel her about her request? (14 marks) (b) What precautions will you take to ensure a safe vaginal delivery? (6 marks)

2. Do you agree that Caesarean section rates in the UK are too high? (20 marks)

3. You are about to perform an elective Caesarean section on a 28-year-old woman having her third baby. She requests that sterilisation be performed at the time of surgery. (a) What factors will you take into consideration during counselling? (12 marks) (b) You agree to perform the procedure. What options are available to you? (8 marks)

4. Critically appraise the management of a woman in her second pregnancy, the first having been delivered by emergency classical Caesarean section for transverse lie. (20 marks)

5. A 30-year-old woman with placenta praevia grade III posterior is scheduled to undergo an elective Caesarean section at 39 weeks' gestation. (a) Outline the steps you will take to minimise complications. (8 marks) (b) After delivery of the baby and placenta, she continues to bleed. What will be your subsequent management? (8 marks) (c) How will you counsel her about her next pregnancy? (4 marks)

1. A 34-year-old teacher, in her third pregnancy, the previous two having been delivered by Caesarean section, presents at 37 weeks' gestation requesting for a trial of vaginal delivery. (a) How will you counsel her about her request? (14 marks) (b) What precautions will you take to ensure a safe delivery? (6 marks)

Common mistakes

- Offer sterilisation
- Cannot delivery vaginally
- Decision can only be made by consultant, so refer
- Discussing the operation of Caesarean section
- Quoting incorrect rates of uterine rupture

A good answer will include some or all of these points

(a) How will you counsel her about her request? (14 marks)

- Traditional practice – after two Caesarean sections, elective Caesarean section
- Rationale – increased risk of uterine rupture
- Increasingly, women are being allowed to deliver vaginally
- Good evidence to indicate safe delivery in well-selected cases
- Why the previous two Caesarean sections? Maybe for recurrent reasons, e.g. contracted pelvis, etc.
- Why does she want a vaginal delivery?
- Type of previous Caesarean section – if classical or inverted-T, unsafe for trial of vaginal delivery
- Allow vaginal delivery if no contraindications
- Place of second opinion
- Exclude contraindications to vaginal delivery, such as abnormal presentation, fetal macrosomia, etc.

(b) What precautions will you take to ensure a safe delivery? (6 marks)

- Cross-match blood or group and save
- Hospital confinement; continuous monitoring in labour – cardiotocographs (CTGs) for early detection of rupture
- Warn patient of potential risks of uterine rupture
- Emergency Caesarean section and other complications
- If goes past dates, prostaglandins (for induction) – relatively contraindicated
- No use of oxytocics in labour

Sample answer

(a) How will you counsel her about her request? (14 marks)

Standard practice after two or more lower-segment Caesarean sections is to recommend delivery by Caesarean section. This is based on the fact that the risk of uterine rupture during labour is significantly greater in these women. Increasingly, this approach has been questioned as there are no randomised trials to justify the reasoning behind this. Many practitioners are allowing a trial of vaginal delivery in well-selected cases after two lower-segment Caesarean sections, and the evidence emerging is in favour of such a pragmatic approach. However, before a patient is offered this choice, careful consideration must be given to her past obstetric history and the current pregnancy. It is only after appropriate counselling about the risks that this option should be allowed.

The first approach in counselling this patient is to establish why she wants a vaginal delivery. It may be her previous experiences or she might have read or heard about this option. The reasons for the previous two Caesarean sections should also be established from the notes and from the patient. If they were for a recurrent problem, such as a contracted pelvis or a congenital malformation of the uterus, this option will be unsafe for her. If this was not the case, the types of Caesarean section performed should be ascertained from her notes. If either of them was a classical or an inverted-T Caesarean section, a trial of vaginal delivery would be considered unsafe. It is also important to establish that the Caesarean sections were not complicated by postoperative infections (especially the second one) which could easily have weakened the scar.

Assuming that there are no contraindications from the past obstetric history, the current pregnancy needs to be evaluated to exclude contraindications to a vaginal delivery. This evaluation will include abnormal lie, placenta praevia and abnormal presentation. In the absence of any of these, the patient should be counselled about the risk of a trial of vaginal delivery. The risk of uterine rupture is significantly greater than that in women with one previous Caesarean section (1:200) or no scars on the uterus. The delivery should therefore take place only in the hospital where blood would be grouped and saved, an intravenous (i.v.) access will be secured during labour, and there are facilities for continuous fetal monitoring, experienced staff and ready access to a theatre should the need for an emergency delivery arise because of a uterine rupture.

In addition, the complications of emergency Caesarean section should be discussed, including the possibility of a hysterectomy were the uterus to rupture. Where there is a rupture, there may be fetal bradycardia, which may require very precipitate delivery when general anaesthesia would be the chosen form of anaesthesia.

Part of the counselling should include the problems that could arise when the pregnancy goes past term. Induction of labour with prostaglandins would be considered unsafe in this patient. If this were to happen, an elective Caesarean section would be the preferred mode of delivery. In addition, if the patient went into labour and required augmentation, syntocinon would be relatively unsafe because of the risk of rupture. Again, were this to be necessary, a Caesarean section will be the better option.

If there are contraindications to a trial of vaginal delivery, or the patient is unprepared to accept these conditions, a second opinion should be sought. She should be referred to someone senior or to another obstetrician. It is very likely that once her reasons for requesting a vaginal delivery have been addressed and information provided in an unbiased way, the patient will opt for the approach that is safest for her baby and herself.

(b) What precautions will you take to ensure a safe delivery? (6 marks)

The precautions that must be taken to ensure a safe delivery include delivery in the hospital with facilities for continuous fetal monitoring (CTG) and quick access to Caesarean section. This must therefore be in a unit with preferably 24-hour anaesthetic cover. When she is admitted in labour, an i.v. line must be secured and blood sent for group and cross-match, or at least serum must be saved. The patient must understand that the risk of uterine rupture is greater than that after one Caesarean section. If she goes past her dates or labour is dysfunctional, there will be real reluctance to use prostaglandins and Syntocinon® respectively. Under these circumstances, she would have to accept a Caesarean section.

2. Do you agree that Caesarean section rates in the UK are too high? (20 marks)

Common mistakes

- Discussing the indications for Caesarean section
- Arguing about the complications of Caesarean section
- Discussing patients' choice for Caesarean section
- Listing the procedure of Caesarean section

A good answer will include some or all of these points

- Incidence of Caesarean section is rising in the UK
- What is the nationally accepted Caesarean section rate? Any internationally acceptable rates, e.g. World Health Organization (WHO) rates?
- Why is the Caesarean section rate rising? Obstetric/medical, social/patient choice and litigious society
- What are the problems with a high Caesarean section rate? Morbidity and mortality, long-term medical complications, cost implications
- Other implications of a high Caesarean section rate – deskilling of junior doctors and other clinicians in vaginal delivery procedures

Sample answer

Caesarean delivery rates are rising in most developed countries. In some parts of the world, up to 50 per cent of women are delivered by Caesarean section. This is not only more expensive for the care provider but is associated with significant morbidity. In the UK, the Caesarean section rate has been rising gradually from less than 10 per cent in the 1970s to current rates of between 20 and 35 per cent (depending on the unit). There is obviously some concern about this trend and, if it continues to rise at this rate, it is possible that within the next two decades over 50 per cent of women will be delivered by Caesarean section.

What is considered a high Caesarean section rate and who determines what the Caesarean section rate should be? This is an issue which is difficult to address. By implication, therefore, an unacceptably high Caesarean section rate is difficult to define. The WHO has attempted to define what an acceptable Caesarean section rate should be. The rationale for this standard is unclear. A few studies from developing countries were used to arrive at the rate of about 10–15 per cent. Although this appears to be the acceptable rate to most in the UK, countries with such rates should be evaluated within that environment rather than on a global perspective.

An important question is – why is the Caesarean section rate rising? Many reasons could be advanced for this, including obstetric, medical, social and legal factors. Neonatal survival has improved significantly so that compromised fetuses at early gestations can now be delivered safely and nurtured to survive in modern neonatal intensive care units. Therefore, a large number of Caesarean sections are performed in early pregnancy when complications such as severe fetal growth restriction and pre-eclampsia require early delivery. In addition, increasing numbers of multiple pregnancies from ever-improving assisted conception techniques increase the rate of Caesarean section.

Although the indications appear to be changing, the experience of medical staff has a significant effect on the rates of Caesarean section. The less experienced the medical staff, the higher the Caesarean section rates. Since training has been restructured to comply with the Calman (now Modernising Medical Careers) timescale and the European Union Working Time Directive, experience will continue to be eroded. Recent evidence and recommendations that all breech presentations at term should be delivered by Caesarean section is also responsible for the rising Caesarean section rates. In a society where litigation is becoming the norm, most obstetricians (junior and senior) are inclined to practise defensive obstetrics, which inevitably means more Caesarean sections. Although there are some women who admonish obstetricians for doing too many Caesarean sections, there are a larger number who elect to have Caesarean section deliveries for fear of uncertainties about vaginal delivery and the complications. It has been argued in the journals and the national press that women should be allowed to chose their method of delivery. This social pressure imposes a significant stress on obstetricians who, for fear of litigation, increasingly allow Caesarean section on demand.

Caesarean delivery is associated with prolonged hospitalisation and recovery, complications of surgery (e.g. adhesions, venous thromboembolism, etc.), most of which have cost implications for the hospital and the family. Often, the management of subsequent pregnancies may be affected. However, it may be argued that since the average family size in the UK has been falling, a scarred uterus will not significantly influence the number of children families have. However, an increasing Caesarean section rate results in the deskilling of doctors in the art of vaginal delivery, especially where there are complications such as breech presentation and deep transverse arrest. Ultimately, all abnormal labours will be resolved by Caesarean section with its accompanying morbidity and mortality.

Although there are no nationally acceptable standards for a Caesarean section rate, the National Sentinel Audit (RCOG, 2001) demonstrated that there are very wide variations in standards nationally. The rate of rise is alarming in some units. Since the factors responsible for this rise are not as dynamic as the rate, there must be intrinsic factors which may be minimised to reduce the rate of rise. This can only be done via national audits, such as the Sentinel Audit, and by re-education of patients, obstetricians and midwives.

Reference

RCOG (2001) National Sentinel Caesarean Section Audit. London: Royal College of Obstetricians and Gynaecologists.

3. You are about to perform an elective Caesarean section on a 28-year-old woman having her third baby. She requests that sterilisation be performed at the time of surgery. (a) What factors will you take into consideration during counselling? (12 marks) (b) You agree to perform the procedure. What options are available to you? (8 marks)

Common mistakes

- Discussing the merits and demerits of sterilisation in general
- Stating that counselling can only be offered if the partner is present
- Making sweeping statements such as 'Reversals will not be done on the NHS', 'Sterilisation is permanent', 'She will not be offered this procedure at this stage', 'It will be performed laparoscopically – at Caesarean section'!

A good answer will include some or all of these points

(a) What factors will you take into consideration during counselling? (12 marks)

- When was the decision to have sterilisation made? Before time of Caesarean section or at time of Caesarean section?
- Ideally should be long before Caesarean section (at least 2 weeks)
- Timing of decision – suboptimal:
  - Emotional period
  - Complications of the procedure
  - Decision may be influenced by fear of Caesarean section, lack of support
- Offer interval procedure – 3 months and effective contraception
- Offer alternative – vasectomy/Mirena® intrauterine contraceptive device
- If patient insists: counsel about failure rate
- Procedure itself – portion of tube to be removed
- High regret rate
- Increased risk of ectopic pregnancy and failure
- Low successful reversal rate

(b) You agree to perform the procedure. What options are available to you? (8 marks)

- Pomeroy's technique
- Uchida's technique
- Modified Pomeroy's technique
- Parkland's (Maryland's) technique
- Salpingectomy
- Tubal clip occlusion

Sample answer

(a) What factors will you take into consideration during counselling? (12 marks)

Sterilisation is regarded as a permanent method of contraception, although under certain circumstances it can be reversed with a good chance of success if the procedure was undertaken with clips or rings. The decision to undergo this procedure must therefore be taken very carefully, especially as about a third of women sterilised live to regret the decision.

Sterilisation during delivery is gradually being discouraged. This is because pregnancy is a very stressful time for most women and decisions could be influenced by experience during the pregnancy. In this patient, it is important to establish when the decision to undergo sterilisation was taken. If it was made just before the time of the Caesarean section, it is unlikely to have been thought through carefully. Of course, the patient might have made this decision long before the pregnancy but only informed her carers before the Caesarean section. Where the decision was made long before the Caesarean section, was documented in the notes and appropriate counselling offered, it could be performed provided all the options were discussed.

Where the decision was made only at the time of the Caesarean section, this must be questioned. However, if there is evidence that the patient is very certain about her decision, further counselling must be offered on the complications of the procedure and the difference between Caesarean section sterilisation and interval sterilisation. She should be offered the option of Depo-Provera® for 3 months after the Caesarean section and an interval laparoscopic sterilisation if she has not changed her mind at that time. Other contraceptive options, such as vasectomy and subdermal implants (Implanon® or Norplant®), should also be discussed. It should be emphasised that the failure rate following sterilisation at Caesarean section is considered to be slightly higher than that after interval procedures with clips or rings, and that reversal is less likely to be successful with such procedures.

If the patient is certain and the decision was made long before the time of Caesarean section, counselling about the risks of failure, the complications of the procedure, the regret rate and increased risk of ectopic pregnancy should be offered.

(b) You agree to perform the procedure. What options are available to you? (8 marks)

The options for Caesarean sterilisation include tubal occlusion with clips, diathermy to the Fallopian tubes, Pomeroy's technique, Uchida's technique, Parkland's or Maryland's technique, salpingectomy or the modified Pomery's technique. Tubal clipping is not advisable as the tubes have undergone the hypertrophy of pregnancy and the clips may not completely obliterate the tubal lumen. Where the decision is to undergo the procedure, a Pomeroy or modified Pomeroy will be the most common approach. Diathermy is an option that may be considered but is associated with a higher morbidity and failure rate. Salpingectomy is one option which certainly guarantees that the tubes are removed. However, it is associated with a higher morbidity, takes longer to perform and does not afford the patient any opportunity to have a reversal if she ever so desired. The Pomery's technique, even the modified version, is the most common approach. The Uchida and Parkland techniques ensure that the fimbrial ends of the tubes are not accessible to the ovaries. The most commonly performed procedure is the Pomeroy's or its modification.

4. Critically appraise the management of a woman in her second pregnancy, the first having been delivered by emergency classical Caesarean section for transverse lie. (20 marks)

Common mistakes

- No place for a vaginal delivery
- Induction
- Repeat classical if cause of transverse lie present
- No need for routine antenatal care
- Any benefit in seeing her frequently on outpatient basis?
- Monitoring lie (not really relevant)
- Not asked to expound on the problems of Caesarean section (morbidity and mortality not really relevant)
- Indications for Caesarean section not relevant

A good answer will include some or all of these points

- Main danger – uterine rupture during pregnancy and labour (silent rupture not usually preceded by labour)
- At booking – consultant unit. Discuss plan of pregnancy care
- Admission
  - When and why? 24, 28, 32 weeks, etc.
- Frequent visits to the hospital? Why?
- Outpatient care? Why?
- Delivery – when?
- 37–38 weeks – advantages and disadvantages
- Repeat Caesarean section – why, how, disadvantages and advantages. Bypasses emergency Caesarean section
- Spontaneous vaginal delivery – advantages/disadvantages
- Augmentation – not an option
- Use of oxytocic agents if vaginal delivery
- Sterilisation?

Sample answer

Since Cragin's dictum that 'Once a Caesarean, always a Caesarean', many women with a previous Caesarean section have successfully been allowed to deliver vaginally. In fact, more than 70 per cent of women with a previous lower-segment Caesarean section will have successful vaginal deliveries in subsequent pregnancies. However, the situation with a classical Caesarean section is different as the risk of uterine rupture is significantly high. This rupture may occur during pregnancy (silent rupture) or during labour. The risk of rupture in these patients is between 30 and 50 per cent. The management of this patient should therefore take into consideration this risk.

If the patient had been counselled properly after the classical Caesarean section, she would be well informed of the potential risk of rupture in this pregnancy. At booking, which must be in a consultant unit, the risks and implications should be discussed. The plan for the pregnancy should be discussed. This should include the need for admission for inpatient observation and the timing of delivery.

There is considerable debate about the need for antenatal admission. Some advocate admission from 24 weeks and others after 28 weeks. The rationale for this is the risk of silent ruptures. Those who advocate admission argue that if rupture occurs in the hospital, the chances of delivering a live baby are better than if it occurred at home. However, early admission may be stressful to the mother (who would leave her other child at home for a long time). If a rupture did occur at 24 weeks, the chances of the fetus surviving would be considerably lower. Therefore, it may not be advisable to admit at this early gestation. However, after 28 weeks rupture is more likely. Although admission may be offered to the patient, she may decline it. In this case, will she benefit from frequent hospital visits? There is no evidence to suggest that such visits will improve the detection of early rupture. It is important that she is counselled about the warning signs of rupture and made to report to hospital immediately should they occur. These include rupture of fetal membranes, abdominal pain, shoulder-tip pain or if she starts contracting or is bleeding per vaginam.

The timing of delivery in this patient is another area of controversy. When should it be? It has been suggested that this could be somewhere between 37 and 39 weeks' gestation. If there have been no complications at 37 weeks, delivery would guarantee a viable matured fetus. However, there is an increased risk of transient tachypnoea of the newborn and respiratory distress syndrome at this gestation compared to delivery at 39 weeks' gestation. However delaying up to 39 weeks may risk uterine rupture and fetal death. Although there are advantages in delivering at 37 weeks, if the decision is to deliver at the latter date, the patient ought to be in hospital.

Delivery should be by a repeat Caesarean section, preferably by the lower segment. This has the advantage of reduced morbidity, although it leaves the uterus with an inverted-T scar. This does not increase the risk of rupture in a subsequent pregnancy. However, if there are contraindications to a lower-segment Caesarean section, a repeat classical incision should be made. After two classical Caesarean sections, sterilisation should be considered in the interest of the mother. This should be discussed with the patient before surgery.

Where the patient requests a vaginal delivery, this must be discouraged. Although there are several reported cases of spontaneous vaginal delivery following classical Caesarean section, a 30–50 per cent risk of uterine rupture and the associated morbidity should discourage any woman from opting for such a delivery. Even if she went into spontaneous labour and wanted to continue, prostaglandins and oxytocic agents should be regarded as contraindicated.

5. A 30-year-old woman with placenta praevia grade III posterior is scheduled to undergo an elective Caesarean section at 39 weeks' gestation. (a) Outline the steps you will take to minimise complications. (8 marks) (b) After delivery of the baby and placenta, she continues to bleed. What will be your subsequent management? (8 marks) (c) How will you counsel her about her next pregnancy? (4 marks)

Common mistakes

- Take a history and do a physical examination
- Discussing the management of placenta praevia antenatally
- Details of the Caesarean section procedure
- Expanding the remit of the question – discussing breech presentation and placenta praevia, previous classical Caesarean section, etc.
- Depends on the parity and the wishes of the patient
- Abdominal pressure – to compress the aorta

A good answer will contain some or all of these points

(a) Outline the steps you will take to minimise complications. (8 marks)

- Group and cross-match at least 4 units of blood; have at least 2 units in theatre and some group O-negative blood
- Ensure at least two large-bore cannulae
- Senior obstetrician and anaesthetist to be present
- Notify blood bank – may require blood at very short notice
- Counsel about the risk of hysterectomy
- If available, inform interventional radiologist – prepare for potential embolisation

(b) After delivery of the baby and placenta, she continues to bleed. What will be your subsequent management? (8 marks)

- Under-running bleeding vessels – not easy but may be effective
- Intramyometrial prostaglandins
- Brace suture (Lynch brace suture)
- Internal iliac artery ligation
- Hysterectomy
- Bakri balloon
- Packing the uterine cavity

(c) How will you counsel her about her next pregnancy? (4 marks)

- Increased risk of placenta praevia

- Increased risk of Caesarean hysterectomy – from placenta accreta
- Should be screened for placenta praevia, and accreta if possible

Sample answer

(a) Outline the steps you will take to minimise complications. (8 marks)

The most important complication is haemorrhage. At least 4 units of blood should be cross-matched and at least 2 units should be available on the delivery suite, if not in theatre. Group O-negative blood should also be available on the unit in case there is a need for massive blood replacement. Prior to Caesarean section, at least two large-bore cannulae should be inserted and the blood bank informed of the surgery. Preferably a senior obstetrician (consultant) and senior anaesthetist (consultant) should be involved in the surgery. The consultant haematologist should also be available in the blood bank in case there is need for massive transfusion. The patient should be counselled about the greater risk of hysterectomy and where available, an interventional radiologist should not only be informed but prepared to provide assistance if necessary.

(b) After delivery of the baby and placenta, she continues to bleed. What will be your subsequent management? (8 marks)

The first step in stemming bleeding from the placental bed is to under-run the bleeding vessels. If this fails, then various oxytocics should be given – initially i.v. but later intramyometrially (starting with Syntocinon® as a bolus dose then ergometrine) followed by intramyometrial prostaglandin $F2_\alpha$. The next approach to stop the bleeding will be the brace suture. If this fails, then internal artery ligation maybe attempted if the expertise is available – usually by a gynaecological oncologist if one has been notified of the surgery. A hysterectomy should be considered if the above options fail and there are no facilities for interventional radiology. Other options that may be considered before resorting to a hysterectomy include packing the uterine cavity, although this tends to give a false sense of security until the pack has soaked through, or using a Bakri or any other type of balloon.

(c) How will you counsel her about her next pregnancy? (4 marks)

With regards to the next pregnancy, there is an increased risk of placenta praevia, placenta percreta and placenta accreta. The risk of Caesarean hysterectomy is much greater and so too are the complications of surgery. There may be a reduction in her chances of having a successful pregnancy because of this complication.

14

Postpartum complications

1. Evaluate the methods of controlling severe postpartum haemorrhage at Caesarean section for placenta praevia. (20 marks)

2. A woman who has just had a vaginal delivery is bleeding profusely from the vagina. (a) Outline your initial management of this patient. (13 marks) (b) Briefly discuss the complications of massive postpartum haemorrhage. (7 marks)

3. (a) Justify the investigations you will perform on a woman 6 days after delivery presenting with a pyrexia of 38.6°C. She is breastfeeding and both breasts are normal. (14 marks) (b) How will you manage her if the cause of the pyrexia is non-infective but localised in the pelvis? (6 marks)

4. The recent confidential enquiries into maternal mortality revealed that psychiatric disorders have become an important cause of maternal mortality. What steps will you take to minimise this preventable cause of maternal mortality? (20 marks)

1. Evaluate the methods of controlling severe postpartum haemorrhage at Caesarean section for placenta praevia. (20 marks)

Common mistakes

- Listing causes of postpartum haemorrhage
- Forgetting the fact that this is following Caesarean section
- Take a history and physical examination!
- Quickly examine the patient to ensure that she is haemodynamically stable
- Remove retained products of conception

A good answer will include some or all of these points

- Most likely cause of postpartum haemorrhage in this patient is bleeding from the lower segment
- This may be from large vessels or from placenta accreta or increta
- Methods of controlling the bleeding will therefore depend on the aetiology
- Bleeding from large vessels – under-run the vessels
- Uncontrollable – Hebamate® (prostaglandins) – unlikely to be effective
- Tamponade procedures – packing or balloons, e.g. Bakri balloon:
  - Packs may provide a false sense of security as they soak up bleeding which then only becomes obvious after it has soaked through
- Brace suture
- Internal iliac artery litigation
- Hysterectomy
- Uterine artery embolisation

Sample answer

Postpartum haemorrhage is a recognised complication of placenta praevia. Anticipation of this complication is essential in reducing morbidity and mortality. The most likely source of the haemorrhage in such patients is the placental bed in the lower segment. The haemorrhage may be recognised at the time of surgery or immediately after.

At the time of surgery, the haemorrhage may be from the placental bed after it has been removed. In some cases the placenta may either be an accreta or an increta, in which case partial separation will be associated with haemorrhage. The first approach to controlling the haemorrhage at this time is under-running the bleeding vessels. This is effective in some cases. The advantage is that it is done under direct vision, ensuring that the major bleeding sinuses are occluded. However, it may not be possible to under-run all the bleeding points.

Parenteral oxytocic agents (bolus doses of ergometrine or continuous infusion of Syntocinon®) may be used to cause contraction of the myometrium. This may not be effective

193

in controlling bleeding from the lower segment as the myometrial constituent is significantly lower in this region. However, with good contraction of the upper segment, it may reduce the blood flowing to the lower segment and therefore reduce the haemorrhage. The bolus doses may be repeated if they are initially not very effective. Intramyometrial prostaglandin (Hebamate®) may be used to stimulate contraction. This is unlikely to be effective with severe haemorrhage, again on the basis that there are fewer muscles in the lower segment. Tamponading techniques are beneficial if applied appropriately. Packing the uterus is useful, except that it may give a false sense of security until the bleeding has soaked through the pack. In addition, packs will require removal, usually after 24–48 hours. The Bakri balloon can be used to provide a similar tamponading effect. Its advantage is that it does not result in any concealed bleeding.

The brace suture would be considered one of the most effective means of controlling the haemorrhage at the time of surgery or even when the patient returns to the theatre. This suture is easy to apply for those who are familiar with it and does not require any expensive material. Various reports have demonstrated its efficacy in most patients. It reduces blood flow to the uterus and therefore controls the haemorrhage.

Where this cannot be applied, or has failed, other options would be internal iliac artery ligation, hysterectomy and embolisation of the uterine artery. Ligation of the internal iliac artery is not a procedure with which most obstetricians are familiar. It is effective when used properly, but because the surgeon may not be familiar with the technique it may be too time consuming. Uterine artery embolisation is a new technique that has been tried and been shown to be effective. It requires a skilled radiologist, the correct equipment, and easy access to the labour ward or radiology department. For a patient who is haemorrhaging this may be technically difficult; however, when available, it is quite effective. A hysterectomy is the last resort; however, there must be no delay in undertaking this procedure. Mortality from haemorrhage, especially that due to placenta praevia, is not uncommon because of a delay in performing a hysterectomy. This procedure is effective but requires considerable counselling afterwards.

If the haemorrhage was noticed after the patient has left the theatre, the same principles will be applicable except that she may have to go back into theatre for a more effective control of the haemorrhage.

2. A woman who has just had a vaginal delivery is bleeding profusely from the vagina. (a) Outline your initial management of this patient. (13 marks) (b) Briefly discuss the complications of massive postpartum haemorrhage. (7 marks)

Common mistakes

- Take a history and do a physical examination – there is no time to do this
- Discussing the details of all the procedures you performed
- Listing the things you do without evaluating
- Being illogical in your approach

A good answer will include some or all of these points

(a) Outline your initial management of this patient. (13 marks)

- Secure an intravenous (i.v.) line. Collect blood for urgent cross-matching and blood grouping (most important step). Explain why the most important step
- Examine uterus – contracting? Stimulate contractions – most common cause – atony, especially if prolonged labour
- Repeat oxytocic agents
- Intravenous Syntocinon®
- Is the placenta complete?
- Examine the genital tract and placenta and membranes
- Uterine hypotonia – oxytocic agents, prostaglandins – intramyometrial
- Surgery – brace suture, internal iliac ligation
- Uterine artery embolisation
- Hysterectomy
- Packing the uterus – not very effective – false sense of security
  - Balloon, e.g. Bakri
- Involvement of haematologist and anaesthetist, senior obstetrician
- Other causes – inversion, ruptured uterus, retained placenta

(b) Briefly discuss the complications of massive postpartum haemorrhage. (7 marks)

- Renal failure
- Death – maternal mortality
- Disseminated intravascular coagulation (DIC)
- Sheehan's syndrome
- Psychological sequelae – stress, depression, nightmares and fear of pregnancies
- Bonding with the baby
- Consequence of massive transfusion – hypothermia, hypocalcaemia, infections – viral

Sample answer

(a) Outline your initial management of this patient. (13 marks)

Severe postpartum haemorrhage is an obstetric emergency, which may be associated with maternal mortality. The management must therefore be aggressive and multidisciplinary, involving the haematologist (as blood may be required), an anaesthetist (examination under anaesthesia and exploration of the uterus or laparotomy may be required) and a senior obstetrician, who may be required to undertake the various surgical procedures.

One of the most important stages in the management of this patient is securing an i.v. line and also cross-matching blood. The i.v. access should be secured with a large-bore Venflon®. This will ensure that resuscitation would be possible if she collapses. It may be advisable to secure a second i.v. access, as rapid replacement of fluid may be required to avoid maternal mortality. This is probably one of the most important steps in the management of this patient.

A quick examination of the abdomen will determine whether the uterus is contracting. If it is not, rubbing it may stimulate contractions and stem the bleeding. This is a simple measure that is effective where the cause of the bleeding is hypotonia of the uterus. If, despite this, the uterus fails to contract, i.v. oxytocic agents should be given – first as a bolus dose and then as a continuous infusion. If hypotonia is the cause, this may be enough to control the haemorrhage. It is important to determine whether the placenta was complete. It may be advisable to ask for it to be re-examined. If a missing lobe or cotyledon or membranes are identified, then efforts must be made to remove them.

If, after all this, the patient continues to bleed, an examination of the genital tract should be undertaken. This will exclude trauma to the vulva, vagina and cervix as the cause of the haemorrhage. In the absence of trauma, and if bleeding continues, an examination of the uterus under anaesthesia should be undertaken. This is to ensure that there are no retained products of conception. This is not uncommon, even when the placenta is thought to have been delivered complete.

For continuing uterine hypotonia and an empty uterus, intramyometrial prostaglandins may be administered. These are effective but may be associated with significant systemic side-effects. Although packing of the uterine cavity has been advocated by some to stem the bleeding, this has the disadvantage that it conceals any blood loss and by the time it has soaked through the gauze, it may be significant. It may be a temporary option but the pack cannot be left *in situ* indefinitely. More recently, the use of balloons (e.g. Bakri) provides the tamponade effect without concealing bleeding.

Where the above steps fail to stop the haemorrhage, a laparotomy would be necessary. At this procedure, a brace stitch could be inserted. This is cheap, easy to insert and very effective. It is easier than internal artery ligation and does not compromise fertility. Internal iliac artery ligation is difficult to perform and may require a gynaecological oncologist as most obstetricians might never have performed this technique. Fertility is also preserved with this step. An alternative is an abdominal hysterectomy. This will certainly stop the haemorrhage but fertility will be affected. It should therefore only be used as the last option. The advent of uterine artery embolisation has provided an alternative to the management of massive postpartum haemorrhage. It is effective and safe but difficult to administer because of availability of radiologist and machine. These difficulties may make its availability for such an emergency difficult.

(b) Briefly discuss the complications of massive postpartum haemorrhage. (7 marks)

The complications of the haemorrhage can be immediate or late. Immediate complications include renal failure, DIC and maternal mortality. The long-term consequences include psychological problems such as depression, nightmares and fear of subsequent pregnancies. It may also affect bonding. If the haemorrhage is severe and persistent, it could result in pituitary necrosis followed by panhypopituitarism (Sheehan's syndrome). This will cause difficulties breastfeeding, amenorrhoea and the side-effects of various hormone deficiencies. The patient is at risk of the side-effects of massive transfusion and these include hypothermia, hypocalcaemia, hypokalaemia, circulatory overload and infections (although this is rare) such as new variant Creutzfeldt–Jakob disease (CJD).

3. (a) Justify the investigations you will perform on a woman 6 days after delivery presenting with a pyrexia of 38.6°C. She is breastfeeding and both breasts are normal. (14 marks) (b) How will you manage her if the cause of the pyrexia is non-infective but localised in the pelvis? (6 marks)

Common mistakes

- Take a history and do a physical examination
- Treatment – details of antibiotics
- For exploration under general anaesthesia
- Laparotomy is indicated

A good answer will include some or all of these points

(a) Justify the investigations you will perform on a woman 6 days after delivery presenting with a temperature of 38.6°C. She is breastfeeding and both breasts are normal. (14 marks)

- Diagnosis is puerperial pyrexia
- Causes – urinary tract infection (UTI), breast infection, genital tract infection, chest infection, venous thromboembolism (VTE), pyrexia of unknown origin (PUO)
- Investigations – state type and give reason(s): full blood count (FBC); sputum; chest X-ray (CXR); midstream specimen of urine (MSU); Doppler scans, blood gases, electro-cardiography (ECG), D-dimers; swabs – wound, vagina and endocervix; blood cultures

(b) How will you manage her if the cause of the pyrexia is non-infective but localised in the pelvis? (6 marks)

- Most likely cause:
  - Deep vein thrombosis (DVT).
  - Treatment:
    - Full anticoagulation with heparin or low-molecular-weight heparin
    - Warfarin treatment
    - Counselling about contraception
  - Lifestyle modifications – smoking, etc.
  - Screening for thrombophilia
  - Advice for next pregnancy
- Exclude tuberculosis (TB)

Sample answer

(a) Justify the investigations you will perform on a woman 6 days after delivery presenting with a temperature of 38.6°C. She is breastfeeding and both breasts are normal. (14 marks)

The causes of this pyrexia include urinary tract and chest infections, wound infections, genital tract infections, pelvic collections, VTE and, in some cases, PUO. The investigations for the cause of this patient's pyrexia will therefore depend on the suspected cause. A FBC will demonstrate leucocytosis in the case of bacterial infection. However, it is important to understand the normal physiological changes occurring in the blood after delivery. There is often a degree of leucocytosis and this must not be confused with that secondary to infection. An MSU for urinalysis and also for microscopy, culture and sensitivity is mandatory. One of the most common causes of puerperal pyrexia is UTI. Urinalysis may indicate the presence of leucocytes, nitrites, proteins or blood, all of which may be suggestive of UTIs.

Other investigations will depend on the suspected cause of the pyrexia. Where an intrauterine infection (endometritis) is suspected, a high vaginal and endocervical swabs for microscopy culture and sensitivity will be most appropriate. However, it is not uncommon to fail to isolate the organism responsible for the endometritis from these swabs. An ultrasound scan may reveal the presence of retained products of conception. However, the presence of retained products will not necessarily imply endometritis as the cause. It is not unusual after delivery to have blood clots within the uterus and ultrasound scan will invariably report these as retained products.

If the patient has chest symptoms, such as cough, or positive signs on clinical examination, sputum for culture and sensitivity and a CXR would be applicable. In some cases, there may be no obvious signs but TB must always be suspected, especially with the recent rising trends in pulmonary TB in the UK. Therefore, in this case, a Mantoux test may be appropriate. Where TB is a possibility, any sputum should be sent for acid-fast bacillus examination. A bronchopulmonary lavage for *Mycobacterium tuberculosis* polymerase chain reaction is the most reliable investigation to diagnose pulmonary TB. If there is a suspicion of a DVT or VTE, investigations such as a venogram of the legs, Doppler scan of the leg vessels and an ECG would be essential. A ventilation–perfusion scan will be necessary if there is suspicion of pulmonary embolism. The level of D-dimers in the maternal blood in the cases of VTE will be raised but this is non-specific.

The patient's temperature is above 38°C; therefore a blood culture is necessary if the cause of the pyrexia is not yet identifiable. This must be for Gram-positive and Gram-negative organisms (i.e. two cultures should be set up). Where the cause of the pyrexia is indeterminable, screening for TB must be undertaken. This will be additional to the investigations outlined above and consist of early morning urine for microscopy culture and sensitivity. Although the breasts may appear normal, they must be examined carefully again and, if there are any features of mastitis, this must be treated accordingly. Other additional investigations will include wound swabs for suspected wound infections, especially following operative deliveries and pelvic ultrasound for localisation of abscesses. This latter investigation will be very relevant if the patient has been suffering from a swinging pyrexia.

(b) How will you manage her if the cause of the pyrexia is non-infective but localised in the pelvis? (6 marks)

If the investigations have excluded a non-infective cause of the pyrexia, then the most likely cause will be pelvic DVT. The diagnosis is difficult and a high index of suspicion will be required. The treatment will consist of full anticoagulation with heparin or low-molecular-weight heparin for a minimum of 4–5 days followed by warfarin for at least 3–4 weeks. This may be continued for up to 3 months. There is no contraindication to breastfeeding on warfarin. Her contraceptive requirements will have to be reviewed, especially if she is not breastfeeding, as the combined oral contraceptive pill will be contraindicated. Appropriate counselling must also be provided with regards to further pregnancies. It may be valuable considering a thrombophilia screen at a much later date. If she is a smoker, it would be advisable for her to stop as this significantly increases the risk of VTE. Additional lifestyle advice, such as modification of excessive alcohol consumption, will be offered.

4. The recent confidential enquiries into maternal mortality revealed that psychiatric disorders have become an important cause of maternal mortality. What steps will you take to minimise this preventable cause of maternal mortality? (20 marks)

Common mistakes

- Listing all the types of psychiatric disorders in pregnancy
- Treatment of psychiatric illnesses
- Being too vague in your answer
- Deliver electively at 38–39 weeks' gestation

A good answer will include some or all of these points

- High-risk group
- Previous puerperal psychiatric disorders
- Known psychiatric illness
- Problem pregnancy
- Domestic violence
- Antenatal measures: education; plan care with psychiatrist; joint care – obstetrician, midwife, general practitioner (GP) and psychiatrist
- Postnatal: treatment of disorder – sooner rather than later; support at home; warning signs; GP; mother and baby units

Sample answer

Psychiatric illness was one of the most common cause of indirect maternal mortality over the last triennium. Most of the mortalities occurred postpartum and after 6 weeks. A large number of them were suicides. An important factor thought to be responsible for this was failure to recognise this problem and deal with it properly. The best approach to reducing this cause of maternal mortality starts with recognition of the high-risk group, and planning care both in the hospital and in the community during pregnancy and after.

Those at risk include women with known psychiatric illness as well as those with previous postnatal psychiatric diseases, such as depression. Women with known psychiatric disorders are also at an increased risk of psychiatric problems, especially after delivery. Other factors that may increase the risk of psychiatric illness include complicated pregnancies, women suffering from domestic violence, poor socioeconomic class, ethnic minorities, those with very little knowledge of English, asylum seekers and single unsupported parents.

Antenatally, appropriate measures should be taken in the management of these high-risk women. Such measures should be taken by a combined effort from psychiatric nurses, GPs and social workers, where applicable. Such education will concentrate on the positive aspects of pregnancy and providing information about how to recognise early signs of postnatal psychiatric diseases.

After delivery, early treatment of the disorders should be instituted. Where this is identified, early involvement of a psychiatrist and community nurses is vital. Admission into dedicated mother and baby units should be offered early. Support should be offered at home and, again, early warning signs should be recognised and treated. It is better to institute treatment early rather than to delay it until severe depression sets in. Where there is poor support at home, this should be provided. It is important to recognise the fact that these illnesses may occur for the first time after the first 6 weeks of delivery and that suicides occur commonly within this time. Surveillance of at-risk women should be continued for at least 1 year after delivery.

Institution of treatment should not be delayed, even if the woman is breastfeeding. There are very few contraindications to breastfeeding and, even if the drug she would benefit from is contraindicated, it is preferable to switch the baby from the breast to the bottle in order to treat the disorder. A positive attitude towards the mother and other members of the family is vital. For those with a history of domestic violence, social workers should be involved.

15

Anaesthetic disorders in pregnancy

1. Mendelson's syndrome is a recognised cause of maternal mortality and morbidity. What steps are normally taken to minimise this complication in pregnancy/labour? (20 marks)

2. Approximately one-third of women delivering in the UK have epidural analgesia in labour. (a) Briefly discuss the complications of epidural analgesia. (10 marks) (b) How may these complications be avoided? (10 marks)

3. Briefly outline the advantages and disadvantages of epidural and general anaesthesia (GA) in labour. (20 marks)

4. In the last confidential enquiries into maternal death, all anaesthetic deaths were related to GA. (a) How may the risk of this complication be minimised antenatally? (8 marks) (b) What appropriate steps must be taken during labour to minimise maternal mortality from GA? (12 marks)

1. Mendelson's syndrome is a recognised cause of maternal mortality and morbidity. What steps are normally taken to minimise this complication in pregnancy/labour? (20 marks)

Common mistakes

- Should be managed only by anaesthetist
- Discussing the management of Mendelson's syndrome
- Process of induction – unnecessary details (drugs, etc.)
- Minimising Caesarean section rates
- No need to define Mendelson's syndrome

A good answer will include some or all of these points

- Definition of condition
- Increased risk in pregnancy – why?
- Measures to minimise complications: diet; antacids; empty stomach: epidural/regional preferred to GA; cricoid pressure; cuffed endotracheal tubes; extubation in lateral position
- Early recognition and treatment

Sample answer

The measures that may be taken to minimise this complication range from preventative to early diagnosis and treatment. Preventative measures must guard against vomiting and aspiration. This complication most commonly occurs at the time of induction of GA. Avoiding or reducing the rate of GA in obstetric units will significantly reduce the risk of this complication. Although it may occur during the administration of regional anaesthesia, the risks are not as high as during GA. Where an operative delivery is planned, as in the case of elective Caesarean section, or anticipated, an empty stomach is essential. However, although this may be practicable for elective cases, it is not feasible in patients during induction of labour. During this process, a light diet should be provided as it is easier for this to be absorbed. Overnight fasting ensures that the stomach is empty before surgery.

    The use of antacids has become universal in labour and before surgery. During labour, every patient should be given an antacid such as sodium citrate. This neutralises the acid in the stomach and reduces the risk of chemical pneumonitis should the patient vomit and aspirate. For those undergoing surgery, this is administered in the form of an H_2-antagonist (Zantac®) overnight and on the morning of surgery. For emergency Caesarean sections, sodium citrate should be given before induction of GA. A combination of this and an antiemetic, such as metoclopramide, will significantly reduce the risk of vomiting and therefore aspiration. In some cases of emergency Caesarean section, intravenous (i.v.) H_2-antagonists may be administered.

An important procedure to minimise the risk of aspiration is the application of cricoid pressure during intubation. This helps prevent vomiting and aspiration. A cuffed endotracheal tube prevents aspiration even if the patient vomits. A suction machine, readily available, will ensure that all vomit is sucked out of the patient's mouth and throat. Vomiting and aspiration can occur during extubation. Therefore, this should be performed preferably with the patient in the lateral position and head down with readiness to suck if there is any vomiting.

Once this complication has occurred, early recognition and prompt treatment will minimise the consequences. Recognising that this complication can occur in normal labouring women is vital. Early symptoms include tachypnoea, cyanosis and rhonchi in the chest. Treatment must include steroids, antibiotics and, if necessary, ventilation. A combination of these measures will reduce the risk of this complication and minimise the consequences when it occurs.

2. Approximately one-third of women delivering in the UK have epidural analgesia in labour. (a) Briefly discuss the complications of epidural analgesia. (10 marks) (b) How may these complications be avoided? (10 marks)

Common mistakes

- Discussing the indications for epidural anaesthesia
- Details of how epidurals are performed
- Counselling patients about complications
- Ensure that appropriate instruments are available

(a) Briefly discuss the complications of epidural analgesia. (10 marks)

- Complications include:
  - Spinal tap
  - Pyrexia
  - Weakness of the legs
  - Unblocked segments
  - Failed epidural
  - Postpartum pain
  - Urinary retention
  - Intrathecal injection of drugs
  - Hypotension with associated fetal bradycardia

(b) How may these complications be avoided? (10 marks)

- Appropriate training and supervision
- Provision of obstetric anaesthetic services – consultant based
- Appropriate patient selection
- Structured services with inclusion of antenatal assessment clinics
- Documentation of management pathways
- Early recognition and treatment
- Counselling prior to the siting of epidurals
- Postnatal follow-up

Sample answer

(a) Briefly discuss the complications of epidural analgesia. (10 marks)

These complications include weakness of the legs, unblocked segments, postpartum pain, retention of urine, hypotension, dural tap and intrathecal injection of local anaesthetic agents.

Fortunately, most of these are uncommon. An unblocked segment is said to occur in about 10–15 per cent of patients. This is easily recognised by persistent pain with each contraction. This pain tends to be located especially in the groin region. It can be ameliorated by changing the position of the patient and increasing the level of the block or the concentration of the anaesthetic agent. Occasionally, the epidural may have to be resited.

Some weakness of the legs is expected with most epidurals. However, where there is muscle paralysis the leg may become very weak. When the patient complains of this, it can be treated by administering a weaker concentration of the local anaesthetic agent. Postpartum pain is often described as excruciating pain in the perineum and especially at the episiotomy site. This may only be treated with local or mild systemic analgesic agents. Urinary retention may occur during labour or afterwards. Often, this is because the loss of sensation during the epidural causes distension of the bladder and subsequent loss of the sensation to void. If this is pro- longed, the patient may suffer from urinary retention after the epidural has worn off. It should be treated with catheterisation and in some cases the catheter should remain *in situ* for at least 24 hours.

Hypotension is a common complication of epidural anaesthesia. This may cause fetal hypoxia and bradycardia associated with decelerations. This is due to reduced venous return to the heart. An epidural anaesthetic blocks the sympathetic and sensory nerves to the lower limbs, and causes vasodilatation and pooling of blood in the lower limbs. This is recognised by a drop in maternal blood pressure and fetal bradycardia.

Another uncommon but potentially fatal complication is intrathecal injection of the local anaesthetic. The greatest risk of this complication is that of complete spinal paralysis with complete apnoea or signs of respiratory insufficiency.

A more common complication is an accidental dural tap/puncture. This occurs in about 1–2 per cent of all cases. It is recognised from the passage of cerebrospinal fluid through the needle, which is larger than spinal needles. The patient may complain of headache.

(b) How may these be avoided? (10 marks)

One of the most effective approaches to minimising the complications of epidural analgesia is appropriate training and supervision of junior staff. It is generally recommended that all obstetric units are staffed by experienced anaesthetists to minimise these complications. Where cover at consultant level is not possible, appropriate supervision of junior anaesthetists is essential. Provision of anaesthetic antenatal services where women who could pose potential challenges during the siting of epidurals or administration of GA, and therefore increased risk of complications (e.g. obese, spina bifida), can be seen and assessed will ensure that care path- ways are documented in notes and that such high-risk groups are covered by consultants, especially obstetric anaesthetic consultants. Where such services are unavailable, considera- tion must be given to referral to tertiary centres.

As for specific complications, preventative measures should be taken as appropriate. For example, preload is often advised to prevent hypotension. When it occurs, the mother should be placed on her left side and i.v. fluid administered. Very rarely, vasopressors may be used.

For most of the other complications, early recognition and urgent intervention is often required to prevent mortality. For example, in cases of intrathecal injection and associated apnoea, quick intubation and ventilation is vital. A clinician experienced in resuscitation should therefore be available when an epidural is being sited. Treatment is either by means of a blood patch or infusing a Ringer's lactate solution into the epidural space with the patient confined to bed for 3–4 days.

Epidural analgesia is recognised to be associated with backache in the long term. This is unlikely to be recognised at the time of siting the epidural and these patients may benefit from physiotherapy and analgesics.

3. Briefly outline the advantages and disadvantages of epidural and GA in labour. (20 marks)

Common mistakes

- Listing the contraindications for either epidural or GA
- Describing in details how to site an epidural anaesthetic
- Details of other methods of pain relief in labour
- Differences between spinal and epidural anaesthesia
- Details of the mobile epidural
- Failing to outline the advantages and disadvantages of both forms of anaesthesia

A good answer will include some or all of these points

- GA:
  - Advantages:
    - Quick to administer; patient relaxed and asleep; surgeon and staff less tense
  - Disadvantages:
    - During induction, blood pressure rises and increases the risk of cardiovascular accident (CVA); recovery risk of aspiration; risk of chest infections; recovery from anaesthesia longer; requires pain relief postoperatively; can only be offered during operative delivery
- Epidural:
  - Advantages:
    - Patient awake; partner available during delivery; risk of aspiration reduced; post-operative recovery shorter; used for analgesia for the immediate postoperative period; used for pain relief during labour
  - Disadvantages:
    - Backache; dural tap; no guarantee that it will work; prolongs first and second stage and therefore increases operative deliveries; where rapid intervention is required, may not be suitable; where there is massive haemorrhage, patient and partner anxiety may affect staff

Sample answer

Epidural analgesia and anaesthesia are increasingly becoming the most potent forms of pain relief in labour, and of anaesthesia for operative deliveries. With the evolution of obstetric anaesthesia as a discipline, most good units in the UK have epidural rates of over 30 per cent. The increasing use of this form of pain relief is mainly due to the advantages it confers over other forms of pain relief, but there are also several disadvantages.

The main advantages of epidural compared to GA include the lesser risk of aspiration, quicker mobility after surgery (and therefore a lower risk of venous thromboembolism), faster postoperative recovery (with some patients eating soon after surgery), continuous use of the epidural anaesthetic for postoperative pain relief, the opportunity for the partner or family member to be present at the time of delivery and, for the patient herself, an opportunity to cherish the very moment of delivery. These are advantages compared to GA for operative deliveries. For pain relief in labour, epidural anaesthetics offer prolonged and effective pain relief, and easy conversion to potent anaesthesia for surgery if necessary. In hypertensive patients, epidural anaesthesia lowers the blood pressure and therefore reduces the risk of CVAs and fits.

Disadvantages include the potential for a dural tap, which may be complicated by headaches, prolonged backache and infection in the spine. Occasionally, it may inadvertently become a spinal block, which may be total, requiring immediate ventilation of the patient. Other disadvantages include the potential psychological distress complications of surgery may cause the patient and her partner or relative, and the pressure that their presence or awareness of these complications may put on staff. When used for pain relief, epidural anaesthesia may cause a delay in the first and second stages of labour and be associated with an increase in the rate of assisted vaginal deliveries.

On the other hand, GA has advantages such as rapid administration whenever there is the need to act quickly, better relaxation and the potential to paralyse the patient, and absence of the external pressure on staff from the patient or her partner. However, GA is associated with the following disadvantages: a rapid rise in blood pressure during induction (which may precipitate a stroke in a hypertensive patient); increased risk of aspiration (Mendelson's syndrome) during induction and waking up from anaesthesia; increased risk of chest infections; the need for additional pain relief during recovery from surgery; and slower postoperative recovery. The risk of VTE is higher because of the slower recovery. It cannot be used for pain relief during labour and requires a more experienced anaesthetist to administer.

4. In the last confidential enquiries into maternal death, all anaesthetic deaths were related to GA. (a) How may the risk of this complication be minimised antenatally? (8 marks) (b) What appropriate steps must be taken during labour to minimise maternal mortality from GA? (12 marks)

Common mistakes

- Discussing all the causes of maternal mortality
- Details of how to administer epidurals
- Discussing the complications of epidurals
- Management of dural tap
- History and examination
- Maternal haemorrhage and management

A good answer will include some or all of these points

(a) How may the risk of this complication be minimised antenatally? (8 marks)

- Ensuring standard obstetric anaesthetic cover is available – reducing isolation of units from anaesthetic back-up and other specialties, especially critical care units (which were judged to be isolated and did not have back-up anaesthetic and critical care services)
- Early consultant involvement essential – should be sought and be appropriate and prompt (in most of the cases, early involvement was not the case and even when involved, it was not prompt).
- Avoid the administration of GA by junior staff (especially senior house officer with no experience in obstetric anaesthesia – deaths due to misplacement of the endotracheal tube)
- Appropriate checking of machines to ensure that they are functioning well and gases are flowing from the correct tubes (in some cases gases were flowing through the wrong tubes) – prechecking by skilled staff (operating department practitioners (ODPs) and anaesthetists)
- Checking of drugs to ensure that they are ready and appropriate
- Need for competency testing for all new anaesthetists
- Capnographs must be available for intubation
- Regular updates on advanced life support for all anaesthetic staff
- Selection of at-risk patients
- Obese – late pregnancy increases the risk of hiatus hernia which also increases the chances of regurgitation, difficulty with tracheal intubation

(b) What appropriate steps must be taken during labour to minimise maternal mortality from GA? (12 marks)

- Multidisciplinary co-operation
- Appreciation of the severity of the illness

- Perioperative care
- Management of haemorrhage
- In young fit women the severity of haemorrhage may not be recognised until the cardiovascular system decompensates suddenly
- Tachycardia will usually indicate hypovolaemia and blood pressure may not fall until the circulating blood volume is very low. However, some patients may not exhibit the normal tachycardic response to haemorrhage, such as women with pregnancy-induced hypertension treated with beta-adrenergic blockers
- Care of women who suffer a major haemorrhage or are at high risk of major haemorrhage must involve consultant obstetric anaesthetists at the earliest possible time
- Help from several anaesthetists may be required for optimal management of massive blood loss
- Blood and a device to rapidly infuse warmed blood must be immediately available in all cases at high risk of major haemorrhage
- Blood is regularly removed from blood bank refrigerators by blood transfusion technicians and therefore a check that the blood is actually available is essential
- Isolated maternity units distant from blood transfusion services and the intensive care unit present a particular risk when major haemorrhage occurs
- Central venous and direct arterial pressure monitoring should be used when the cardiovascular system is compromised by haemorrhage or disease
- When difficulty is encountered, ultrasound guidance for the insertion of a central venous catheter is recommended
- Surgical compression with packs and aortic compression may allow time to restore the circulating volume while waiting for more senior surgical and anaesthetic help
- The anaesthetist may need to request this from the obstetrician. The anaesthetist should be aware that surgical manoeuvres that may be considered include the B-Lynch suture, uterine or internal iliac artery ligation, or hysterectomy
- The placement of bilateral iliac artery balloon catheters under portable image intensifier control may also help to control haemorrhage in an emergency. Arterial embolisation is also an option but may be more difficult to deliver where haemorrhage has occurred without warning or if the woman's condition does not permit safe transfer to the radiology department
- Postoperative care frequently needs to be provided in an intensive care or high dependency unit
- Stabilisation of cardiovascular parameters prior to transfer is necessary and improvement of a metabolic acidosis can be a helpful indication of success. Hands-on help from an intensivist, such as providing appropriate inotropic support, in theatre before transferring the patient may be life saving
- A plan of management for women at high risk of placenta accreta, such as those with an anterior placenta praevia after a previous Caesarean section, should be evident
- These women require particular preparation, as they are at very high risk of major haemorrhage. The placement of bilateral iliac artery balloon catheters immediately prior to Caesarean section should be considered in high-risk elective cases
- The use of a 'cell saver' is something that could be considered for a woman having a Caesarean section who declines homologous blood transfusion on religious grounds

(a) How may the risk of this complication be minimised antenatally? (8 marks)

Maternal mortality from GA can be minimised in several stages. The first of this is ensuring that there is support for the provision of standard obstetric anaesthetic service. Units should not be isolated from anaesthetic back-up and other specialties such as critical care units.

During the antenatal period, attempts should be made to select the patients at risk who should then be seen and assessed by consultant anaesthetists. These may well require additional plans for pain relief or Caesarean section. Care pathways should be documented in the notes of these patients and arrangements made for supportive facilities, e.g. bed for a very obese woman.

Efforts should be made to improve on the general health of the women by counselling them on adverse lifestyle factors such as smoking and drugs. Those with medical disorders that are likely to increase morbidity and mortality should be referred to the appropriate specialists for support and advice on management in labour.

With regard to machines, these must be checked regularly to ensure that they function well and that the gases are flowing from the correct tubes. In some of the cases where mortality was reported, gases were flowing through the wrong tubes. Prechecking by skilled staff such an ODP and anaesthetists will minimise this risk. Adequate staffing and training must be maintained for each unit with suitable level supervision and support when necessary.

(b) What appropriate steps must be taken during labour to minimise maternal mortality from GA? (12 marks)

The causes of anaesthetic deaths included misplaced endotracheal tubes, isolated sites (with delay in obtaining help), aspiration of gastric contents and anaphylaxis. Some of these causes were combined with morbid obesity, poorly functioning machines and delay in obtaining help in isolated sites. Common themes amongst these causes include lack of multidisciplinary cooperation, lack of appreciation of the severity of the illness, lack of perioperative care and poor management of haemorrhage.

To minimise these causes, every effort should be made to reduce the number of GAs in obstetric patients. This can be done by ensuring that those at risk of failed epidurals are seen prenatally and their epidurals are sited by consultants. In addition, these women (especially those who are morbidly obese) should be given antacids during labour and prior to induction to minimise the risk of aspiration.

Regular checking of machines to ensure that they function appropriately will reduce the risk of hypoxia secondary to failed flow of oxygen. Checklists for equipment should be introduced and such a list must be completed before a machine is used. In addition, no trainee should induce GA without a capnograph. Junior staff should avoid administering GA (especially the most junior trainees in obstetric anaesthesia). This will reduces the risk of death from misplaced endotracheal tubes.

Drugs to be used should also be checked by the anaesthetists and the ODPs, ensuring that they are available and also appropriate. All new anaesthetic machines should be competency tested while capnographs must be available for intubation. Finally, with regards to the selection of patients, those most likely to have difficult procedures should be referred to the consultant. These will include obese women, and those with hiatus hernia and various other medical disorders.

Where units are isolated, high-risk patients such as the morbidly obese should be referred to tertiary centres or adequate back-up should be available. There must be no delay in seeking this help. Every unit should have the right equipment, including drugs, for the resuscitation of cardiac arrest and all trainees should be familiar with the principles of advanced life support.

Multidisciplinary team work (consisting of an anaesthetist, an ODP and an obstetrician) will ensure that a well co-ordinated approach is adopted in case of an emergency.

Finally, there must be regular fire drills on recognition and management of potentially fatal complications such as massive haemorrhage and sepsis, especially in the young woman.

Consultant involvement is essential and should be sought early and be appropriate and prompt. In most cases of mortality, this was not the case and even when consultant involvement was sought, this was not prompt.

Further reading

CEMACH (2007) *Saving Mothers' Lives – Reviewing Maternal Deaths to Make Motherhood Safer, 2003–2005.* London: Confidential Enquiry into Maternal and Child Health. Available from: http://www.cemach.org.uk/getattachment/927cf18a-735a-47a0-9200-cdea103781c7/Saving-Mothers—Lives-2003-2005_full.aspx

Clyburn PA (2004) Early thoughts on 'Why Mothers Die 2000–2002'. *Anaesthesia* 12: 1157.

Cooper GM, McClure JH (2005) Maternal deaths from anaesthesia. An extract from *Why Mothers Die 2000–2002*, the Confidential Enquiries into Maternal Deaths in the United Kingdom. *Br J Anaesth* **94**: 417–23.

Ngan Kee WD (2005) *Confidential Enquiries into Maternal Deaths*: 50 years of closing the loop. *Br J Anaesth* **94**: 413–16.

Weindling AM (2003) The confidential enquiry into maternal and child health (CEMACH). *Arch Dis Child* **88**: 1034–7.

16

Neonatology

1. A diabetic mother attends for a discussion in preparation for pregnancy. (a) What complications may her baby suffer from in the neonatal period? (10 marks) (b) How will you minimise these complications? (10 marks)

2. Critically appraise your management of a neonate with hypothermia on the postnatal ward. (20 marks)

3. A newborn baby has been noticed to be jaundiced. (a) Briefly discuss the causes of this baby's jaundice. (5 marks) (b) Justify the investigations you will undertake on the baby. (10 marks) (c) What factors will influence the treatment of the baby? (5 marks)

4. A mother complains that her baby has refused feeds on the first day after delivery. (a) Outline your management of the baby, including how you will counsel the mother. (16 marks) (b) What complications may the baby suffer from? (4 marks)

1. A diabetic mother attends for a discussion in preparation for pregnancy. (a) What complications may her baby suffer from in the neonatal period? (10 marks) (b) How will you minimise these complications? (10 marks)

Common mistakes

- Discussing antenatal complications
- Intrapartum complications
- Congenital malformations
- Risks of maternal infections and polyhydramnios

A good answer will include some or all of these points

(a) What complications may her baby suffer from in the neonatal period? (10 marks)

- Most are related to macrosomia and intrauterine hyperglycaemia
- Difficulties with siting Venflon®
- Metabolic – hypoglycaemia
- Respiratory – respiratory distress syndrome (RDS), especially if preterm
- Haematological – polycythemia, neonatal jaundice, hyperviscosity, thrombosis
- Thermoregulation – hypothermia
- Others – biochemical (hypocalcaemia, hypomagnesaemia – tetany)

(b) How will you minimise these complications? (10 marks)

- Good control before embarking on the pregnancy (Glycosylated haemoglobin (HbA1c) <7 per cent)
- Multidisciplinary care – obstetrician, physician, midwife, dietitian – to ensure tight control during pregnancy and prompt identification and treatment of complications
- Monitoring of fetal growth and pregnancy – for early signs of pre-eclampsia, polyhydramnios, etc.
- Intrapartum care – well supervised to minimise complications and time interventions
- Decision to deliver must be informed by clinical reasons rather than social (not all should be induced at 38 weeks)
- Vaginal delivery better than Caesarean section
- Postnatal – monitor blood glucose, metabolic status

Sample answer

(a) What complications may her baby suffer from in the neonatal period? (10 marks)

The complications include biochemical, respiratory, metabolic and haematological problems and those of macrosomia. Where there has been birth trauma, the effects may extend into the neonatal period.

The most common biochemical complications are hypoglycaemia and RDS. Hypoglycaemia is seen in babies whose mother had poor diabetic control during pregnancy. In these babies, insulin levels are high as a result of the hyperglycaemia *in utero*. When the source of glucose is removed with separation from the mother, the high insulin levels continue to convert glucose in the neonate to glycogen, with a resultant hypoglycaemia. Early feeding reduces this complication. The hypoglycaemic baby may become jittery, hypothermic and will feed poorly.

Biochemical complications that may occur in the neonate from a diabetic mother include hypomagnesaemia and hypocalcaemia, both of which may manifest as tetany. Temperature control may be a problem. Although macrosomic, the proportion of brown fat in the baby is small. Since babies do not undergo shivering thermogenesis, and depend entirely on brown fat for heat generation, they are more likely to suffer from hypothermia.

Respiratory distress syndrome is associated with a diminished production of phospholipids. Their production is inhibited by high glucose levels. This complication is more common with poorly controlled diabetes mellitus. The baby of a diabetic mother is said to be a few weeks less mature than one from a non-diabetic mother. Consequently, RDS is more common in diabetic babies delivered after 38 weeks' gestation.

Haematological complications which may occur in the neonates are related to polycythaemia. These include neonatal jaundice, increased blood viscosity and thrombosis, especially of the superior sagittal sinus.

(b) How will you minimise these complications? (10 marks)

These complications can be minimised by ensuring a better control of the mother's diabetes, preferably before pregnancy (ideally pregnancy should be avoided until the glycosylated haemoglobin (Hb) is <7.0 per cent) and involving an experienced multidisciplinary team of physician, obstetric physician, diabetic midwives/nurses) in her antenatal care. During pregnancy, her diabetes should be well supervised and episodes of hypoglycaemia and hyperglycaemia minimised. Whenever complications arise, they should be identified early and prompt intervention instituted. Since fetal macrosomia, growth restriction and polyhydramnios are complications that reflect poor control, regular ultrasound scans should be offered, including a detailed scan at 20 weeks and a fetal echo at 24 weeks' gestation.

The timing of delivery should be when maximum benefit has been derived from intrauterine existence. Where delivery is to be effected before 36 weeks' gestation, betamethasone should be given to accelerate pulmonary maturity. Where appropriate, a vaginal delivery is preferred. Since shoulder dystocia is more common, skilled manpower should be available for delivery. Regular fire drills will ensure that this expertise is regularly updated.

Immediately after delivery, the baby's blood sugars should be checked and early feeding introduced. Temperature control should be tight and well monitored. A period of observation is essential to reduce the risk of late identification of any complications. Finally, educating the parents on these complications will ensure early presentation.

2. Critically appraise your management of a neonate with hypothermia on the post-natal ward. (20 marks)

Common mistakes

- Refer to neonatologist
- Take a history and do a physical examination
- Describe the method of keeping the labour ward/delivery suite warm
- Education of staff on how to manage hypothermia
- Early recognition

A good answer will include some or all of these points

- Identify the at-risk fetus:
  - At-risk fetus: preterm; intrauterine fetal growth restriction (FGR); baby of diabetic mother
- Prevention: kangaroo approach; thermoneutral environment; early feeding; wrapping with warm clothes
- Treatment: provide warmth; transfer to neonatal unit; feed early; monitor closely

Sample answer

Neonatal temperature control is mainly by means of energy generation from brown fat. This is located over the scapula and the axilla. Since the production of heat from this fat is dependent on oxygen consumption, it is the fetal metabolic rate that determines temperature control in the neonatal period. It is therefore advisable to nurse the neonate in a thermoneutral environment where the amount of energy required to maintain body temperature is minimal and therefore oxygen consumption and, by implication, metabolic rate are low.

Hypothermia is likely to occur in situations where there is inadequate brown fat to generate heat (as in fetal growth-restricted (FGR) fetuses, fetuses of diabetic mothers and premature babies). The management of hypothermia must start with the identification of the babies at risk. These are those from the high-risk groups defined above. At the time of delivery, these babies need to be wrapped in warm clothing to minimise their surface area heat loss. This is especially important in the preterm neonate as the ratio of body weight to surface area is disproportionate in favour of more heat loss.

Neonates at risk of hypothermia should be nursed in an environment where the temperature is more than room temperature. The thermoneutral environment is ideal for nursing. An open ward is not ideal for neonates. Therefore, for preterm babies, nursing in an incubator is ideal. However, the FGR neonate who does not require incubator nursing should be nursed in a warm environment and early feeding initiated. Unfortunately, some of them have difficulties feeding and may have to be tube fed.

The disadvantage of wrapping neonates warmly is the danger of overheating, especially of preterm and FGR neonates. If the temperature is too high, and the baby is unable to control it properly, it could have a febrile convulsion. Although incubators are readily available in developing countries, in some parts of the world they are uncommon. Adopting the kangaroo approach (body-to-body contact) between the mother and baby may provide an ideal thermoneutral environment to maintain body heat. It is cheap and effective. However, there is an increased risk of infection, especially in preterm babies.

3. A newborn baby has been noticed to be jaundiced. (a) Briefly discuss the causes of this baby's jaundice. (5 marks) (b) Justify the investigations you will undertake on the baby. (10 marks) (c) What factors will influence the treatment of the baby? (5 marks)

Common mistakes

- Treatment of neonatal jaundice
- Complications of neonatal jaundice
- Take a history and do a physical examination
- Do a cholangiography
- Screen for chromosomal abnormalities

A good answer will include some or all of these points

(a) Briefly discuss the causes of this baby's jaundice. (5 marks)

- Physiological
- Infections
- Haemolytic:
    - Glucose-6-phosphate dehydrogenase deficiency
    - Rhesus incompatibility
    - ABO incompatibility
    - Congenital spherocytosis
- Hypothyroidism
- Breastfeeding
- Obstruction:
    - Biliary atresia
    - Cholelodochal cyst
    - Other congenital malformations

(b) Justify the investigations you will undertake on the baby. (10 marks)

- Haemotological investigations – full blood count (FBC), blood groups, Coombs' test, G6PD status
- Biochemical – urea and electrolytes (U&Es), liver function tests (LFTs)
- Immunological
- Radiological – ultrasound
- Infection screen – midstream urine, swabs from umbilicus, throat, eyes
- Metabolic – thyroid function test

(c) What factors will influence the treatment of the baby? (5 marks)

- Gestational age at delivery
- The cause of the jaundice
- The levels of the total and unconjugated bilirubin
- Birth weight of the baby
- Facilities available for treatment

Sample answer

(a) Briefly discuss the causes of this baby's jaundice. (5 marks)

Jaundice is a common manifestation in the neonatal period. It is often physiological, although in some cases it is secondary to pathology. The causes of neonatal jaundice include prematurity, physiological jaundice, obstruction of the biliary system, infections (e.g. hepatic or generalised septicaemia), ABO incompatibility, Rhesus isoimmunisation, haemolysis (e.g. in cases of G6PD deficiency or hereditary spherocytosis) and congenital malformations such as choledochal cysts and biliary atresia. Other causes include hypothyroidism and breastfeeding. Identification of the cause will depend on the history, findings on physical examination and, more importantly, the results of various investigations. In some cases the cause is unknown.

(b) Justify the investigations you will undertake on the baby. (10 marks)

Investigations include a FBC for Hb and differential count. In severe haemolysis, the Hb drops, whereas in infections the white cell count rises and the differential count may indicate whether it is a viral or bacterial infection. Reticulocytosis will indicate how the fetus is responding to haemolysis or anaemia. Blood for culture will identify an infective organism in cases of suspected septicaemia. A LFT will estimate the total and unconjugated bilirubin, the liver enzymes and serum albumin. The level of bilirubin often determines the type of treatment to be offered, whereas raised transaminases, for example, will suggest some hepatocellular damage.

The baby's blood group, Rhesus typing, presence of atypical antibodies and its G6PD status are important and must be determined. Associated with this investigation is a Coombs' test. This allows for the identification of antibodies that are responsible for the haemolysis in Rhesus isoimmunisation. A thyroid function test will exclude hypothyroidism. It is essential to check U&Es as part of an infection screen. Infection screening must focus not only on the obvious bacterial infections but also on atypical organisms, including viruses. Blood must be collected for hepatitis, cytomegalovirus and rubella screening. Urinalysis for the presence of proteins, nitrites, blood and culture will exclude infections. Very rarely, a liver biopsy should be performed to rule out obstruction. However, ultrasound of the liver and gallbladder will identify obstruction.

(c) What factors will influence the treatment of the baby? (5 marks)

The factors that will influence treatment include the level of bilirubin, especially the unconjugated component. Other factors will include the cause of the jaundice, the gestational age of the baby, its birth weight and the facilities available in the unit. Any associated complications or consequences of the cause of the jaundice will also influence the treatment offered.

Irrespective of the cause, treatment should be determined by the bilirubin levels, especially the unconjugated values. Other investigations include an ultrasound scan of the liver and gall-bladder.

4. A mother complains that her baby has refused feeds on the first day after delivery. (a) Outline your management of the baby, including how you will counsel the mother. (16 marks) (b) What complications may the baby suffer from? (4 marks)

Common mistakes

- Assume that it is mechanical
- Investigate with ultrasound – what are you investigating?
- Offer X-rays – of what?
- Surgical treatment – Duhamel's operation for duodenal stenosis or congenital atresia of the duodenum
- Intravenous (i.v.) fluids the only means of treatment

A good answer will include some or all of these points

(a) Outline your management of the baby, including how you will you counsel the mother. (16 marks)

- Discuss the symptom and possible causes
- Obtain information from the mother and notes
- Treat according to first principles
- Causes of refusal of feed
- Infections
- Hypoglycaemia
- Hypothermia
- Structural abnormalities

(b) What complications may the baby suffer from? (4 marks)

- Hypoglycaemia
- Electrolyte imbalance
- Failure to thrive
- Death

Sample answer

(a) Outline your management of the baby, including how you will you counsel the mother. (16 marks)

Refusal of feeds on the first day of life is an important symptom and one that could distress parents. A sensitive approach to investigating and treating this symptom is vital in order not to frighten the parents. The aetiology of this symptom varies from physiological, metabolic and infective to anatomical problems. To manage this problem, its cause must be sought carefully.

Information from the parents is vital. It is essential to know whether the baby took and tolerated feeds before, or had not really been fed. If the former is the case, a congenital malformation is unlikely, especially if there was no regurgitation or vomiting. An infective or physiological cause may therefore be considered. A quick review of the antenatal and birth record may reveal additional information, e.g. there might have been polyhydramnios or suspicion of bowel obstruction. It is unlikely to be the case here, unless the baby had vomited its first feeds and this was not recognised.

The possible causes of this baby's problem, assuming that it was able to tolerate feeds before, could be hypoglycaemia, hypothermia or infections. Hypoglycaemia is more likely to occur in babies of diabetic mothers. This information should be available in the mother's records. If this is not possible, a simple blood glucose estimation (mother and baby) would indicate whether this is the case. Hypothermia is more common on an open ward, often associated with a draught and poor temperature control. Septicaemia, especially associated with meningitis, would be the most worrying cause for the parents. They must therefore be advised about the investigations and management. This must include an infection screening and initiation of i.v. antibiotics.

Usually, this situation settles within a few days. However, if feeds continue to be refused, the ultimate treatment of this baby is to offer i.v. nutrition or tube feeding. The advantage of tube feeding is that it bypasses the risk of introducing infections and also ensures that, if there is any upper gastrointestinal obstruction, the tube will identify it. The surface area of a baby is large compared to its body weight and failure to adequately rehydrate a baby which has not fed for a day may have important consequences.

Finally, sedation should be excluded by information about medication from the mother. Some of these drugs, especially those that cross the placenta, may be responsible. Such babies require observation and possibly tube feeding until the effects of the drugs wear off.

(b) What complications may the baby suffer from? (4 marks)

The complications will be related to the refusal of feeds and their causes. Those related to refusal of feeds include hypoglycaemia, which may then result in coma or fits, and electrolyte imbalance, which if uncorrected will eventually result in renal failure. Poor temperature control is another complication, especially as newborn infants are unable to undergo shivering thermogenesis and therefore depend on the metabolism of ingested food for heat generation.

If refusal to feed is only partially corrected, the baby will suffer from failure to thrive. Eventually, if refusal of feeds persists, the baby will die.

Section Two

Part Two: Gynaecology

1

Paediatric and adolescent gynaecology

1. Justify your management of a newborn who, on examination, is found to have ambiguous external genitalia. (20 marks)

2. A 25-year-old woman, whose pregnancy was uncomplicated, unexpectedly delivered a baby suspected to have Down's syndrome. The antenatal serum screening test had been normal (1:1500) and no markers had been identified on ultrasound scan. (a) Critically appraise your management prior to discharge from the hospital. (15 marks) (b) How will you counsel her at the postnatal visit? (5 marks)

3. A 6-year-old girl has been referred to the gynaecology clinic with persistent vaginal discharge. (a) Discuss critically your initial approach to her management. (14 marks) (b) How will you treat the discharge? (6 marks)

4. A mother brings her 7-year-old daughter to you because she has been menstruating regularly for the past 4 months. (a) Briefly discuss the possible causes of this girl's problems. (6 marks) (b) Outline your initial steps in her management (excluding treatment). (8 marks) (b) Assuming that no cause is found, what will your management be? (6 marks)

5. Evaluate your management of a 10-year-old girl presenting with vaginal bleeding of 1 week's duration. (20 marks)

1. Justify your management of a newborn who, on examination, is found to have ambiguous external genitalia. (20 marks)

Common mistakes

- Listing the causes of external ambiguous genitalia
- Discussing in detail the various chromosomal and genetic factors regulating the differentiation of the internal and external genitalia
- Undertaking a physical examination after taking a history – failing to address the problem as it is presented (a newborn and not anyone with external ambiguous genitalia)
- General discussion of the management of ambiguous genitalia – failing to justify (i.e. give reasons for all the steps you take in the management of this neonate)
- Referring the patient to a psychosexual counsellor!
- Involving a plastic surgeon in the management
- Listing investigations (again without justification) is not enough

A good answer will include some or all of these points

- The importance of assigning the correct sex at birth
- Communication with the parents about the uncertainty in the assignment
- Need to exclude congenital adrenal hyperplasia (CAH) of the salt-losing type – if missed may result in mortality
- Investigations:
    - Urea and electrolytes (U&Es)
    - Adrenal hormones – urinary 17 ketosteroids or serum 17α-hydroxyprogesterone
    - Karyotype
    - Pelvic ultrasound scan – to confirm the presence of uterus and ovaries (confirms the diagnosis of CAH)
- Involvement of different teams – paediatricians, geneticists if necessary, and clinical psychologist to support the parents
- Definitive management at birth and later:
    - CAH – salt-losing type – correct electrolyte derangement and replace cortisol deficiency, e.g. with deoxycorticosterone acetate (DOCA)
    - Long-term – continuation of cortisol replacement
- Implications for ambiguous external genitalia:
    - Surgical correction of the clitoris within 18 months, any labial fusion correction (e.g. by simple posterior incision around 3–4 years)
- Psychological support – mainly to parents at the outset but later to the child
- Involve a clinical geneticists if CAH – autosomal recessive condition
- Information leaflet and contact details of support groups and websites

Sample answer

The finding of ambiguous external genitalia must be managed sensitively and tactfully, as assignment of the wrong sex to a child will have long-term implications both for the child and the family. Once the diagnosis is made, the parents must be informed of the uncertainty. An important step must be to exclude CAH of the salt-losing type, as failure to recognise this may be associated with mortality. This is excluded by serum measurement of U&Es and various adrenal hormones (e.g. urinary 17 ketosteroids or serum 17α-hydroxyprogesterone).

A detailed drug history from the mother may identify exogenous virilising causes, although this is uncommon. The involvement of a neonatologist will help with a more thorough examination, aimed at locating the gonads, if present, in the inguinal region or as abdominal masses.

The karyotype must be determined (either from a cord blood sample or from a sample collected from the neonate) to help assign the genetic sex. This is essential as it will be useful in defining the underlying cause and sex of rearing. For example, this could be a 46XX neonate with CAH (the most likely cause), whereas a 46XY neonate may be related to other factors. An ultrasound scan of the pelvis looking for the presence of a uterus and ovaries is essential as their presence will confirm the likelihood of CAH.

Following the genetic studies, subsequent management will depend on the evaluation of the best possible sex of rearing for the child. Assessment must be with this in mind. Where CAH is the cause, if the salt-losing type, then urgent correction of any electrolyte imbalance is paramount followed by cortisol replacement. This can be in the form of DOCA although other forms may be used. This replacement would be continued for life.

With regards to the external genitalia, reduction in the size of the clitoris is recommended within the first 18 months. If there is fusion of the labia, attempts to separate them should be made at 3–4 years. This may involve posterior incision. Other genital abnormalities should be dealt with accordingly; some of these may involve the creation of a neovagina. Irrespective of the treatment, counselling and psychological support, initially for the parents and later for the child, will be required. This may be offered by a clinical psychologist. It may be necessary to involve a clinical geneticist if this is CAH, as it is an autosomal recessive condition.

If information leaflets are available, these should be given to the parents. Contact numbers of support groups or specialised web sites (if known) should also be provided. Finally, a follow-up appointment should be arranged with the various specialties including obstetrics.

Further reading

Edmonds K (2003) Congenital adrenal hyperplasia. In: Shaw RW, Soutter WP, Stanton SL (eds) *Gynaecology*, 3rd edn. Edinburgh: Churchill Livingstone, pp. 191–3.

2. A 25-year-old woman, whose pregnancy was uncomplicated, unexpectedly delivered a baby suspected to have Down's syndrome. The antenatal serum screening test had been normal (1:1500) and no markers had been identified on ultrasound scan. (a) Critically appraise your management prior to discharge from the hospital. (15 marks) (b) How will you counsel her at the postnatal visit? (5 marks)

Common mistakes

- Discussing the prenatal diagnosis of Down's syndrome
- Discussing the various test for prenatal diagnosis – advantages and disadvantages
- No need to critically appraise amniocentesis or chorionic villus sampling
- It is irrelevant to say that this ought not to have happened
- Shortfalls of serum screening and ultrasound screening – unnecessary
- Criticism of the screening procedure
- Discussing risk management
- Giving the parents advice on how to sue the hospital for compensation!

A good answer will include some or all of these points

(a) Critically appraise your management prior to discharge from the hospital. (15 marks)

- Recognise that parents and staff will be shocked at this diagnosis
- A truthful, careful and sensitive approach must be adopted to inform the parents
- They must be given time to assimilate the news
- Paediatrician to be involved to inform the couple of the neonatal problems of Down's syndrome. Examination of the neonate to exclude malformations (especially those associated with Down's syndrome, e.g. cardiac)
- Need to confirm the diagnosis – chromosomes from blood
- Involvement of a geneticist
- Explanation about why the diagnosis was missed
- Giving information to the couple about various support groups and the society
- The general practitioner (GP) and community midwife should be informed

(b) How will you counsel her at the postnatal visit? (5 marks)

- Reiterate the possible explanation as to why the diagnosis was missed – screening is expected to miss some cases (most cases of Down's syndrome babies are delivered to women below the age of 35 years in the UK for this reason)
- Most likely sporadic Down's syndrome
- Recurrence risk approximately 1 per cent if karyotype of parents is normal
- Parents may wish to be karyotyped to exclude balanced translocation
- Long-term support at home and when complications arise

● Discussion about prenatal diagnosis in subsequent pregnancy, including the risk of recurrence

Sample answer

(a) Critically appraise your management prior to discharge from the hospital. (15 marks)

The unexpected diagnosis of Down's syndrome at birth is a shock, not only to the parents but also to the staff. Therefore, the approach has to be sensitive, empathic and multidisciplinary. The first step must be to inform the parents of the diagnosis. By this stage, paediatricians would have been involved and they are most suited to inform the parents. Honesty must be paramount. The parents will no doubt be shocked and angry, and staff must be prepared to support them to come to terms with the diagnosis.

Where a paediatrician is not already involved, one should be asked to examine the neonate, to confirm the diagnosis and then to exclude other congenital malformations that may be associated with Down's syndrome, especially cardiac abnormalities. No matter how certain the diagnosis is from this physical examination, the parents must be made to understand the importance of confirming the diagnosis by karyotyping. The presence of associated malformations will certainly have an effect on the quality of life of the newborn. It is also necessary for the paediatrician to counsel the couple on the immediate neonatal and long-term care of the baby. It may be appropriate at this stage to mention some possible complications associated with this problem. However, care must be taken not to give too much information to the parents at this early stage.

A blood sample is essential for chromosomal analysis to confirm the diagnosis of Down's syndrome. Involvement of the clinical geneticist will provide genetic support and counselling, whereas social workers, the patient's GP and midwife will provide support in the community. It may not be necessary at this stage to involve the geneticist, but he or she needs to be informed. The geneticist may only see the couple if they wish to do so.

Once the couple have come to terms with the diagnosis, a plan needs to be made about the immediate care of the neonate. Some parents may be too shocked to take the baby home. Under such circumstances, arrangements should be made for the immediate care of the baby in the hospital. If the couple decide to take the baby home, information must be provided on the possible complications that such babies may have and how to recognise the early symptoms (e.g. recurrent chest infections).

Pamphlets should be given to the parents – those prepared by the Down's Syndrome Association contain details about where to get help, the problems and how to cope with a Down's syndrome baby. The obstetrician, neonatologist and geneticist must arrange to follow-up the couple.

(b) How will you counsel her at the postnatal visit? (5 marks)

The objective of this is, first, to explain how the diagnosis was not made antenatally and, second, to answer all questions that the couple may have. Most cases of Down's syndrome babies are delivered to women under the age of 35 years. This is because the screening test is not

100% sensitive. The option of having their karyotypes determined should be discussed. This will exclude translocations and therefore allow a more accurate estimation of the recurrence risk. For most cases the recurrence risk is approximately 1 per cent, but this may be altered if their karyotype is abnormal. In any subsequent pregnancy, antenatal diagnosis would be discussed and offered. Chorionic villus sampling and amniocentesis are the two options to be discussed.

Although most couples will opt to take the baby home, some may reject it and the option of late acceptance must be available, but simultaneously, plans must be made for adoption. Finally, it is important to confirm that the parents have had access to all the sources of information and support that they will require, including education on the complications and what to do when these arise.

3. A 6-year-old girl has been referred to the gynaecology clinic with persistent vaginal discharge. (a) Discuss critically your initial approach to her management. (14 marks) (b) How will you treat the discharge? (6 marks)

Common mistakes

- Listing the causes of vaginal discharge in this menstruating young girl – who said she is menstruating?
- Assuming it is due to sexual abuse and involving the police and social workers without justification
- Undertaking a vaginal and rectal examination
- Taking a high vaginal swab in the clinic
- Referring the girl to the genitourinary medicine unit
- Treating with oestrogen creams and triple antibiotics, irrespective of the cause
- Failure to provide critical appraisal of management
- Discussing competence to give consent to treatment (Fraser or Gillick)

A good answer will contain some or all of these points

(a) Discuss critically your initial approach to her management (14 marks)

- A good candidate will recognise that this is a distressing problem to the young girl and her parents
- Recognise the sensitivity involved and the implications
- Recognise that sexual abuse may be a cause and that suspicions of this must be handled with care because of the sensitivity and the implications of attaching such a label
- Take a good history to exclude associated symptoms of pruritus, bloody discharge, change of clothing or soap. Any known allergies?
- Other investigations, such as examination under anaesthesia (EUA), swabs, stool examination, etc.
- Causes – atrophic vaginitis predisposing to infections, foreign body, threadworms, sexual abuse and, rarely, tumours
- Gentle inspection of the vulva and anus, looking for signs of trauma and noting atrophic changes. Taking swabs from the introitus and external urethra and rectum if necessary
- Gentle rectal examination may be necessary with the little finger – identify foreign body in vagina (but best avoided in the clinic and undertaken under general anaesthesia (GA))
- EUA – using a paediatric laryngoscope. Remove foreign body and gently cleanse vagina. Offer oral antibiotics if any infection or suspicion of infection

(b) How will you treat the discharge? (6 marks)

- Atrophic vaginitis – treat with sparing topical application of oestrogen cream to the vulva for about 2 weeks

- Foreign body – remove
- Allergic reaction – remove allergen and offer antihistamines
- Antibiotics for suspected infection – alone or with a foreign body
- General hygiene
- Anthelmintics for threadworm

Sample answer

(a) Discuss critically your initial approach to her management. (14 marks)

Vaginal discharge in a young girl is distressing not only to her, but to her parents. The way it is managed is important as it may cause further distress to families, especially if sexual abuse is suspected as a possible cause of the discharge.

The first step in her management will be to take an appropriate history from the girl and her parents. Although this may provide important clues to the cause of the discharge, information from this young girl may not be forthcoming. For example, a history suggestive of the insertion of foreign body or sexual abuse may not be obtained easily. The nature of the discharge (bloody, foul smelling, purulent, etc.) should be determined. However, if there is any associated itching then the discharge may be related to threadworms. On the other hand, a sudden change in bathing soap, underwear or other agents that may cause an allergic reaction must be excluded.

After this, a physical examination must be performed. In a 6-year-old this is difficult as an internal examination may not only be difficult but may be very distressing. Such an examination needs to be performed by a doctor experienced in adolescent gynaecology so as to recognise tell-tale signs of sexual abuse. During the investigations, swabs for bacteriology and virology should be obtained to exclude infections. However, these may not be very reliable in view of the fact that these will be mainly from the introitus. The presence of excoriations in the vulvoperineal region should heighten the suspicion of sexual abuse. If this is the case, an expert must be notified to come and examine the child, and if possible, to take photographs. Unfortunately, this action will cause enormous distress to the family. The way it is handled must therefore be very tactful. It will not be necessary at this stage to involve the police and social workers unless the evidence is overwhelming.

Further investigations include an ultrasound scan and an abdominal X-ray. Abdominal X-rays will identify radio-opaque foreign bodies in the vagina, although if one is present as the cause of the discharge, it will need removal – probably under GA. Ultrasound scan may similarly identify the cause (e.g. a foreign body) but, again, another procedure will be necessary for its removal. Examination under anaesthesia will not only allow diagnosis, but also allow the removal of any foreign bodies. However, this procedure, in the absence of radiological support, may miss hidden foreign bodies.

(b) How will you treat the discharge? (6 marks)

The treatment options will depend on the identifiable cause. Where a foreign body has been identified, this will be removed and broad-spectrum antibiotics prescribed if there is superimposed infection. She should be dewormed if there is a suspicion of threadworm infection. Where the treatment is a simple improvement in hygiene, education of the parents may be all that is needed. It is important not to be seen to be judgemental, and some parents may become resentful at the thought of being accused of negligence, to the distress of their daughter. If the cause is an allergic reaction, then the allergen should be identified and removed. It may be necessary to institute antihistamines for a short period. Finallly, where sexual abuse is the cause, the appropriate gynaecologist/paediatrician must take over the care of this young girl.

4. A mother brings her 7-year-old daughter to you because she has been menstruating regularly for the past 4 months. (a) Briefly discuss the possible causes of this girl's problems. (6 marks) (b) Outline your initial steps in her management (excluding treatment). (8 marks) (c) Assuming that no cause is found, what will your management be? (6 marks)

Common mistakes

- Ascertaining competence before history and treatment
- Treating this girl as an adult
- Taking a history from the girl and performing a physical examination, such as vaginal and speculum examination – are these really relevant?
- Failing to recognise the need to involve paediatricians
- Failure to recognise the psychological implications and the other consequences, such as pregnancy
- Assuming that the cause is pathological and therefore concentrating on the diagnosis and treatment of the various pathological causes

A good answer will include some or all of these points

(a) Briefly discuss the possible causes of this girl's problems. (6 marks)

- Central (true) precocious puberty:
  - This is gonadotropin dependent
  - Familial (idiopathic)
  - Intracranial lesions (e.g. encephalitis, abscesses, tumours, trauma, irradiation, hydrocephalus)
  - Gonadotropin-secreting tumours
  - Autoimmune hypothyroidism
  - Congenital brain defects, arachnoid cysts, suprasellular cysts, third ventricular cysts, neurofibromatosis, harmatomas
- Gonadotropin independent (pseudo-precocious puberty)
  - CAH
  - Cushing's syndrome
  - McCune–Albright syndrome
  - Exogenous oestrogen ingestion/administration
  - Sex-steroid-secreting tumours of the ovary or adrenals, chorionepithelioma

(b) Outline your initial steps in her management (excluding treatment). (8 marks)

- Her management must be approached sensitively – it may not only be embarrassing to the girl but also to her parents

- History:
  - Drugs
  - Family history
  - Personal history – trauma or infections, symptoms of other syndromes such as Cushing's syndrome, etc.
- Physical examination:
  - Secondary sexual characteristics
  - Height and weight
  - *Café au lait* spots
- Investigations:
  - Biochemistry:
    - Follicle-stimulating hormone (FSH), luteinising hormone (LH), oestradiol, androgens (testosterone), dehydroepiandrosterone (DHEA), dehydroepiandrostendione sulfate (DHEAS), 17-hydroxyprogesterone and tests of CAH if indicated
    - Gonadotropin levels – FSH, LH
    - Free thyroxine (T4) and thyroid-stimulating hormone (TSH)
  - Imaging:
    - Ultrasound scan of the pelvis and abdomen
    - Magnetic resonance imaging (MRI)/computerised tomography (CT) scan of the brain
    - X-ray of the wrist to determine bone age

(c) Assuming that no cause is found, what will your management be? (6 marks)

- Recognise and mention the consequences of precocious puberty
- Bone development
- Risk of pregnancy and sexual abuse
- Psychological consequences on the child, especially when she compares herself with her peers
- Offer treatment – medical and otherwise
- Need for follow-up in the appropriate clinic

Sample answer

(a) Briefly discuss the possible causes of this girl's problems. (6 marks)

This girl most likely has precocious puberty, which may not only be embarrassing to her, especially among her peers, but also to her parents. The possible causes can be grouped under two headings – the central (true) precocious type and the gonadotropin-independent (pseudo-precocious puberty) type. Included in the first group are those that are constitutional (familial), secondary to intracranial lesions (e.g. encephalitis, abscesses, irradiation, hydrocephalus, tumours and trauma), gonadotropin-secreting tumours, autoimmune hypothyroidism and congenital brain defects (arachnoid cysts, suprasellular cysts, third ventricle cysts and neurofi-bromatosis and harmatomas). For most of these, there may be unrelated symptoms. The causes within the second group include CAH, Cushing's syndrome, McCune–Albright's syndrome, exogenous oestrogen ingestion and sex-steroid-secreting tumours.

(b) Outline your initial steps in her management (excluding treatment). (8 marks)

Her management must be approached with sufficient sensitivity and understanding. In most cases, it is usually accompanied by pubarche, thelarche and adrenache, although their absence does not exclude it. In the first instance, information will be obtained from the parents about the sequence of events that preceded the first period. Associated symptoms of hypothyroidism must be excluded. A personal history of trauma to the skull, previous encephalitis or symptoms of endocrine disorders such as Cushing's syndrome and hypothyroidism may provide clues as to the cause. Other associated important factors that must be excluded include infective encephalitis, headaches, visual disturbances and fractures of the skull. These will point to possible aetiological factors for the precocious puberty. In constitutional cases, there may be a family history of precocious puberty. A careful drug history will exclude exogenous steroids as a cause.

Following the detailed history, a thorough search for signs would be undertaken. The presence of these may suggest the cause of the precocious puberty. The presence of *café au lait* spots, for example, suggests neurofibromatosis. Other signs include an enlarged thyroid gland, hydrocephalus, visual field abnormalities, abdominal masses and an abnormal ratio of the various long bones. Investigations such as thyroid function test (free T4 and TSH), FSH and LH, prolactin, testosterone, oestradiol, DHEAS, screening for Cushing's syndrome and ultrasound scan of the ovaries and adrenal glands would further help in the identification of the cause. An MRI/CT scan of the brain will be helpful in excluding the intracranial lesions that may cause precocious puberty. The bone age should be determined by an X-ray of the wrist.

(c) Assuming that no cause is found, what will your management be? (6 marks)

Where the cause is constitutional (no obvious explanation is found), the treatment of choice is gonadotropin-releasing hormone analogues. These will inhibit the pituitary function and therefore suppress ovarian activity. Exogenous oestrogens should be avoided, as these are responsible for the premature closure of the epiphyses. Cyproterone acetate has been used in some cases with reasonable success. The advantage of this is that the anterior pituitary is not completely suppressed. Although medroxyprogesterone acetate has been tried it does not appear to be associated with much success.

The implications for this condition must also be addressed. If the girl is ovulating, the possibility of pregnancy if she is sexually exposed must be considered. Sensitive counselling must be offered in this regard. The second consequence of precocious puberty is premature closure of the epiphyses. Although the girl may initially be tall for her age, her ultimate height will be shorter. Treatment must not only be aimed at the cause but also at preventing premature closure of the epiphyses.

Whatever treatment the girl is offered, it must be accompanied by adequate psychological support. This will depend on her age and her needs. In other words, psychotherapy must be tailored to the needs of the patient.

Further reading

Duncan SLB (1997) Disorders of puberty. In: Shaw RW, Soutter PW, Stanton S (eds) *Gynaecology*. Edinburgh: Churchill, pp. 188–99.

Swaenepoel C, Chaussain CL, Reger M (1991) Long-term results of long-acting luteinising hormone-releasing hormone in the central precocious puberty. *Horm Res* **36**: 126–30.

5. Evaluate your management of a 10-year-old girl presenting with vaginal bleeding of 1 week's duration. (20 marks)

Common mistakes

- Assuming that she has cancer and ignoring all other causes of bleeding per vaginam
- Treating her as an adult
- Taking a detailed sexual history and excluding features of pregnancy
- Performing a physical examination – general, vaginal and speculum, taking swabs for cervical smear and microbiological investigations
- Failing to recognise that infections and sexual abuse may be a cause
- Assuming she has precocious puberty and investigating for all the causes of this condition
- Treating her for menstrual problems

A good answer will include some or all of these points

- Recognise that this is a young patient and therefore a sensitive approach is required
- The co-operation of her parents is essential and, where possible, paediatricians may be involved
- Need to take a careful history (from the girl and her parents) to exclude: trauma; sexual abuse; infections; foreign body
- Investigations to include: EUA if possible; ultrasound scan; high vaginal swabs/rectal swabs; hormonal investigations
- If any tumours – biopsy
- Treatment – depending on the identified cause

Sample answer

The management of this young girl requires understanding of the psychological consequences of various investigations and treatment of the bleeding, on both the girl and her parents. An important first step is to take a thorough history. This will provide possible clues to the aetiology of the bleeding, e.g. trauma, a foreign body and menarche. Chronological development of secondary sexual characteristics culminating in vaginal bleeding suggests menarchial bleeding. Other possible causes include infections, sexual abuse and malignancies. Although information about sexual abuse is difficult to obtain, efforts must be made in a sensitive and non-threatening way to gauge whether this could be the cause. Often, this can only be suspected after a pelvic examination.

Physical examination is essential to eliminate possible causes of the abnormal vaginal bleeding. In the first instance, characteristics of puberty should be identified if present. These will include breast development, height, pubic hair and other features of puberty. An abdominal examination may identify masses in the pelvic area, such as oestrogen-secreting ovarian tumours, which may be responsible for the vaginal bleeding. Where infection is the suspected cause, swabs must be obtained from the vagina and other suspected sites, such as the urethra and rectum. A restrictive pelvic examination starting with a gentle inspection of the vulval and perianal area may point to an infection or trauma, which may be sexually related. A gentle rectal examination with the little finger may identify a foreign body in the vagina. It may also identify a tumour in the vagina, which may be responsible for the bleeding.

Where there is no obvious cause identified, further investigations should be performed. These will include an EUA. A paediatric laryngoscope may be used to examine the vagina. Where there is a tumour, a biopsy should be taken. The most common type of tumour in this age group is sarcoma botryoides. This has a fleshy appearance and is of vaginal origin. Although the appearances of such a lesion are characteristic, it is necessary to confirm the diagnosis by a biopsy under GA. An ultrasound scan of the abdomen and the lower genital tract will not only identify any ovarian pathology but may be able to identify foreign bodies in the vagina. A pregnancy presenting as threatened miscarriage can also be excluded by ultrasound scan.

Following these simple and extremely important stages, subsequent management will depend on the suspected cause of the bleeding. Where atrophic changes are thought to be the cause, simple but sparing application of topical oestrogen will suffice. However, this should not be offered for more than 2 weeks. If it is an infection such as threadworms, there will be associated pruritus and deworming may be all that is needed with appropriate education about hygiene. The diagnosis of a vaginal malignancy will require surgery, but this needs to be undertaken by an adequately skilled surgeon.

2

Menstrual disorders

1. A 37-year-old woman presented to you with regular and heavy periods. (a) Outline with reasons the investigations you will undertake on her. (6 marks) (b) Briefly evaluate the options (excluding hysterectomy) available for her treatment. (14 marks)

2. A 33-year-old woman with menorrhagia wishes to have surgery. (a) Evaluate the various surgical options you will consider for her. (14 marks) (b) If she has associated abdominal pain, what factors will influence which treatment you offer her? (6 marks)

3. Critically appraise your management of a woman with cyclical secondary dysmenorrhoea. (20 marks)

4. A 31-year-old para 2 + 1 presents with secondary amenorrhoea. A pelvic examination was normal. (a) What additional useful information will you obtain from the patient about her complaint? (8 marks) (b) Briefly outline the investigations you will undertake on her. (6 marks) (c) How will you treat her if the cause is found to be non-endocrinological? (6 marks)

5. How will you justify your management of a 37-year-old teacher presenting with suspected severe premenstrual syndrome? (20 marks)

1. A 37-year-old woman presented to you with regular and heavy periods. (a) Outline with reasons the investigations you will undertake on her. (6 marks) (b) Briefly outline the options (excluding hysterectomy) available for her treatment. (14 marks)

Common mistakes

- Discussing the management of uterine fibroids
- Assuming that she has an infection
- Listing the causes of bleeding in this woman
- Assuming that she has completed her family
- Offering her a hysterectomy as the best treatment – you have been told to exclude this option
- Discussing hysteroscopy, endometrial biopsy and ultrasound as part of your management
- Failure to give reasons for your answer

A good answer will include some or all of these points

(a) Outline with reasons the investigations you will undertake on her. (6 marks)

- Physical examination if history is suggestive of pathology (NICE, 2007)
- Full blood count (FBC) to exclude anaemia, blood group and save if surgery is contemplated or transfusion if severely anaemic
- Thyroid function test – only if symptomatic
- Coagulation screen – if heavy menstrual bleeding dates back to menarche, or there is a personal or family history suggestive of coagulation defect
- Pelvic ultrasound scan – uterus enlarged, failed medical treatment, e.g. at general practitioner's (GP's)
- Hysteroscopy – if ultrasound scan is inconclusive (e.g. the precise location of a fibroid is unclear), or there is suspicion of malignancy – persistent intermittent bleeding

(b) Briefly evaluate the options (excluding hysterectomy) available for her treatment. (14 marks)

Treatment options:

- Medical/hormonal:
  - Combined oral contraceptive pill
  - Antifibrinolytic agents; prostaglandin synthetase inhibitors
  - Progestogens:
    - Norethisterone
    - Levonorgestrel intrauterine system (Mirena®)
  - Anti-oestrogens; gonadotropin-releasing hormone (GnRH) analogues

- Non-steroidal anti-inflammatory drugs (NSAIDs)
- Surgical:
  - Ablation of the endometrium
  - Second generation devices – balloon/microwave ablations

Sample answer

(a) Outline with reasons the investigations you will undertake on her? (6 marks)

A physical examination is the first investigation. This will identify clinical anaemia and any potential causes of the heavy periods such as thyroid masses and pelvic/abdominal masses. A tender pelvis with induration will be suspicious of endometriosis.

A FBC will determine whether she is anaemic or not. It may be necessary to transfuse her if she is very anaemic or requires surgery, in which case grouping and saving serum should be undertaken. Other investigations will be undertaken if there is an indication. If she has symptoms of thyroid dysfunction, then a thyroid function test (free thyroxine (T4) and thyroid-stimulating hormone (TSH)) should be undertaken. A coagulation test is indicated if her menorrhagia started at menarche, or there is a personal or family history suggestive of a coagulation defect.

A pelvic ultrasound should be performed if the uterus is palpable or there is an adnexal mass palpable per abdomen. In addition, if the GP had tried medical treatment and this had failed, then an ultrasound will be indicated even if there are no palpable masses. Saline infusion sonography is not routinely indicated but may be helpful in the diagnosis of endometrial polyps. A hysteroscopy and or endometrial biopsy would be required if she has an inconclusive ultrasound scan (e.g. one that fails to locate fibroids precisely) or there is persistent associated intermittent bleeding. At the hysteroscopy, an endometrial biopsy would be performed if there is a suspicion of hyperplasia or malignancy.

(b) Briefly evaluate the options (excluding hysterectomy) available for her treatment. (14 marks)

The combined oral contraceptive pill is the first medical therapeutic option. It is cheap, efficacious and provides the additional benefit of contraception. However, in view of the patient's age it may not be very suitable, especially if she is a smoker, overweight, or is at risk of venous thromboembolism (VTE). An additional disadvantage is the need to take the pill regularly. Even if she has no need for contraception, this will still be an appropriate therapeutic option.

Antifibrinolytic agents are the second medical option. The most effective is tranexamic acid. A randomised controlled trial (Bonnar and Sheppard, 1996) concluded that this was the most effective treatment for menorrhagia. Its main advantage is that of proven efficacy. It is also cheap and does not increase the risk of venous VTE. However, the patient needs to take this medication during menstruation and unless her periods are as regular as clockwork, she may find the occasional early period unacceptable. Although the NSAID mefenamic acid is not as effective as tranexamic acid, it is an acceptable option. In addition, it reduces the pain that may accompany heavy periods. These and other prostaglandin synthetase inhibitors are not as effective as tranexamic acid and may be associated with gastric ulceration.

The levonorgestrel intrauterine system (Mirena®) is an option that has many advantages. It is administered once every 5 years. It is effective and provides additional contraception if necessary. It reduces menstrual blood loss by about 80 per cent within 6 months of insertion. Although expensive, it is more cost effective than the other options in the long term. It may be associated with irregular vaginal bleeding, especially during the first 6 months, and in a woman who has multiple sexual partners may increase the risk of pelvic inflammatory disease (PID). It may also cause headaches, acne, breast tenderness and functional ovarian cysts. It requires skill to insert and, if ineffective, will need to be removed.

The use of anti-oestrogens or GnRH analogues in this patient will, in most cases, produce excellent results. These drugs are very effective when administered regularly. The nasal sprays have to be taken regularly, whereas the depot injections have to be administered monthly. Depot GnRH analogues are administered by qualified persons only and therefore compliance is not an issue. They are expensive and are associated with menopausal symptoms. If used for more than 6 months, they may cause osteopenia unless combined with add-back therapy.

Cyclical progestogens, in the form of norethisterone 15 mg given on day 5–26, are the least effective medical option in this patient. In a randomised trial (Bonnar and Sheppard, 1996) norethisterone was found to be the least effective in controlling menorrhagia (reducing blood loss in less than 40 per cent of patients), although it is the most commonly prescribed. It is cheap but has side-effects, such as breakthrough bleeding, breast tenderness and mood swings. Again, it has to be taken daily and failure to do so may be associated with unwanted side-effects, such as breakthrough bleeding.

Surgical options include ablation of the endometrium and for this, the second generation devices are recommended. These techniques require skill and special equipment. Most are undertaken in hospitals, although many are treated as day cases. Recognised complications include haemorrhage, perforation and infections. Interventional radiology in the form of embolisation is an option for fibroids if her family is complete. This requires expertise and appropriate equipment. Complications include: persistent vaginal discharge; postembolisation syndrome – pain, nausea, vomiting and fever (not involving hospitalisation) and less commonly need for additional surgery; premature ovarian failure; and haematoma. Very rarely, the patient may have haemorrhage, non-target embolisation causing tissue necrosis, and infection causing septicaemia.

References

Bonnar J, Sheppard BL (1996) Treatment of menorrhagia during menstruation: randomised controlled trial of ethamsylate, mefenamic acid and tranexamic acid. *BMJ* **313**: 579–82.
NICE (2007) *Clinical Guideline 44. Heavy Menstrual Bleeding.* January 2007. London: National Institute for Health and Clinical Excellence.

Further reading

Dwyer N, Hutton J, Stirrat GM (1993) Randomised controlled trial comparing endometrial resection with abdominal hysterectomy for the surgical treatment of menorrhagia. *BJOG* **100**: 237–43.

> 2. A 33-year-old woman with menorrhagia wishes to have surgery. (a) Evaluate the various surgical options you will consider for her. (14 marks) (b) If she has associated abdominal pain, what factors will influence which treatment you offer her? (6 marks)

Common mistakes

- Listing the treating methods and discussing the details of how they are administered
- Discussing the medial therapeutic options of this patient
- Stating that she ought not to have surgery without first trying the medical options – this may well be the case, but the question is not asking you to critically appraise the decision to offer her surgical treatment
- Failing to evaluate the options listed
- Taking a history and doing a physical examination. Although this is not irrelevant, it is unlikely to earn you many marks
- The definition of menorrhagia is standard; therefore, irregular menstrual periods should not be considered in the management of this patient
- Assuming that she has polycystic ovary syndrome (PCOS) and listing the treatment for this condition
- Discussing treatment for infertility
- Considering a uterine malignancy as a differential diagnosis; although this is possible, it is very unlikely in this patient – remember, common things occur commonly

A good answer will include some or all of these points

(a) Evaluate the various surgical options you will consider for her. (14 marks)

- Surgical options include:
  - Endometrial ablation – balloon/diathermy endometrial ablation
  - Myomectomy
  - Hysterectomy
  - Laparoscopic ablation of endometriosis
  - Transvaginal ligation of the uterine arteries
- Endometrial ablation – balloon, etc. less expensive; day case procedure, cheaper; however, offered mainly by specialists, effective
- Hysterectomy – final, expensive, etc.
- Myomectomy – if fibroids
- Polypectomy – day case, cheap and easy to perform
- Laparoscopic laser/diathermy ablation of endometriosis/endometrioma – effective for endometriosis but may need combined medical treatment

(b) If she has associated abdominal pain, what factors will influence which treatment you offer her? (6 marks)

- Nature of the pain – menstrual or perimenstrual
- Associated pathology
  - Endometriosis adenomyosis, fibroid polyp, PID
- Treatment must aim to eliminate menorrhagia and pain

Sample answer

(a) Evaluate the various surgical options you will consider for her. (14 marks)

The surgical options available to this patient will depend on several factors, the most important of which is her desire to have children, or more children, and also on the cause of her menorrhagia. Causes that will require specific surgical treatment include uterine fibroids, adenomyosis and endometriosis.

If she has dysfunctional uterine bleeding (i.e. her menorrhagia is idiopathic), surgical options include endometrial ablation and a hysterectomy. Endometrial ablation is easy to perform and associated with a lower morbidity. This should be done with the second generation devices which include microwave, thermal and the balloon. Most are only performed in hospitals (as day cases) by gynaecologists under general anaesthesia (GA), although increasingly these are being performed under local anaesthesia. Because of the short operative time and early postoperative recovery, they have a significant advantage in a patient who is at a significant risk of VTE from prolonged surgery. In good hands, 70–80 per cent of patients are very satisfied with the results. When it fails it must be considered as an expensive option as it has to be superseded by a hysterectomy or a repeat procedure. A local destructive procedure will only be considered in this patient if she has completed her family.

The second surgical option, hysterectomy, is appropriate for idiopathic menorrhagia and that secondary to uterine fibroids, PID, adenomyosis and endometriosis. The advantage of this is that it is the definitive treatment of menorrhagia. It is cost effective and completely eliminates the problem. However, it is expensive and may be associated with complications, including mortality. Although very effective, it can only be performed in hospital and is associated with a prolonged recovery when compared to that of an ablative/destructive procedure. Its main advantage is the effectiveness of the treatment.

If the cause of the menorrhagia in this patient is uterine fibroids, another other option for her treatment would be a myomectomy. This surgical procedure is associated with complications, such as bleeding, adhesion formation and, in some cases, progression to a hysterectomy. It is the best option if the patient has not completed her family. Myomectomy is expensive and has to be performed by an experienced surgeon. The possible drawback is the fact that not all the fibroids may be removed. Therefore the patient may re-present with menorrhagia and require a repeat procedure.

Lastly, if endometriosis is the cause of the patient's menorrhagia, destruction of the endometriosis and laparoscopic uterosacral nerve ablation with laser or diathermy may reduce the menorrhagia. The success of these procedures is poor, although when combined with

247

medical treatment there is significant benefit. These procedures may also be associated with complications, such as damage to the bladder, bowel and ureters.

More recently, there is evidence that transvaginal ligation of the uterine arteries in such patients is associated with a significant reduction in menstrual loss. However, this is not widely available and more evidence is required to confirm its effectiveness.

The nature of the pain and its relationship with menstruation will determine the associated pathology and hence treatment. If the pain is primarily related to the heavy periods, treating it will be enough; however, if secondary to endometriosis or PID, the appropriate treatment for the pathology must be offered. A hysterectomy or ablation would be accompanied by hormonal therapy. It should be recognised that medical options alone may be inadequate.

3. Critically appraise your management of a woman with cyclical secondary dysmenorrhoea. (20 marks)

Common mistakes

- Taking a history and undertaking a physical examination – although this is important, you do not need to spend too much time on this
- Defining different types of cyclical dysmenorrhoea – primary and secondary. The question has already stated that the patient has secondary dysmenorrhoea, so focus on this only
- Devoting most of the essay to the causes of secondary dysmenorrhoea
- Detailed discussion on the differential diagnoses – these should only be mentioned
- Why is it important to make a diagnosis – trying to justify the distinction in the management approach between primary and secondary dysmenorrhoea
- Not critically appraising your answer but simply outlining or discussing the management

A good answer will include some or all of these points

- Definition of secondary dysmenorrhoea
- Common causes of cyclical secondary dysmenorrhoea – only briefly mentioning these: endometriosis; adenomyosis; chronic PID; no identifiable cause (idiopathic)
- Diagnosing the cause of dysmenorrhoea: specific symptoms may help diagnosis – limitations of history-taking; physical examination – limited but may exclude other pathologies; diagnostic laparoscopy – will exclude the main causes – expensive and will not exclude all causes, e.g. adenomyosis; ultrasound scan – will exclude adenomyosis and fibroids
- Treatment – depends on the cause: adenomyosis – gestrinone (Dimetriose®), GnRH analogues, etc.; endometriosis – treat accordingly; PID – often difficult to treat
- Supportive care

Sample answer

Cyclical secondary dysmenorrhoea in this patient could be due to endometriosis, chronic PID, adenomyosis, an intrauterine contraceptive device, cervical stenosis or it may be idiopathic. Some of these conditions may be suspected from a well-directed history. The clinical symptoms of some of them are unique. For example, in the presence of endometriosis there may be an associated deep dyspareunia. However, while history may be useful in suspecting some causes, it is unlikely to provide a definitive diagnosis. In addition, some of the causes of secondary dysmenorrhoea listed above may present with similar symptoms.

A physical examination may identify some signs of the pathologies causing the patient's dysmenorrhoea. These include retroversion with or without fixation, bilateral adnexal tenderness, adnexal masses, and a bulky uterus. The value of a clinical examination in the diagnosis of the cause of her symptoms is limited. The presence of these signs does not necessarily diagnose the cause of the dysmenorrhoea. However, it will exclude major pelvic pathologies. A stenosed cervix, especially in a patient who has had a cone biopsy, will be suggestive of cervical stenosis. In some patients, a bulky uterus with a doughy consistency will suggest adenomyosis. Although a physical examination may be helpful, it may not be very accurate.

Specific investigations will, therefore, have to be performed to make a definitive diagnosis, or to exclude all the suspected causes of the dysmenorrhoea. A diagnostic laparoscopy will exclude endometriosis and PID and suggest adenomyosis. Unfortunately, the absence of obvious endometriosis does not exclude endometriosis. Similarly, the diagnosis of chronic PID may not be conclusive at laparoscopy. Laparoscopy is expensive and has to be performed in the hospital – usually under GA (although it can also be performed under conscious sedation). This procedure may be complicated by bowel and bladder injuries, haemorrhage or air embolism. It will, however, be the most important investigation in the management of this patient.

Another investigation of importance is ultrasound scan of the pelvis. This investigation depends on the expertise of the operator and the quality of the machine being used. Ultrasound scan will exclude adenomyosis and uterine fibroids. Ovarian endometriomata may also be diagnosed; however, the absence of pathology on scan does not exclude it. Thus, whilst this investigation is expensive and may provide hints on the possible cause of the dysmenorrhoea, it will only diagnose a cause in some cases.

The value of taking swabs from the cervix to exclude PID is debatable. However, PID as a cause of dysmenorrhoea is difficult to diagnose from swabs from the endocervix or vagina. Although this may be useful in the diagnosis of acute infections, it will be ineffective in the diagnosis of chronic PID.

The treatment of this patient will depend on the cause of the dysmenorrhoea. For endometriosis, the treatment options include the combined oral contraceptive pill, progestogens and GnRH analogues. The combined oral contraceptive pill is effective in a premenopausal patient with no contraindications. It has to be taken continuously and has the advantage of being an effective contraceptive; however, it may cause breakthrough vaginal bleeding. Another alternative is a progestogen. Again, this needs to be taken daily and may be associated with acne, weight gain and irregular vaginal bleeding. If the woman is older and a smoker, the combined oral contraceptive pill will be an unacceptable option. Gestrinone (Dimetriose®), a testosterone derivative, is effective in the treatment of endometriosis, adenomyosis and dysmenorrhoea of unknown aetiology. The GnRH analogues are probably the most effective but are associated with menopausal side-effects, which may also affect tolerance. Where the cause of the dysmenorrhoea is PID, attempting to treat the cause may be impossible. However, suppressing ovulation and providing NSAIDs may be effective.

The last option before surgery is supportive care. Simply explaining the nature of the patient's symptoms and the diagnosed cause will go a long way towards increasing the success rate. Where all the options discussed above have failed, hysterectomy must be considered. This is an expensive major procedure, associated with short- and long-term complications, but it is cost effective in the treatment of secondary dysmenorrhoea. The patient must have completed her family before considering this option.

4. A 31-year-old para 2 + 1 presents with secondary amenorrhoea. A pelvic examination was normal. (a) What additional useful information will you obtain from the patient about her complaint? (8 marks) (b) Briefly outline the investigations you will undertake on her. (6 marks) (c) How will you treat her if the cause is found to be non-endocrinological? (6 marks)

Common mistakes

- Enumerating all the causes of secondary amenorrhoea
- Defining amenorrhoea and classifying it into primary and secondary
- Listing all the investigations of secondary amenorrhoea
- Ignoring the facts given and doing a pelvic examination (it has already been stated that a pelvic examination was normal)
- Inducing ovulation – assuming that the patient's other problem is infertility (after investigating the male partner)
- Detailed discussion about infertility treatment including offering advice about *in vitro* fertilisation and gamete intrafallopian transfer
- Assuming the problem is ovarian in nature and concentrating your answer on this

A good answer will include some or all of these points

(a) What additional useful information will you obtain from the patient about her complaint? (8 marks)

- Weight loss – stress-induced, exercise, anorexia
- Hyperprolactinaemia – inappropriate galactorrhoea, headaches
- Drugs – steroids, antihypertensives
- Features of hyperandrogenism – acne, hirsutism, weight gain, voice change
- History to exclude causes such as Asherman's syndrome, from an evacuation after a miscarriage or delivery, myomectomy and infections (e.g. tuberculosis (TB)) and the intrauterine contraceptive device
- Symptoms of thyroid dysfunction or Cushing's syndrome

(b) Briefly outline the investigations you will undertake on her. (6 marks)

- Pregnancy test
- Hormone profile – follicle-stimulating hormone (FSH), luteinising hormone (LH), prolactin, testosterone, sex-hormone-binding globulin, TSH, free T4, androstenedione
- Endoscopy – value – identify cause and may be therapeutic, e.g. division of adhesions
- Imaging:
  - Hysterosalpingography – identify cause but not therapeutic

- Chest X-ray
- Ultrasound scan of the pelvis – PCOS and hormonal profile; computerised tomography (CT) scan of the brain – if suspicious of tumour (prolactinoma)
- Others:
  - Karyotype
  - Screen for TB (e.g. tuberculin skin test – Mantoux test)

(c) How will you treat her if the cause is found to be non-endocrinological? (6 marks)

- The most likely cause will be Asherman's syndrome:
  - Treatment – division of adhesions, intrauterine contraceptive device, oestrogens (poor results)
- TB of the genital tract – treat with systemic medication but gynaecological prognosis is poor
- If desires future pregnancies – counsel

Sample answer

(a) What additional useful information will you obtain from the patient about her complaint? (8 marks)

The additional information to be obtained may help unravel the possible causes of the secondary amenorrhoea. Pregnancy should be excluded and for this, symptoms of pregnancy and a sexual history including contraception are important. A history of weight loss either induced by exercise or anorexia will suggest a hypothalamic cause. Similarly, information about stress and a sudden change in her circumstances may also suggest a hypothalamic cause.

Hyperprolactinaemia may present with a whitish/milky discharge from the breast or only with amenorrhoea. An enquiry should be made about drugs that may cause hyperprolactinaemia, e.g. Rauwolfia alkaloids, methyldopa, antipsychotic drugs (phenothiazines) and H_2-receptor antagonists and others that may cause amenorrhoea such as Depo-Provera® and danazol.

Symptoms such as hirsutism, acne, weight gain, and voice changes will be suggestive of PCOS or an adrenal tumour. If she has had a surgical treatment of a miscarriage or management of postpartum haemorrhage, termination or myomectomy, then Asherman's syndrome must be considered a possibility. Finally, symptoms of thyroid dysfunction and Cushing's syndrome should be excluded.

(b) Briefly outline the investigations you will undertake on her. (6 marks)

Investigations must aim to exclude possible causes and to make a definite diagnosis. These will include a pregnancy test and a hormone profile (FSH, LH, prolactin, testosterone, sex-hormone-binding globulin, androstenedione, TSH and free T4). Other investigations to be performed will depend on the suspected cause of the amenorrhoea and include a hysteroscopy or hysterosalpingography to diagnose Asherman's syndrome, ultrasound scan of the pelvis to exclude PCOS, a CT scan of the brain if a tumour is the suspected cause and karyotype, especially if premature menopause is suspected. If TB is suspected as a possible cause, then a tuberculin skin test such as the Mantoux test should be performed as well as a chest X-ray.

(c) How will you treat her if the cause is found to be non-endocrinological? (6 marks)

The most likely cause is Asherman's syndrome, although other causes such as TB and premature menopause must be considered as differential diagnoses. If it is Asherman's syndrome, the treatment is hysteroscopic division of the adhesions, insertion of an intrauterine device to prevent reformation and oestrogen stimulation of regeneration of the endometrium from glands. Unfortunately, this treatment is not very successful. If the patient does not want any more children, reassurance is all that is needed. If she desires pregnancy, appropriate counselling will be required. Unless she resumes normal menstruation, the chances are slim. In addition, the risks of miscarriage, premature labour, placenta accreta and percreta are high with pregnancy.

For TB, the treatment is chemotherapy with antituberculosis agents in conjunction with a chest physician. The prognosis for this cause is also poor and she is unlikely to become pregnant. If she has premature menopause as a result of an autoimmune or karyotypic abnormality, then counselling and hormone replacement therapy (HRT) would be the treatment options.

5. How will you justify your management of a 37-year-old teacher presenting with suspected severe premenstrual syndrome? (20 marks)

Common mistakes

- Offering treatment before confirming diagnosis
- Physical examination to confirm diagnosis
- Hormone profile to confirm diagnosis
- Ultrasound – an important investigation
- Premenstrual syndrome may be a differential diagnosis of large uterine fibroids, PID and endometriosis – discussing these differentials and their management
- Avoid vague phrases, such as 'Various drugs can be tried'!
- Failure to justify (give reasons) your answer

A good answer will include some or all of these points

- Diagnosis needs to be confirmed: best from a symptoms chart/diary/calendar; therapeutic trial with GnRH analogues
- Management – multidisciplinary team approach, including psychologist/psychiatrist
- General comment about treatment methods – high placebo effect
- Treatments of proven benefit: suppress ovulation – combined oral contraceptive pill; progestogens; oestrogens; GnRH analogues; surgery – bilateral oophorectomy; selective serotonin reuptake inhibitors (SSRIs)
- Unproven benefits: evening primrose oil; vitamin E, pyridoxine
- Quality of life assessment of success

Sample answer

Premenstrual syndrome is common at the extremes of reproductive life. Confirming the diagnosis is paramount and this is best done from a symptom diary/calendar or chart; however, a therapeutic trial with a GnRH analogue maybe more precise and effective in some cases. Once the diagnosis is confirmed, subsequent management should ideally be multidisciplinary, involving gynaecologists, psychologists or psychiatrists where it is deemed necessary.

There are various treatment options for premenstrual syndrome. It also has a high placebo effect. In fact, placebo effects have been reported in excess of 90 per cent in some studies. The treatment of choice will be influenced by the patient's desire for contraception or contraindications to the various options. In the absence of contraindications, the combined oral contraceptive pill will be the drug of first choice. It suppresses ovulation but may still be associated with symptoms of premenstrual syndrome. This is more so with Trisequens®, which contains high progestogens in the second half of the packages. The combined oral contraceptive pill may completely relieve the symptoms, limit them to 1–2 days premenstrually, or it may be ineffective.

The second therapeutic option will be progestogens only. Taken in form of tablets or pessaries during the second half of the menstrual cycle, these may improve symptoms in some patients. Monthly or 3-monthly progestogen injections may also be effective. The exact physiological basis for the effectiveness of this option is unclear. It is probably the least likely of all the hormone therapies to be effective.

Gonadotropin-releasing hormone analogues are probably the most effective medical option for this patient. They suppress ovarian activity by downregulating the pituitary gland. In this patient, not only may they alleviate the symptoms but they may enable the determination of what proportion of the symptoms are of ovarian/endocrine origin, and therefore whether she would benefit from bilateral oophorectomy. Although this treatment may be accompanied by menopausal symptoms, these could be overcome by including add-back therapy to the treatment. Where this combination is effective, therapy could be prolonged beyond 6 months.

More recent therapeutic regimens include SSRIs. This option is based on the report of altered serotonergic function in patients with premenstrual syndrome. In these women, it is thought that serotonin deficiency possibly makes them more sensitive to their endogenous ovarian steroids and boosting serotonin should therefore improve symptoms. The use of SSRIs, such as clomipramine and fluoxetine, has been shown to be effective in some patients. What is uncertain is precisely who will benefit from SSRIs. In this patient, this option may be tried and only after assessing her response will it then be possible to assess any benefits from the treatment. In recommending this treatment option, it should be remembered that the patient may develop the severe side-effect of suicidal depression which has been associated with SSRIs.

Oestradiol implants and transdermal patches may also be tried in this patient. These suppress the ovarian cycle and have been demonstrated to benefit some patients. However, the risks of endometrial hyperplasia may require combining them with a progestogen, which may cause premenstrual symptoms and subsequent poor compliance. Combining the implants with the levonorgestrel intrauterine contraceptive device, which theoretically has fewer systemic side-effects, may overcome this problem. This option should only be considered if her premenstrual syndrome is very severe and other options have failed.

An effective option is bilateral oophorectomy. This is effective but will require oestrogen HRT, which, being unopposed, should not be associated with reoccurrence of the symptoms. The selection of patients for this radical procedure is important and GnRH analogues may be useful in this regard. If her symptoms are eliminated over a period of 3 months on this regimen, then oophorectomy would be successful.

Non-SSRI antidepressants and anxiolytics have been shown to alleviate one or more symptoms but a significant number of women discontinue treatment because of the unwanted side-effects such as drowsiness, nausea, anxiety and headaches.

The use of treatment regimens such as evening primrose oil, vitamin E and pyridoxine may alleviate her symptoms, but the efficacy of these non-hormonal regimens is unpredictable. However, a combination of these with psychotherapy may be associated with better results.

Further reading

O'Brien PM, Ismail KMK, Dimmock P (2003) Premenstrual syndrome. In: Shaw RW, Soutter WP, Stanton SL (eds) *Gynaecology*, 3rd edn. Edinburgh: Churchill Livingstone, pp. 401–13.

3

Termination of pregnancy and early pregnancy complications

1. Critically appraise the methods of contraception you may offer a 21-year-old woman following a termination of pregnancy at 12 weeks' gestation. (20 marks)

2. You suspect that a 26-year-old nulligravida has had an incomplete septic miscarriage. (a) Describe the important clinical signs that will support your diagnosis. (5 marks) (b) What investigations will you undertake? (4 marks) (c) How will you treat this patient? (7 marks) (d) What complications may she develop if not properly managed? (4 marks)

3. Miss O wishes to have a termination of pregnancy. She has read that this can be done either surgically or medically. How will you counsel her about the (a) surgical (6 marks) and (b) medical (8 marks) options? (c) Describe how you will medically terminate her pregnancy if she is 10 weeks. (6 marks)

4. Women undergoing a termination of pregnancy are at an increased risk of complications of genital *Chlamydia trachomatis*. (a) Explain the rationale for screening and treating for this infection. (8 marks) (b) Discuss the benefits of screening all these women for *C. trachomatis* at the time of the procedure. (6 marks) (c) Critically appraise the various approaches to its therapeutic prevention. (8 marks)

5. A 26-year-old woman presents with 6 weeks' amenorrhoea and a slight vaginal bleed. She had an ultrasound scan which did not show any free fluid in the peritoneal cavity but identified a complex right adnexal mass with a fetal heartbeat seen. These appearances were diagnostic of an ectopic pregnancy. Critically appraise your management of this patient. (20 marks)

1. Critically appraise the methods of contraception you may offer a 21-year-old woman following a termination of pregnancy at 12 weeks' gestation. (20 marks)

Common mistakes

- Listing all the methods of contraception available and failing to make references to the patient
- Discussing sterilisation as the only method
- Discussing every method of contraception
- Referring the woman to a family-planning specialist for advice

A good answer will include some or all of these points

- Combined oral contraceptive pill:
  - Effective with several advantages:
    - Regulates periods and effective if having heavy periods (menorrhagia)
    - Requires motivation as needs to be taken daily
    - Reduces the risk incidence of pelvic inflammatory disease (PID)
  - Contraindications have to be excluded:
    - Thrombophilia
    - Focal migraine headaches
    - Previous venous thromboembolism (VTE)
    - VTE on the pill
    - Active or recent oestrogen-dependent cancer
- Barrier methods:
  - Provide immediate contraception
  - Best if not in a regular relationship
  - Efficacy depends on how they are used – high failure rate linked to method failure
  - Protect against sexually transmitted infections (STIs)
  - Contraindicated in those with allergies to the materials used in the barrier methods
- Intrauterine contraceptive device:
  - Inserted at the time of termination or a month after with the next period
  - Advantage – efficacy is independent of patient (does not have to remember)
  - May be associated with menstrual irregularities, which could result in removal
  - Perforation and expulsion rates high with insertions at termination
  - Increased risk of PID
- Progestogen-only contraceptives:
  - Mini-pill – effective but requires patient's compliance
  - May be associated with unacceptable irregular bleeding
  - Side-effects – progestogens

- Long-acting reversible hormonal contraceptives – Mirena®, Implanon® or Norplant® depending on availability, depot medroxyprogesterone acetate (Depo-Provera®):
  - Effective, no need to remember to take daily
  - Monthly injections require going for injection
  - Menstrual abnormalities
  - Progestogenic side-effects
- Surgery – sterilisation – unsuitable for this 21-year-old

Sample answer

The type of contraception offered to this patient will depend on her needs, her perceived ability to comply with the method and any contraindications. The range of options available includes barrier methods, the combined oral contraceptive pill, the progestogen-only contraceptive pill, intrauterine contraceptive devices and sterilisation. Each of these methods must be considered within the context of its advantages, potential complications or disadvantages and the anticipated problems in this young woman, especially those of compliance and suitability.

The first method is the combined oral contraceptive pill. This is effective, but requires the patient to take the pills daily. Compliance is therefore an important factor in its effectiveness. Contraindications to the use of the combined oral contraceptive pill must initially be excluded. These include focal migraine headaches, thrombophilia and VTE. The advantage of this method of contraception is its ability to regulate irregular cycles, ameliorate the problem of menorrhagia and reduce the incidence of PID. This patient could start to take the oral contraceptive pill before her discharge from the hospital. However, if she is not well motivated this may not be the best method of contraception for her.

The second option is the barrier method of contraception. In this young woman this may be adequate, provided it is acceptable to her and her partner. The barrier method will provide immediate contraception, but the failure rate is high. The barrier method may be the patient's most suitable method of contraception if she is not in a regular relationship and therefore has no need for regular contraception. The added advantages of the barrier method are protection against STIs, no need to comply with daily administration and no systemic side-effects. In this patient, it could also be started immediately. The low efficacy of this method of contraception may be related to its application or to method failure itself. It is a method that is suitable for any couple, unless they have an allergy to the substances used in the device. This patient may depend on her partner for the success of this method and such a lack of complete control may present a disadvantage.

Although the intrauterine contraceptive device may be an option, it must be considered in the context of an increased risk of PID in a young woman. However, if the patient is married or in a stable relationship and is unable to tolerate any other method of contraception, this may be her only option. The main advantage is that she does not have to remember to take anything. It only has to be fitted once. In addition to the increased risk of PID if the patient has multiple sexual partners, there may also be an increased risk of menstrual abnormalities and an increased incidence of ectopic pregnancies (both independently of PID which may also present with these disorders). If this is her chosen method, the intrauterine contraceptive device could be inserted before the patient is discharged from hospital. However, inserting it at the time of termination is associated with higher perforation and expulsion rates.

Although sterilisation is an option, it is likely to be unsuitable, especially if the patient has not completed her family. If she has, this could be performed at the same time as the termination. It is an effective method, which does not require motivation on the part of the patient. However, she must understand that it is not always reversible and that the risk of ectopic gestation if it fails is higher. For a patient of this young age, this option should not be considered unless she demands it.

The last option is the progestogen-only contraceptive pill. The pill must be taken at the same time every day. The failure rate is higher and it is also associated with irregular vaginal bleeding. However, it may be used in patients who have a contraindication to oestrogens. Again, it may be started before the patient is discharged from hospital. Other progestogens, e.g. Depo-Provera® administered 3 monthly or subdermal implants (Norplant® or Implanon®) confer significant advantages over the mini-pill. There is no need for daily administration. However, the side-effects are similar and the implants require special skills for their insertion and removal. The Mirena® device is another progestogen option which, once inserted and tolerated, can remain effective for 5 years.

2. You suspect that a 26-year-old nulligravida has had an incomplete septic miscarriage. (a) Describe the important clinical signs that will support your diagnosis. (5 marks) (b) What investigations will you undertake? (4 marks) (c) How will you treat this patient? (7 marks) (d) What complications may she develop if not properly managed? (4 marks)

Common mistakes

- Defining/classifying miscarriages
- Listing all the methods available
- Treating a hypothetical patient
- Discussing the treatment of miscarriages in general
- Discussing the diagnosis of miscarriage

A good answer will include some or all of these points

(a) Describe the important clinical signs that will support your diagnosis. (5 marks)

- General examination findings:
  - Pyrexia, hypothermia
  - Hypotension, tachycardia, tachypnoea, delerious
  - Sweaty, cold and clammy extremities
- Abdomen:
  - Distended
  - Tender, guarding, rebound
- Pelvis:
  - Vagina – foul-smelling discharge, hot vagina, cervical os – opened with/without products, adnexal tenderness

(b) What investigations will you undertake? (4 marks)

- Full blood count (FBC)
- Group and save
- Urea and electrolytes
- Liver function test (LFT)
- Blood cultures if indicated
- Ultrasound scan – may not be necessary
- Swabs for microscopy culture and sensitivity (M/C/S)
- Products of conceptions – for histology

(c) How will you treat this patient? (7 marks)

- Intravenous fluids
- Broad-spectrum antibiotics – intravenously to cover Gram-negative, Gram-positive organisms and anaerobes (e.g. cefuroxime, metronidazole and gentamicin)
- Arrange evacuation (preferable after the start dose of antibiotics – precautions for haemorrhage; appropriate counselling about the risk of haemorrhage and proceeding to hysterectomy
- Observe in intensive care unit/high dependency unit (ICU/HDU) for at least 4–6 hours after evacuation – risk of Gram-negative septicaemia
- Continue with antibiotics for at least 5–7 days

(d) What complications may she develop if not properly managed? (4 marks)

- Treatment related – Asherman's syndrome
- Gram-negative septicaemia and septic shock
- Liver and renal failure
- Haemorrhage and disseminated intravascular coagulation (DIC)
- PID
- Infertility

Sample answer

(a) Describe the important clinical signs that will support your diagnosis. (5 marks)

The important clinical signs that will support the diagnosis include pyrexia on general examination. However, this may be absent and indeed some of the patients may be hypothermic if they have Gram-negative septicaemia. Other signs include tachycardia, hypotension and tachypnoea – features of shock. The patient may also be found to be delerious, sweaty, shivering (having rigors) or may have cold and clammy extremities.

The abdomen may be distended, tender and tympanic on percussion. There may be localised guarding with some rebound. Very occasionally there may be evidence of a collection, especially in the paracolic gutters.

A pelvic examination may reveal a foul-smelling vaginal discharge, a hot vagina and products of conception within the vagina or cervical os. The uterus may be enlarged and tender. Bilateral adnexal tenderness is a common sign and fullness in the posterior fornix and lateral fornices may be present.

(b) What investigations will you undertake? (4 marks)

These include a FBC (checking her haemoglobin as she may require blood transfusion), and the white cell count, which is likely to be raised. Blood should be grouped and saved. In some cases, there may be the need to cross-match at least 3–4 units of blood. The risk of haemorrhage following evacuation is higher than that following a non-septic miscarriage. Other investigations include urine for M/C/S, swabs of any discharge or products for M/C/S, blood cultures and a LFT. An ultrasound scan will confirm that the uterus contains products and may identify a pelvic collection.

(c) How will you treat this patient? (7 marks)

Once the diagnosis is confirmed, the potential complications and the need to be meticulous and aggressive in the management must be recognised. There is no place for conservative management of a septic incomplete miscarriage.

The definitive management of this patient is to evacuate the infected retained products of conception. Before the evacuation, she must be given broad-spectrum antibiotics to cover Gram-positive and Gram-negative organisms and anaerobic bacteria, and an aminoglycoside. The most commonly used antibiotics are a combination of metronidazole and a cephalosporin (cefalexin) and gentamicin. Before their administration swabs should be sent for M/C/S. These antibiotics must be administered intravenously and preferably for at least 8 hours before surgical evacuation. This is to minimise the risk of generalised septicaemia following the evacuation.

Because of the potential complications of a surgical evacuation in this patient, the procedure is best performed under general anaesthesia (GA). Prior to this, the patient should be counselled about potential complications, including septicaemia, haemorrhage (which may require transfusion and occasionally a hysterectomy) and Asherman's syndrome, which may be due to overzealous scraping of the endometrium.

The surgical procedure should be performed by an experienced clinician because of the danger of overzealous curetting. Ideally, it should be performed by suction rather than by curettage. It is also important to cover the procedure with intravenous Syntocinon® or Syntometrine®. This reduces the risk of haemorrhage and therefore the need for blood transfusion and, very occasionally, a hysterectomy.

Following the evacuation, the antibiotics should be continued for at least 5–7 days. It may be necessary to monitor her in an ICU/HDU for a few hours to days.

(d) What complications may she develop if not properly managed? (4 marks)

The complications of incompletely evacuating the uterus or not treating with appropriate antibiotics include generalised septicaemia, PID with associated tubo-ovarian abscess, infertility and chronic pelvic pain.

The surgical evacuation may result in a perforation or be followed by uncontrollable haemorrhage and a resulting hysterectomy. She may develop Gram-negative septicaemia and shock, liver and renal failure and ultimately may die. Haemorrhage may be secondary to DIC, perforation or infection penetrating the myometrium, making it difficult for it to contract and stem bleeding. Where the evacuation is poorly undertaken, the patient may develop Asherman's syndrome.

3. Miss O wishes to have a termination of pregnancy. She has read that this can be done either surgically or medically. How will you counsel her about the (a) surgical (6 marks) and (b) medical (8 marks) options? (c) Describe how you will medically terminate her pregnancy if she is 10 weeks. (6 marks)

Common mistakes

- Discussing the following
  - Complications of termination of pregnancy
  - Advantages of surgical termination
  - Use of oxytocic agents and ergometrine
  - Methods of cervical priming before surgical termination
  - Conservative methods

A good answer will include some or all of these points

How will you counsel her about the (a) surgical (6 marks) and (b) medical (8 marks) options?

- Surgical option:
  - Upper limit of gestation – 12–13 weeks in most units and not before 7 weeks
  - Legally can be done before 24 weeks but most units will not and specialised units may go up to 20 weeks. Recent debate in the UK about lowering the age of legal abortions to about 12 weeks, hence few units will undertake terminations after 12 weeks
  - Requires GA but can be done under regional
  - Preparation of cervix with prostaglandins (gemeprost or misoprostol, approx. 3 hours prior to surgery)
  - Dilatation and suction evacuation if not more than 12 weeks
  - Advantages:
    - Single procedure
    - No need for prolonged stay in hospital
    - Asleep and not conscious of procedure of abortion
  - Complications:
    - Trauma to the cervix
    - Perforation
    - Haemorrhage
    - Incomplete evacuation and infections
- Medical option:
  - Available to women up to 9 weeks' (63 days') gestation but not recommended for 9–14 weeks as incidence of incomplete abortion high
  - Antiprogestogen – RU486 (mifepristone) and cervical prostaglandins/oral prostaglandins
  - Need at least 36–48 hours for prostaglandin to be added

- Stays at home until need for prostaglandins
- Complete abortion achieved in over 95 per cent of cases
- Risk of incomplete abortion and need for surgical evacuation in 2–3 per cent of cases
- Risk of infections and haemorrhage from retained products, bleeding may continue for up to 20 days after the abortion
- Allergic or unexpected reaction from drugs
- Skilled staff to offer counselling and undertake procedure – specialised nurses
- No need for anaesthesia except analgesia for severe pain which may accompany the abortion
- Require a follow-up appointment around 2 weeks after the administration of prostaglandins (especially for the 5 per cent who do not pass an identifiable fetus and/placenta)

(c) Describe how you will medically terminate her pregnancy if she is 10 weeks. (6 marks)

- RU486 (mifepristone) 200 mg – antiprogesterone
- 36–48 hours later, admitted for misoprostol – 600–800 μg orally or vaginal gemeprost – 3 mg
- Admit onto day ward for misoprostol and monitoring
- After abortion, ultrasound to confirm uterus empty
- Counselling
- Ultrasound to confirm gestational age

Sample answer

(a) How will you counsel her about the surgical option? (6 marks)

Surgical termination of pregnancy may be performed in all units up to the gestational age of 12–13 weeks. It is not advisable to perform a surgical termination before 6 weeks as there is a significant risk of missing the pregnancy (i.e. the pregnancy continues after the procedure). Legally, a termination can be performed surgically up to 24 weeks but recent debate in the UK has been critical of the liberal attitude towards termination and there is an increasing recognition that the legal limit may be reduced. In a selected number of units surgical terminations may be performed up to 20 weeks by experts in late terminations. Although GA is commonly offered, this is not invariable. In this procedure, the cervix is dilated and products evacuated by use of a vacuum pump.

Complications include perforation of the uterus, cervical trauma and haemorrhage. Before surgical evacuation, prostaglandins, such as gemeprost, may be used to soften the cervix and therefore reduce the risk of complications such as cervical trauma. Although less likely, the uterus may not be completely evacuated. Where there is a bicornuate or double uterus only one horn may be evacuated and, if the pregnancy is in the other horn, it may continue. For this operation, expertise is required.

The advantages of surgical over medical termination include no need to stay in hospital for long periods, a guarantee that the procedure will be performed, in most cases completely, and the less likely risk of a second evacuation. However, if the patient has an infection in the lower genital tract, this may spread easily into the upper genital tract.

(b) How will you counsel her about the medical options? (8 marks)

The medical method of termination is effective, but case selection is vital. It is recommended for pregnancies up to 93 days (9 weeks) and after 12 weeks but not recommended for 9–12 weeks. However, in practice it is possible to medically terminate pregnancies at this gestational age range. This is achieved with a combination of misoprostol (prostaglandin) and RU486 (mifepristone) – an antiprogestogen. Usually, the mifepristone is administered 36–48 hours before the misoprostol, which may be administered orally or vaginally. The dose of the misoprostol varies from 200 to 600 µg. This vaginal administration commonly starts off the contractions. This method is associated with a success rate of over 95 per cent.

The main advantage of this method is that the patient stays at home after the mifepristone until she attends for the prostaglandin. In addition, there is no need for GA.

The disadvantage of this method is that of time spent in hospital waiting for the process to be completed. This may take a few hours or sometimes a day or two. There is no guarantee that the patient will not proceed to surgery. A surgical procedure (often under GA) to complete the process may be required in less than 5 per cent of cases. Other complications include bleeding secondary to incomplete evacuation of the uterus, infections and allergic reaction to the medication. Medical termination requires skilled nursing staff to support the service and counsel the women. In addition, there should be provision for follow-up to ensure that there are no added complications. For most cases, this can be arranged 2 weeks after the procedure.

(c) Describe how you will medically terminate her pregnancy if she is 10 weeks. (6 marks)

The first step will be confirmation of the gestational age by ultrasound scan. She is then counselled about the procedure and following consenting, will be given mifepristone (200 mg) to be taken in the hospital. An appointment is then made for a visit to the unit 36–48 hours later when she is given 600 µg of misoprostol vaginally. She is observed on the unit where she will remain until products of conception have passed and bleeding has settled. On discharge, she is provided with an information leaflet containing details of when to report back to the unit or to call for emergency services. Such information will include bleeding, abdominal cramps and temperature. It is good practice to perform an ultrasound scan to confirm that the uterus is indeed empty but this may not be necessary if she is clinically well.

4. Women undergoing a termination of pregnancy are at an increased risk of complications of genital *Chlamydia trachomatis.* (a) Explain the rationale for screening and treating for this infection. (8 marks) (b) Discuss the benefits of screening all these women for *C. trachomatis* at the time of the procedure. (6 marks) (c) Critically appraise the various approaches to its therapeutic prevention. (8 marks)

Common mistakes

- Discussing the screening for *C. trachomatis* in general
- Enumerating the complications of *C. trachomatis* infection and how to recognise them
- Discussing all the World Health Organization criteria for screening for *C. trachomatis*
- Discussing the procedure for termination of pregnancy
- Aseptic precautions to avoid the risk of ascending infections

A good answer will include some or all of these points

(a) Explain the rationale for screening and treating for this infection. (8 marks)

- *C. trachomatis* is the most common STI in the UK and is associated with tubal infertility
- Common in single women
- Prevalence could be as high as 10–15 per cent of single women undergoing termination of pregnancy
- Surgical procedures such as termination increase the risk of ascending infections and pelvic inflammation
- Most are asymptomatic
- Treatment is cheap and effective
- Spread by men who are asymptomatic

(b) Discuss the benefits of screening all these women for C. trachomatis at the time of the procedure. (6 marks)

- Screening a high-risk group – ensures that those with the infection are identified
- Opportunity for treating those with infection
- Eliminates treating everyone, irrespective of whether infected or not
- Cost effective
- Recall or contact tracing – possible since treatment will be offered only to those who are screened positive
- Resources targeted to screen positive individuals
- Implications of a positive test – may result in break-up of relationships

(c) Critically appraise the various approaches to its therapeutic prevention. (8 marks)

- Options:
  - Single dose of azithromycin prior to termination to all
  - Treating only those who screen positive – identified at first consultation
  - Screen and then offer a single dose of azithromycin
- Single dose at the time of termination of pregnancy:
  - Advantages – ensures that everyone with the infection is treated
  - Expensive as many uninfected will be treated
  - Without screening, contact tracing will be impossible and the risk of reinfection high
  - Lost opportunity to educate on the risk of STI to those infected
- Treating only those who screen positive:
  - This involves screening at the first consultation
  - Positive cases treated prior to termination of pregnancy to reduce the risk of ascending infection
  - Positive cases – contact tracing before termination of pregnancy
  - Education on consequences
- Screen and then offer single dose of azithromycin:
  - Ideal as ensures targeted treatment
  - At the time of termination of pregnancy, contact tracing would have been undertaken and treatment also offered
  - Education on consequences and prevention

Sample answer

(a) Explain the rationale for screening and treating for this infection. (8 marks)

Chlamydia trachomatis is the most common STI in the UK. It commonly affects the young and it is associated with PID and tubal infertility in a large proportion of these patients. The prevalence of this infection in populations undergoing termination of pregnancy has been reported to vary between 10 and 15 per cent. In some populations, especially in the inner cities, this may be as high as 25–30 per cent. During termination there is the added risk of ascending infection, which may result in tubo-ovarian disease and infertility. In randomised controlled trials where screening for this infection before termination has been performed, the incidence of operative morbidity has been reduced drastically. Therefore, the question is whether all women attending for a termination of pregnancy should be screened for this infection. Most men as well as a large number of women are asymptomatic. Screening therefore has the potential to identify these subgroups – especially as treatment is cheap and effective.

(b) Discuss the benefits of screening all these women for C. trachomatis at the time of the procedure. (6 marks)

Universal screening is justified if the condition is sufficiently common and there is a recognised diagnostic technique. There also has to be a therapy for the condition and its sequelae must be well recognised. The screening method must also be reliable and the risk of false-positive or false-negative tests must be low. In addition, the test must do no harm. In the case of *C. trachomatis*, it is sufficiently common, there are well recognised sequelae if infection goes untreated and the test itself is sensitive and specific. If identified, the treatment is effective and causes minimal harm. Therefore, the case for screening is made.

Screening all women before termination allows infected patients to be identified and treated and, therefore, postoperative morbidity of ascending infections minimised. It also provides an opportunity for counselling about protection against other STIs and their sequelae. For the screen-positive patients, there is the added advantage of contact tracing and treatment, especially as this infection is notoriously asymptomatic in males and sometimes in females. Treatment is effective and cheap; screening and treating will significantly reduce not only morbidity but spread by contact tracing and treatment.

Screening at the time of termination is cost effective because the patients are more likely to comply. It is best to do the screening when the patients are first seen for consultation, so that by the time they come for the procedure, the results are available. However, with pressure on services for quick delivery of termination services, the results may not be available at the time of termination. This will require additional manpower to follow up the patients and make appointments for contact tracing and treatment. This may be the disadvantage of screening before treating but treating everyone will ensure that no case is missed.

Whether screening should be available before termination is debatable. There is an argument for the procedure to be undertaken and an antibiotic against *C. trachomatis* administered after having screened the patient, but before the results are available. This may not be very cost effective, as over 50 per cent of patients will receive expensive antibiotics without needing them. However, it has been argued that this reduces morbidity from surgery. The ideal set-up would be to screen patients on their first visit and ensure that results are available before termination. This way, those who are screen positive will receive antibiotics and also be channelled to the appropriate genitourinary medicine clinic for contact tracing. The main disadvantage of universal screening is cost. Advantages include reducing morbidity, prevention of tubal infertility (and therefore the cost of its subsequent treatment) and contact tracing and treatment, especially for those who are asymptomatic. Taking all these advantages into consideration, it may be argued that this approach is cheap and cost effective.

The other option would be to offer antibiotics against *C. trachomatis* to every woman attending for termination of pregnancy. Although this may overcome the problem and cost of screening, it would inevitably result in failure to trace contacts and, therefore, would not reduce the spread of the disease, even to the same individual by her male counterpart. Even if it is argued that both partners should be treated, an assumption is made that the partner is the source of the infection and so there will certainly be many cases missed. Although there may be some value in this approach, especially as the cost of treating the infection with tetracycline or its derivative is very cheap, it is not justifiable.

Although screening, treating and contact tracing are ideal, they may also pose some problems. Contact tracing, for example, is a very sensitive problem and one that may result in broken relationships, especially if the male partner is screen negative. In addition, additional resources will be required to trace contacts and to provide adequate education and treatment. If the screening of all women is not to be advocated, what is the alternative? Selective screening of at-risk groups will definitely identify a large proportion of affected women and their partners. However, the assumption that low-risk populations are not at risk must be discounted. Although the prevalence of this infection in the low-risk population is low, it must be recognised that only a small proportion of women attending for termination of pregnancy come from this low-risk population. It may, therefore, be argued that selective screening could be seen as discriminatory, and since the proportion from the low-risk group is small, it may be beneficial to screen everyone. One option would be to screen everyone, to give antibiotics to the high-risk group, but to delay treating the low-risk group until test results are available. Whatever the argument, screening for *C. trachomatis* has more benefits than disadvantages and therefore, on balance, it is best offered to all women attending for termination of pregnancy.

(c) Critically appraise the various approaches to its therapeutic prevention. (8 marks)

The options for therapeutic interventions include a single dose of azithromycin to everyone prior to the termination of pregnancy (with or without screening), treating only those who are screen positive or screening and then offering treatment to those who are screen positive.

A single dose of azithromycin at the time of termination ensures that everyone with the infection is treated. If this is done with screening, it will ensure that contacts of those who are positive are traced and treated. However, this may be difficult as some of those with positive results may refuse to return for follow-up. This universal approach to prophylaxis is expensive as a large number of uninfected patients will be treated. Additionally, failure to contact trace and treat, effectively results in failure to break the infection cycle and the patient is more likely to be reinfected by her partner or others.

5. A 26-year-old woman presents with 6 weeks' amenorrhoea and a slight vaginal bleed. She had an ultrasound scan which did not show any free fluid in the peritoneal cavity but identified a complex right adnexal mass with a fetal heartbeat seen. These appearances were diagnostic of an ectopic pregnancy. Critically appraise your management of this patient. (20 marks)

Common mistakes

- Take a history and perform a physical examination
- Confirm the diagnosis of ectopic pregnancy
- Serial beta-human chorionic gonadotropin (βhCG) estimation
- Perform a transvaginal ultrasound scan
- Offer conservative observational treatment

A good answer will include some or all of these points

- The diagnosis is clearly that of an ectopic pregnancy
- Counselling must be the first step – inform the patient of the diagnosis, the consequences and the management plans
- Treatment options:
  - Surgery – salpingectomy/salpingotomy or milking it out; injection of hyperosmolar solutions, prostaglandins:
    - Laparoscopic
    - Laparotomy
    - Where the surgical approach is salpingostomy or milking, this must be followed up by serial serum βhCG
  - Methotrexate; intramuscular (i.m.) injection of methotrexate:
    - Follow-up with βhCG and ultrasound scan whenever it is indicated – may later require surgery (laparotomy)
- Follow-up
- Contraception:
  - Avoid the intrauterine contraceptive device
  - Combined oral contraceptive pill appropriate
  - Mirena® can be used as well
- Recurrence risk:
  - Risk of recurrence increased 10-fold
  - Missed period, should report early for an opportunity to confirm an intrauterine pregnancy and also if ectopic, allow early surgery

Sample answer

The diagnosis of an ectopic pregnancy in this patient has been confirmed by an ultrasound scan showing an adnexal mass with a fetal heartbeat seen. Her management must focus on treating the ectopic gestation and should include adequate counselling and discussion of the treatment options available to her.

The first important step in this patient's management is adequate counselling. The diagnosis must be explained to her. She needs to have a diagnostic laparoscopy. This procedure will allow assessment of the size of the pregnancy, the other Fallopian tube and may, in fact, allow treatment to be offered. It could be argued that diagnostic laparoscopy should only be undertaken if laparoscopic treatment or conservative medical treatment are options acceptable to the patient. If she elects to have a laparotomy, or if the expertise for laparoscopic surgery is unavailable, there is some justification in proceeding straight to a laparotomy. The advantage of this is that it bypasses prolonged anaesthesia and the added complications of laparoscopy, which include bowel injury, gas embolism and damage to major arteries resulting in massive haemorrhage.

If the patient has completed her family or has been sterilised, the option for her will be a salpingectomy. This can be performed laparoscopically or at laparotomy. The advantages of laparoscopic surgery include reduced hospital stay, reduced morbidity from large abdominal incisions and reduced risk of complications, such as wound infection. However, the patient must understand that not every case may be treated laparoscopically. If, for example, the ectopic pregnancy is cornual or is too large to be dealt with laparoscopically, a laparotomy must be performed. If she has not completed her family, attempts at conserving the Fallopian tubes will be advisable. The treatment of choice will be a salpingotomy. This involves incising the antemesenteric site of the Fallopian tube and removing the ectopic pregnancy. Any bleeding from the bed of the pregnancy may then be coagulated. There is no need to close the linear incision on the Fallopian tube. Although this has the advantage of preserving the Fallopian tube, the patient must be followed up with serial βhCG measurements to ensure that all the trophoblastic tissues have been removed.

Another conservative option for this patient is injection of the ectopic pregnancy with methotrexate or a hyperosmolar solution, such as prostaglandins or 50 per cent glucose. However, for this to be performed the gestational sac diameter should be less than 2 cm. In this case this is unlikely, as the fetal heartbeat was seen on ultrasound scan. If, indeed, a decision is made to offer this treatment, serial monitoring with βhCGs must be offered. The patient must also understand that with this type of treatment there is a chance that she may have to undergo a further laparotomy if the gestational sac does not gradually resolve. If this patient elects for medical treatment of her ectopic gestation, she could be offered i.m. methotrexate, but it is likely that the size of the gestational sac may negate this type of treatment. However, if it is offered, the patient must be prepared to undergo serial βhCG monitoring and, if necessary, repeat methotrexate or subsequent laparoscopic or laparotomy treatment for persisting disease.

The last option is a laparotomy if the ectopic pregnancy is not suitable for laparoscopic surgery. At surgery, she may either have a salpingectomy, a salpingotomy or milking of the ectopic pregnancy. Whichever option is offered will depend on her need for further pregnancies, the state of the Fallopian tube and the size of the ectopic gestation. Salpingectomy will be performed if she does not desire children or the Fallopian tube is significantly damaged. However, the other Fallopian tube must be assessed to ensure that salpingectomy is not performed on the better tube and a severely damaged one left behind. This treatment has the advantage of better exposure and an opportunity of dealing with other pelvic pathologies, such as ovarian cysts and adhesions. Although it may not be advisable to deal with adhesions at the time of surgery, this may be performed, depending on the type and location of the adhesions.

Whichever treatment option the patient is offered, she must be counselled about recurrence and advised on contraception. The intrauterine contraceptive device is contraindicated, whereas the recurrence risk is about 10 per cent. She must be advised about the need to report early in her next pregnancy and to use a barrier method of contraception if she is not in a regular relationship.

4

Benign uterine lesions and endometriosis

1. A 26-year-old nulligravida is diagnosed with multiple uterine fibroids. (a) Discuss the factors that will influence her treatment. (6 marks) (b) Comment critically on her options. (9 marks) (c) How will your management differ if she is found on examination to have a 4×5 cm fibroid polyp protruding through the cervix? (5 marks)

2. A 33-year-old woman presents with a 26-week size uterine fibroid. (a) What additional symptoms may she have presented with? (4 marks) (b) Justify your investigations of this patient. (5 marks) (c) Critically appraise her subsequent management if she has completed her family. (11 marks)

3. A 42-year-old human immunodeficiency virus (HIV) positive nulliparous woman presenting with menorrhagia is, on examination, found to have an 18-week size uterine fibroid and a haemoglobin (Hb) of 9.7 g/dL. (a) What issues must you take into consideration in planning her treatment? (6 marks) (b) Critically appraise her options. (10 marks) (c) If she elects to have uterine preserving surgery, how will you minimise blood loss at surgery? (4 marks)

4. Justify your management of a 41-year-old woman presenting with right iliac fossa cyclical pain of 2 years' duration. She had a hysterectomy and left salpingo-oophorectomy for endometriosis 3 years ago. (20 marks)

5. A diagnosis of endometriosis has been made in a 33-year-old nulligravida whose main symptom is painful and heavy periods. (a) Discuss briefly her management options. (14 marks) (b) How will her desire for pregnancy influence your choice of options? (6 marks)

6. A 30-year-old woman presents with a 2-year history of menorrhagia and deep dyspareunia. She is found on examination to have a uniformly bulky uterus with no other palpable masses. A pregnancy test is negative. (a) Justify the investigations you will undertake in this patient. (6 marks) (b) Discuss her management options, assuming that fibroids have been excluded. (14 marks)

1. A 26-year-old nulligravida is diagnosed with multiple uterine fibroids. (a) Discuss the factors that will influence her treatment. (6 marks) (b) Comment critically on her options. (9 marks) (c) How will your management differ if she is found on examination to have a 4×5 cm fibroid polyp protruding through the cervix? (5 marks)

Common mistakes

- Taking a history and performing a physical examination
- Assuming that the patient must have symptoms
- Listing the symptoms of uterine fibroids
- Simply listing the treatment options available for this patient
- Concentrating on the treatment of menstrual dysfunction only
- Listing the investigations that you will perform on a patient with uterine fibroids

A good answer will include some or all of these points

(a) Discuss the factors that will influence her treatment. (6 marks)

- Symptoms:
  - Asymptomatic and diagnosed incidentally?
  - Associated with menstrual problems – menorrhagia or polymenorrhagia, etc.
  - Pressure symptoms – bowel, urinary tract
  - Abdominal mass – increase in size – cosmetic, etc.
  - Associated with fertility – miscarriages, etc.
- Size and location of fibroids:
  - Single large fibroid, multiple
  - Subserous, intramural, submucous, cervical, etc.
- Desire for fertility:
  - Completed family or not?
- Expertise available for surgery:
  - Is myomectomy an option within the unit?
- Associated pathology:
  - Ovarian pathology, endometriosis, pelvic inflammatory disease (PID), adenomyosis, malignancies, etc.

(b) Comment critically on her options. (9 marks)

- Myomectomy:
  - Major surgery – risk of hysterectomy, adhesion formation, significant morbidity, recurrence, risk of anaesthesia, fibroids removed

- Hysterectomy:
  - Radical – removes all fibroids
  - Risk of anaesthesia
  - Must be with completion of family
  - Resultant amenorrhoea
- Uterine artery embolisation:
  - Available in specialised centres
  - Not suitable for those who have not completed family
  - Interventional radiology
  - May require surgery/has complications including infections
- Medical treatment: gonadotropin-releasing hormone (GnRH) agonists:
  - Only temporary effect
  - Risk of regrowth after stopping treatment
  - Side-effects – oestrogen deficiency
  - May be used as adjuvant to surgery

(c) How will your management differ if she is found on examination to have a 4 × 5 cm fibroid polyp protruding through the cervix? (5 marks)

- Treatment preferred – polypectomy if pedunculated (base possible to transfix)
- Otherwise – laser myomectomy, hysteroscopic myomectomy
- May require tamponade with balloon to stem haemorrhage

Sample answer

(a) Discuss the factors that will influence her treatment. (6 marks)

First, the symptoms she presented with will determine whether she has treatment or not. If fibroids were identified incidentally (e.g. during a routine examination for another gynaecological or non-gynaecological problem), then the best option may simply be observation. If on the other hand she was symptomatic, then the severity of the symptoms will influence the treatment she has and how soon this is offered. Heavy periods associated with anaemia, too frequent and heavy periods, pressure symptoms on the renal tract especially if associated with obstruction (hydronephrosis), associated infertility and the cosmetic effect of the fibroids are important factors that will not only influence the timing but type of treatment she is offered.

Other factors that will influence the timing and type of treatment include the size, number (single or multiple) and location (subserous, intramural or submucous) of the fibroids (i.e. the ease with which they could be removed surgically), her desire for fertility or whether her family is complete, the expertise available for conservative or radical surgery, associated pelvic pathology (e.g. endometriosis, PID, adhesions, adenomyosis and malignancies) and availability of facilities and expertise for interventional radiology (embolisation).

(b) Comment critically on her options. (9 marks)

If the patient is asymptomatic, there will be no need to offer her any treatment other than reassurance. This option avoids the side-effects of surgery and medical treatment. As the fibroids are likely to grow bigger, definitive treatment should be a future option, depending on symptoms.

If she has symptoms, definitive treatment will depend on the size and location of the fibroids, her desire to have (more) children and the facilities available in the unit. The first option will be surgery. This is more cost effective in a young patient, as medical treatment will only delay further growth of the fibroids. The different surgical options are myomectomy, hysteroscopic resection and a hysterectomy. Myomectomy, which can be performed by laparotomy or laparoscopy in a few centres, will remove most of the big fibroids and leave the uterus intact. The risk of this procedure is that of progression to a hysterectomy if there is severe and life-threatening haemorrhage. In addition, it may be complicated by adhesions, which may further compromise fertility in a woman who desires more children. Although this is expensive (requiring inpatient stay and general anaesthesia (GA)), it is an effective treatment option. It must be recognised that myomectomy may not remove all the fibroids and those left behind may regrow. For most patients, the operation will be laparotomy, but where the fibroids are small and are subserous, this may be performed through laparoscopy at some highly specialised centres.

Where the patient is unsuitable for surgery or is reluctant to have surgery, anti-oestrogens such as danazol or GnRH analogues (Zoladex® or Decapeptyl®) will be the treatment of choice. These are associated with menopausal side-effects but can result in a reduction in the size of the fibroids of between 40 and 60 per cent. Danazol has several side-effects including poor compliance and is generally not recommended for use in the UK. The severe side-effects of GnRH agonists may make them unacceptable. If the patient wants to have a family, treatment has to be completed before she embarks on a pregnancy. For this young woman, this may not be an effective treatment option. It may, however, be used preoperatively to minimise blood loss at myomectomy and to reduce the size of the fibroids. Unfortunately, it may make the myomectomy difficult.

The last option is uterine artery embolisation. Although this technique is in the early stages and the Royal College of Obstetricians and Gynaecologists only recommend it as a treatment option in units as part of research, preliminary results indicate that it is an effective treatment and one that will not compromise the fertility of the patient. However, there are reported fatalities with this option and its long-term effects have yet to be evaluated.

(c) How will your management differ if she is found on examination to have a 4 × 5 cm fibroid polyp protruding through the cervix? (5 marks)

Where there is a cervical fibroid polyp, she should be offered a polypectomy alone or with a myomectomy (hysteroscopic or laparotomy) if there are other symptomatic fibroids. The polypectomy could be performed by simple surgical excision after tying the base, or with laser. The latter option will require a hysteroscopy which may be technically difficult with a large polyp protruding through the cervix. A complication of the polyp is erosion and infection.

Where this is the case, a broad-spectrum antibiotic must be offered to offset the risk of infections. Where the patient is anaemic or unable to tolerate surgery immediately, she could be given a GnRH agonist. Whatever the surgical approach, bleeding from the base is a common complication which may be managed with a balloon tamponade.

2. A 33-year-old woman presents with a 26-week size uterine fibroid. (a) What additional symptoms may she have presented with? (4 marks) (b) Justify your investigations of this patient. (5 marks) (c) Critically appraise her management if she has completed her family. (11 marks)

Common mistakes

- Assuming the patient has completed her family
- Management depends on whether or not the fibroids are symptomatic!
- Offering laparoscopic myomectomy/hysteroscopic resection – morcellation
- Use of antifibrinolytic agents to treat fibroids
- Assuming that she has menstrual problems
- Prostaglandin synthetase inhibitors – ineffective
- Failure to justify in part (b) and critically appraise in part (c)

A good answer will include some or all of these points

(a) What additional symptoms may she have presented with? (4 marks)

- These fibroids are very large and are therefore likely to be symptomatic
- Symptoms include menorrhagia, pressure symptoms, miscarriage (spontaneous or recurrent), infertility or subfertility (information to be gleaned from a brief history)
- Pain – from torsion or infarction or infection

(b) Justify your investigations of this patient. (5 marks)

- Hb – anaemia
- Blood group and save serum – will require surgery and may be transfused if anaemic from heavy bleeding
- intravenous urogram (IVU)/ultrasound scan – to exclude urinary tract obstruction; midstream specimen of urine – to exclude urinary tract infection (UTI)
- Urea and electrolytes (U&Es) – if obstructive (pressure effects on ureters, may be associated with early renal insufficiency)

(c) Critically appraise her subsequent management if she has completed her family. (11 marks)

- Completed family and accepts option: total abdominal hysterectomy – curative, but associated with morbidity and mortality; GA and the risks
- Conservative: myomectomy – unlikely to remove all fibroids; associated morbidity; may proceed to total abdominal hysterectomy; preoperative treatment with GnRH analogues – reduces vascularity and size. Makes shelving difficult. Side-effects of GnRH analogues

- Embolisation – interventional radiology offered on outpatient basis and without GA. Complications include failure to reduce the size of the fibroid, recurrence, infections, pain, haemorrhage and death.

Sample answer

(a) What additional symptoms may she have presented with? (4 marks)

The fibroids in this woman are large and therefore unlikely to be asymptomatic. The symptoms with which she may have presented include menorrhagia, pressure on her bladder, ureter, bowel or blood vessels, infertility/subfertility or an abdominal mass. If the fibroids are complicated then they may present with pain secondary to infection, torsion or infection. Very rarely, fibroids may present for the first time with pressure symptoms on the leg veins (oedema of the legs) or pelvic and/or deep vein thrombosis.

(b) Justify your investigations of this patient. (5 marks)

A full blood count (FBC) will exclude anaemia and polycythaemia, which may complicate fibroids and increase the risk of thromboembolism during surgery. The absence of anaemia does not exclude this condition, especially if the patient has been receiving iron supplementation. Blood should be grouped and saved as she may require transfusion to correct either anaemia or haemorrhage during surgery. Urine microscopy will exclude UTIs, whereas U&Es will exclude kidney compromise. The latter may be secondary to ureteric obstruction, the presence of which will necessitate early intervention to avoid further renal compromise. However, a normal renal function test does not exclude obstruction. This can easily be identified by ultrasound scan or magnetic resonance imaging (MRI) of the abdomen, specifically of the kidneys.

(c) Critically appraise her management if she has completed her family. (11 marks)

Having completed her family, the treatment of choice will be an abdominal hysterectomy. This will remove the fibroids with no risk of recurrence. She will need to have a midline incision with the associated risk of incisional hernia. Hysterectomy is associated with a significant morbidity related to the surgery and GA, although there is no reason why the procedure cannot be undertaken under regional anaesthesia.

A myomectomy is an option where she does not wish to lose her uterus. In view of the size of the fibroids, this cannot be done laparoscopically. A laparotomy will be necessary. This procedure will only remove the obvious fibroids (visible and palpable ones). There is, therefore, the risk of smaller fibroids growing to a significant size to cause more symptoms. At the time of surgery, there is always the danger of proceeding to a hysterectomy if there is a life-threatening haemorrhage. Consent for a hysterectomy must therefore be obtained before a myomectomy. This procedure may be complicated by adhesions, which may further compromise fertility. The use of medical regimens such as danazol or GnRH analogues prior to myomectomy has been reported to minimise blood loss, but these may be associated with difficulties with shelving the fibroids and thus an increase in the risk of progression to hysterectomy.

If this woman is unsuitable for surgery, an interim measure may be the option of medical treatment with GnRH analogues or danazol. These agents will reduce the size of the fibroids by up to 60 per cent, but once treatment is discontinued the fibroids regrow. In addition, this treatment is likely to be discontinued after 6 months in view of the side-effects of anti-oestrogens on the musculoskeletal, genital, cardiovascular, metabolic and haematological systems, although add-back therapy may obviate some of these symptoms. Unfortunately, these treatment regimens cannot be continued indefinitely.

The last option for this patient is uterine artery embolisation. This will be a more acceptable option if she is a surgical risk. It does not require GA and can be performed as an outpatient procedure. The patient must accept the risk of failure and recurrence of the fibroids. Complications include abdominal pain, pyrexia, infections haemorrhage and, occasionally, death.

3. A 42-year-old HIV positive nulliparous woman presenting with menorrhagia is, on examination, found to have an 18-week size uterine fibroid and an Hb of 9.7 g/dL. (a) What issues must you take into consideration in planning her treatment? (6 marks) (b) Critically appraise her options. (10 marks) (c) If she elects to have uterine preserving surgery, how will you reduce blood loss at surgery? (4 marks)

Common mistakes

- Management of HIV/counselling pre-pregnancy
- List treatment options – without critically appraising
- Debate treatment/management options: no need to mention MRI/IVU; ineffective medical treatments, such as mefenamic acid, tranexamic acid, Mirena® coil, resection, vaginal hysterectomy
- Unhelpful: history and duration of symptoms/intermenstrual bleeding, duration of HIV, etc.; critically appraise – what is the question asking?

A good answer will include some or all of these points

(a) What issues must you take into consideration in planning her treatment? (6 marks)

- Anaemia:
  - Caused by heavy periods related to the fibroids
  - Treatment of fibroid will improve anaemia but surgery should be undertaken with an improved Hb
- HIV infection:
  - Risk of transmission to staff
  - Immunocompromised status increases risk of morbidity – infections, etc.
- Parity:
  - May require children – natural or assisted – risk of HIV to children
- Size of fibroids:
  - Quite big and may be causing pressure effects on ureter – hence need for urgent treatment

(b) Critically appraise her options. (10 marks)

- Medical treatment:
  - GnRH agonist, danazol
  - Temporary effects only – may allow bleeding to reduce and therefore improve prior to surgery
  - Could be used prior to myomectomy
  - Duration – 6 months and effect is temporary – fibroids tend to regrow. Unlikely to be very effective for fibroid of this size

- Since fibroids shrink after menopause, in this 42-year-old, this option may be acceptable until menopause sets it
- Interventional radiology:
  - Uterine artery embolisation – not for women who are still planning to have a family
  - May not be effective, especially for such large fibroids
  - Requires expertise
  - Associated complications – infection
- Myomectomy:
  - Removes all the fibroids that are obvious (usually >1 cm)
  - Associated with increased risk of hysterectomy, haemorrhage
  - Fibroids not removed may regrow

(c) If she were to have uterine preserving surgery, how will you minimise blood loss at surgery? (4 marks)

- Preoperative GnRH agonist/danazol – problems with shelving fibroids
- At the time of surgery:
  - Shirodkar's clamp, Bonney's myomectomy clamp
  - Rubber tourniquet
  - Vasopressins
  - Transfixing of the uterine arteries

Sample answer

(a) What issues must you take into consideration in planning her treatment? (6 marks)

Amongst the important considerations in planning her treatment are her anaemia, her HIV status, parity and the size of her fibroids. The anaemia is likely to have been caused by the heavy periods secondary to her fibroids. Treating the fibroids will undoubtedly correct the anaemia. The best approach to removing the fibroids will be surgery and for this her anaemia needs some form of correction. Her HIV status poses an important dilemma for the clinician. She presents a significant risk to staff and, as she is likely to be immunocompromised, she will have an increased risk of acquired infections, especially in hospital following invasive management.

She is nulliparous and is desirous of children; conserving the uterus will have to be considered in planning her treatment. The size, number and location of her fibroids will determine not only the type of treatment but the ease with which this can be offered, especially surgery or interventional radiology.

(b) Critically appraise her options. (10 marks)

The definitive treatment will depend on the complications that require urgent treatment, and the patient's fertility needs. As her Hb is low, the first and most important stage in her management will be the provision of haematinic agents to effectively correct her anaemia.

In view of the HIV, anaemia and the size of the fibroids, medical options will be the best approach in the first instance. These could be in the form of danazol (not recommended in the UK) or GnRH analogues. GnRH analogues will downregulate the pituitary gland and therefore induce amenorrhoea. This treatment is expensive but, if effective, provides the best cost effective treatment for this condition. Therefore, this will be the first line of management for this patient. However, she may discontinue this treatment because of menopausal symptoms. If this is the case, add-back therapy could be added. GnRH analogues are not advised for longer than 6 months unless combined with add-back therapy, as taking them may induce osteopenia. However, they could reduce the size of the fibroid by as much as 60 per cent, which will benefit further surgery if it is considered. As the woman is 42, it is possible to maintain her on this regimen and avoid surgery. Unfortunately, once the GnRH therapy is discontinued, the fibroids will regrow.

If medical management fails, surgery will be the option of choice. The definitive surgery will depend on the patient's fertility needs. If she does not want children, a hysterectomy will be the operation of choice. However, prior to this, her anaemia must be corrected. This could be through a combination of GnRH analogues to reduce the size of the fibroids and vascularity, and also to create a state of amenorrhoea therefore allowing her Hb to rise. The advantage of hysterectomy is that it is straightforward with a reduced risk of transmitting the disease to staff compared to the risk involved with myomectomy. It is the operation of choice as it will remove the fibroids and avoid recurrence of the anaemia. Myomectomy will be the operation of choice if she desires children. However, apart from the increase risk of transmitting HIV to staff, there is always the risk of proceeding to a hysterectomy.

In this patient, uterine artery embolisation is probably one of the best options. It is associated with minimal risk of transmitting HIV to staff and reduces the risk of cross-hospital infection to the patient. Unfortunately, this procedure does not have long-term follow-up data to assess its efficacy. It is also mainly available in tertiary centres where research is continuing. In this patient, this treatment will be offered as the first option if medical options fail. Whatever treatment, the genitourinary medicine team must be involved in her care.

(c) If she elects to have uterine preserving surgery, how will you minimise blood loss at surgery? (4 marks)

Blood loss at surgery could be minimised by treating her with GnRH agonist for 3 months prior to surgery. This has been shown not only to shrink the fibroids but also to reduce vascularity and therefore blood loss at the time of surgery. Unfortunately this is associated with an increased difficulty in shelving the fibroids and therefore a greater risk of hysterectomy. At the time of surgery, the options are ligating the uterine arteries, or using a Shirodkar or Bonney's myomectomy clap to apply temporary occlusion of the uterine arteries until after the fibroids have been removed and the cavity obliterated. Where none of these is available, a rubber tourniquet could be applied in the same way. Finally, or using vasopressins injected round the fibroids has been shown to reduce the blood loss. Meticulous attention to haemostasis and losing the cavity of the enucleated fibroids is an effective option at the time of surgery.

4. Justify your management of a 41-year-old woman presenting with right iliac fossa cyclical pain of 2 years' duration. She had a hysterectomy and left salpingo-oophorectomy for endometriosis 3 years ago. (20 marks)

Common mistakes

- Taking a history and physical examination to exclude PID
- Managing the patient as if she had chronic pelvic pain syndrome
- Treating her for bowel problems
- Ignoring the information about previous endometriosis
- Assuming that a pelvic examination and other investigations have been made and the diagnosis confirmed
- Asking about the history of sexually transmitted infections and discussing their differentials
- Failing to consider differential diagnoses
- Not justifying

A good answer will include some or all of these points

- Most likely recurrent endometriosis
- Confirmation of diagnosis:
  - Is the pain cyclical?
  - Examination – why? To detect masses, tenderness and induration – all clinical signs of endometriosis
  - Ultrasound – why? – diagnostic laparoscopy
  - ? Therapeutic trial of GnRH analogues
- Consider the differential diagnoses:
  - Ovarian cysts with or without either haemorrhage or torsion
  - Adhesions
  - Other pelvic pathology
- Treatment:
  - Medical – analgesics, reassurance, drugs for endometriosis (GnRH agonists, aromatase inhibitors)
  - Endometrioma (ovarian) – surgery
  - Ovarian cystectomy, oophorectomy
  - Surgery; hormone replacement therapy (HRT) if oophorectomy
  - Complications of surgery – risk of ureteric and bladder injuries

Sample answer

The most likely diagnosis in this patient is recurrent endometriosis. However, other differential diagnoses, such as ovarian pathology, bowel disorders and adhesions must be considered.

The diagnosis of the cause of the cyclical pain in this patient needs to be confirmed. In the first instance, more information about the nature of the pain is required. For endometriosis, a cyclical pain is typical, although not exclusive. Other associated symptoms of endometriosis that have to be excluded include cyclical urinary symptoms, bleeding from other possible endometriotic sites and, of course, symptoms of abdominal pathologies, such as irritable bowel syndrome.

A physical examination to identify signs of endometriosis or other pathologies will be undertaken next. The presence of an adnexal mass, adnexal tenderness or induration will be highly suggestive of endometriosis. Following this examination, investigations have to be undertaken to confirm the diagnosis and exclude other possible causes of pain. The two relevant investigations for this patient are ultrasound scan and a diagnostic laparoscopy. An ultrasound scan will identify an ovarian endometrioma or other ovarian pathologies which are not endometriotic, for example, a haemorrhagic ovarian cyst. The renal tract should also be assessed as there may be a ureteric obstruction secondary to endometriosis over the ureters.

A diagnostic laparoscopy will have to be undertaken to locate any recurrent endometriosis and ovarian endometriomata. The main concern with such a procedure in this patient is the risk of bowel injury. This is more likely in a patient who has had surgery for endometriosis. The laparoscopy will also exclude other ovarian pathologies, such as benign ovarian cysts, which may have other complications. Unfortunately, a diagnostic laparoscopy may not provide the diagnosis in this patient if she has adhesions, which may render the ovary inaccessible. Consideration must therefore be given to a therapeutic trial for endometriosis in the form of GnRH analogues for 2–3 months. If her symptoms improve during this time, the most likely cause of the cyclical pain is endometriosis. If it fails to rid the patient of her symptoms, the diagnosis is unlikely to be endometriosis.

Once the diagnosis is confirmed, the treatment of choice will be surgery. Where the patient is unsuitable for surgery, GnRH analogues should be offered for 6 months. These may be offered in the first instance without add-back therapy, although there is no evidence that such a combination at the outset reduces efficacy in endometriosis. The surgical options will be oophorectomy and adhesiolysis (if adhesions are present). Before surgery, the patient must be counselled appropriately on the complications associated with adhesions and the importance of HRT, which in her case will be long term. Symptomatic treatment may be useful if the patient is unsuitable for hormonal or surgical treatment. It is important to consider symptomatic relief, as this may be adequate in some cases. Potent analgesics may be sufficient, in which case other forms of therapy would be unnecessary. However, it is very likely that the patient's general practitioner will have tried this option unsuccessfully before referring her to the hospital.

5. A diagnosis of endometriosis has been made in a 33-year-old nulligravida whose main symptom is painful and heavy periods. (a) Discuss briefly her management options. (14 marks) (b) How will her desire for pregnancy influence your choice of options? (6 marks)

Common mistakes

- Discussing the symptoms of endometriosis and how to make a diagnosis
- The value of diagnostic laparoscopy in making a diagnosis
- The need for *in vitro* fertilisation and gamete intrafallopian transfer
- Total abdominal hysterectomy as treatment for her endometriosis
- Presentation with an abdominal mass – discussing the diagnosis and treatment
- Assuming that the endometriosis is mild/severe or moderate!
- Investigating for infertility

A good answer will include some or all of these points

(a) Discuss briefly her management options. (14 marks)

- The severity is important in tailoring treatment for this patient
- Options – symptom relief:
  - Medical treatment
  - Surgical treatment
- Symptom relief – best option – tranexamic acid and androgens: decrease menstrual loss (most effective treatment) and therefore may be combined with analgesics
- Medical treatment:
  - Combined oral contraceptive pill – provided no risk factors. Effective, cheap and provides contraception. However, side-effects
  - GnRH analogues – best value. Sprays/3-monthly depot – compliance not an issue with depot injections. Side-effects. Expensive
  - Danazol – side-effects, compliance may be poor. This is no longer a recommended treatment option in the UK because of side-effects on the ovaries
- The levonorgestrel intrauterine system (Mirena®)
- Surgery – laparoscopy:
  - Laser, diathermy, oophorectomy, uterosacral nerve division/excision
  - If heavy periods secondary to endometriosis, total abdominal hysterectomy
  - Treatment may achieve pregnancy

(b) How will her desire for pregnancy influence your choice of options? (6 marks)

- Medical treatment will not be an option except for symptom relief

- Surgery – treatment of choice for all stages of endometriosis
- Laparoscopic the best option
- Symptomatic relief – tranexamic acid and mefenamic acid
- Pregnancy will improve symptoms

Sample answer

(a) Discuss briefly her management options. (14 marks)

The management of this patient will depend to a large extent on the severity of her symptoms. She has two treatment options – surgery and medical therapy. The choice of treatment will be determined by the wishes of the patient, contraindications to some of the options, availability and acceptability.

For symptom relief alone, the best option will be the antifibrinolytic agent tranexamic acid, given as 1 g four times a day during menstruation. It is effective in decreasing menstrual loss (Bonnar and Sheppard, 1996). Although it may reduce blood loss, tranexamic acid is unlikely to reduce the severity of pelvic pain secondary to endometriosis. Combining it with a potent analgesic may therefore be more effective in symptom control. The only drawback of this option is the need to continue with the therapy for an indefinite period as it is symptomatic therapy rather than treatment for endometriosis. It may, therefore, not be the most cost-effective therapeutic regimen for this patient.

A combination of tranexamic acid and an androgen, such as danazol or gestrinone, may overcome the need to continue treatment indefinitely. The androgen acts at the level of the pituitary gland, hypothalamus and ovary to counteract the effect of oestrogens on the endometriosis. It may therefore lead to a significant regression of the endometriotic lesions and eventually to a significant improvement in clinical symptoms. The side-effects of androgens and poor compliance have resulted in its not being recommended for use in the UK; however, the less-androgenic alternative, gestrinone (Dimetriose®), may be associated with fewer side-effects and therefore better compliance. This combination is effective and negates the need for surgery. Given for 6 months, adequate response may be achieved in up to 70 per cent of patients. However, like other forms of treatment for endometriosis, the recurrence risk of the symptoms is approximately 40 per cent.

The combined oral contraceptive pill taken continuously (without the pill-free interval) is an effective, cheap alternative for this patient. It has the added advantage of offering contraception if it is necessary. There have to be no contraindications for this treatment. These include thrombophilias, focal migraines and previous venous thromboembolism. For this regimen, the patient has to be well motivated, as compliance is an important factor in its success. Side-effects, such as breakthrough bleeding, may affect its efficacy.

The most cost-effective medical treatment for this patient is GnRH analogues in the form of daily nasal sprays or monthly or 3-monthly depots. These will downregulate the pituitary gland and thus cause the endometriosis and associated biochemical changes in the peritoneum to regress. Treatment is usually for 6 months. Beyond this time limit, it is associated with oestrogen deficiency effects, such as osteopenia. To counteract this, add-back therapy in the form of oestrogens or Livial® maybe included and treatment prolonged. More recently, this combination is being offered from the outset and there is no evidence to suggest that it reduces the efficacy of GnRH analogues. Menopausal symptoms and preparations requiring frequent administration may affect compliance; however, with depot preparations, compliance tends not be an issue.

The levonorgestrel intrauterine system (Mirena®) is a suitable non-surgical option. This has been shown to be effective in approximately 70 per cent of minimal to moderate endometriosis, although the side-effect of irregular vaginal bleeding especially in the first 3–4 months may affect continuation rates. This device has the advantage that there is no need to remember to take drugs or injections on a regular basis and it is an effective contraception.

The surgical option (for this patient) is laparoscopic laser/diathermy of the endometriosis, division or total excision of the uterosacral ligaments or oophorectomy. Laparoscopic destruction of the endometriotic lesions is not typically considered a very effective treatment. This is because it is unlikely that all the lesions will be destroyed, especially as the clinical absence of endometriotic lesions does not exclude disease. Additionally, lesions on surfaces that do not lend themselves to destructive therapy are unlikely to be destroyed. A combination of these surgical and medical therapeutic options is likely to achieve the best results. Surgery is expensive, associated with complications and not very effective in isolation. Bilateral oophorectomy is the most effective treatment. In this 33-year-old woman, this should be considered as the last option. It should be offered with or without a hysterectomy. If she does not want children, a hysterectomy should be considered. Although at the outset, it is the most expensive option, it certainly produces the best results. However, the patient must be counselled on the need for prolonged HRT. Since this will take the form of continuous oestrogen, the risk of recurrence of the endometriosis is minimal.

(b) How will her desire for pregnancy influence your choice of options? (6 marks)

For this patient, medical treatment is not a suitable option. If she wishes to have medical options that may reduce disease severity and symptoms, then she cannot be pregnant during treatment. If she elects to have surgery, this will not only help with the symptoms but will improve the chances of a successful pregnancy. Surgery is recognised to improve fertility even in those with minimal to mild disease. In those with moderate to severe disease, surgery remains the best option.

Where radical surgery such as bilateral oophorectomy alone is contemplated she must understand that future pregnancies will require ovum donation. It is currently possible to superovulate followed by ova retrieval and storage but the subsequent successful pregnancy rates from this is estimated to be around 5 per cent. This is in its early stages and is likely to improve with time.

An alternative that must not be forgotten in this patient is pregnancy. If there is no reason for her to delay pregnancy, she could be encouraged on the basis that pregnancy will significantly improve her symptoms. This must be done with extreme caution, as difficulties in conceiving due to the endometriosis may cause extreme anxiety and generate more problems.

Reference

Bonnar J, Sheppard BC (1996) Treatment of menorrhagia during menstruation: randomised controlled trial of ethamsylate, mefenamic acid, and tranexamic acid. *BMJ* **313**: 579–82.

6. A 30-year-old woman presents with a 2-year history of menorrhagia and deep dyspareunia. She is found on examination to have a uniformly bulky uterus with no other palpable masses. A pregnancy test is negative. (a) Justify the investigations you will undertake in this patient. (6 marks) (b) Discuss her management options, assuming that fibroids have been excluded. (14 marks)

Common mistakes

- Take a history and do a physical examination
- Discussing the management of fibroids even though it clearly states that this has been excluded
- Discussing the differential diagnoses and how these can be excluded
- Managing the patient as if she has a pelvic abscess
- Discussing the treatment for endometrial carcinoma
- Listing the investigations and not discussing them – failure to justify these investigations
- Discussing the management of pregnancy – as a differential diagnosis

A good answer will include some or all of the following points

(a) Justify the investigations you will undertake in this patient. (6 marks)

- FBC – Hb may indicate anaemia
- Group and save serum
- Ultrasound scan of the pelvis – fibroids or adenomyosis (poor at diagnosing adenomyosis)
- MRI/computerised tomography scan – best option at making a diagnosis

(b) Discuss her management options, assuming that fibroids have been excluded. (14 marks)

- Most likely diagnosis is adenomyosis
- Management – symptomatic and treatment of adenomyosis
- Symptomatic:
  - Analgesics – mefenamic acid
  - Menorrhagia – tranexamic acid
  - Combination
- Adenomyosis treatment:
  - GnRH agonists
  - Combined oral contraceptive pill
  - Mirena®
  - Surgery – hysterectomy if family complete

Sample answer

(a) Justify the investigations you will undertake in this patient. (6 marks)

A FBC will exclude anaemia, especially as she presents with heavy periods. In addition, the blood film will help identify the type of anaemia, which in this case is likely to be iron deficient. Blood should be grouped and saved. She may require transfusion to correct any resulting anaemia (especially if she has atypical antibodies which make cross-matching difficult). If she were to have surgery, cross-matching blood will ensure that if transfusion is required at the time of surgery, appropriate blood is available.

An important investigation that will help in the diagnosis is an MRI of the pelvic organs. This will help differentiate causes of a uniformly enlarged uterus, such as fibroids from adenomyosis. In addition, an ultrasound scan will be useful in excluding the pressure effects of this pelvic mass of the urinary tract. A significant obstruction will mean urgent surgery to alleviate the obstruction is necessary.

(b) Discuss her management options, assuming that fibroids have been excluded. (14 marks)

The most likely diagnosis in this patient is adenomyosis. The treatment options include medical treatment, surgery and interventional radiology. Medical treatment can be in the form of simple analgesics and antifibrinolytics such as tranexamic acid. When this is combined with a non-steroidal anti-inflammatory drug such as Ponstan Forte®, it may not only reduce the heavy periods but also the pain of endometriosis.

Medical treatment of adenomyosis includes GnRH agonists, which are the gold standard. They induce amenorrhoea and hopefully reduce the size of the adenomyosis. The disadvantages are the side-effects and the fact that once treatment is discontinued, the adenomyosis is likely to regrow. Other medical options include the combined oral contraceptive pill. This has an added advantage where there is need for an effective contraception.

The levonorgestrel intrauterine system (Mirena®) is an alternative to non-surgical treatment. It has been shown to reduce the heavy periods and size of the adenomyosis. The disadvantages of this system include irregular vaginal bleeding, especially within the first 3–4 months, and mild progestogenic side-effects.

Surgery in the form of an abdominal hysterectomy and bilateral salpingo-oophorectmy is considered the ultimate and most aggressive treatment of adenomyosis. If this woman has not completed her family, this option will not be acceptable. An alternative to surgery if she has completed her family is uterine artery embolisation. This has been shown to reduce the heavy periods associated with adenomyosis.

5

Benign ovarian lesions

1. A 38-year-old woman presents to the gynaecology clinic with a swelling in the lower abdomen. You suspect that she has an ovarian cyst. (a) What clinical features will help you in making a diagnosis? (10 marks) (b) Evaluate the investigations you will perform on her. (4 marks) (c) How will you treat her? (6 marks)

2. A 27-year-old woman presents with intermittent lower abdominal pain. She has also noticed that she has been putting on weight and her clothes have been getting tighter. On examination, you find an abdominal mass consistent with a 36 weeks' gestation. The origin of the mass is uncertain but you suspect that it is ovarian. (a) Which clinical features will indicate that the cyst is benign? (8 marks) (b) Outline with reasons the investigations you will undertake on her. (8 marks) (c) Justify your subsequent management of the patient. (4 marks)

3. A young girl of 17 years presents as an emergency with intermittent lower abdominal pain of 3 days' duration. The pain is now constant and is mainly on the right side and radiating to her back. Her last menstrual period of a 28-day regular cycle was 1 week ago. (a) Critically discuss the investigations you will undertake to help make a diagnosis. (6 marks) (b) Justify your management of the patient. (8 marks) (c) What advice will you give her before she is discharged from hospital? (6 marks)

1. A 38-year-old woman presents to the gynaecology clinic with a swelling in the lower abdomen. You suspect that she has an ovarian cyst. (a) What clinical features will help you in making a diagnosis? (10 marks) (b) Evaluate the investigations you will perform on her. (4 marks) (c) How will you treat her? (6 marks)

Common mistakes

- Restating the information given in the question
- Discussing the management of malignant ovarian tumours
- Omitting to obtain more information from a history
- Treatment depends on parity – without first defining the type of ovarian tumour she has
- Assuming that she has an ovarian malignancy and treating her as such
- Refer to a tertiary centre with gynaecological oncologist because such patients should not be managed in the district hospital!
- Diagnostic laparoscopy as an investigation – you need to explain when it will be useful
- Failure to evaluate your answer in part (b)

A good answer will include some or all of these points

(a) What clinical features will help you in making a diagnosis? (10 marks)

- History:
  - Onset of symptoms – duration and associated pains?
  - Nature of pains
  - Any gastrointestinal symptoms – dyspepsia, weight loss
  - Pressure symptoms on the bladder, e.g. frequency of micturition and constipation
- Physical examination:
  - General appearance – cachectic? Suspicion of malignancy
  - Abdomen:
    - Fullness/distension
    - Characteristics of mass:
      - Size, location, solid/cystic or both, fixity, mobility, can get below
      - Associated ascites
    - Pelvis:
      - Bilateral
      - Fixed to pelvis
      - Consistency – solid, cystic or both

(b) Evaluate the investigations you will perform on her. (4 marks)

- Undertaking various investigations to confirm the diagnosis:
  - Ultrasound scan

- Role of magnetic resonance imaging (MRI) in the identification of malignancies and secondaries in the liver and abdominal lymph nodes
- CA125 and other tumour markers
- Urea and electrolytes (U&Es) – if suspicion of urinary tract obstruction
- Laparoscopy – diagnostic but may also be used for therapy at the same time

(c) How will you treat her? (6 marks)

- Treatment – depends on the diagnosis:
  - Laparotomy and oophorectomy or cystectomy
  - Laparoscopic oophorectomy/cystectomy
  - More extensive if malignant – total abdominal hysterectomy, bilateral salpingo-oophorectomy, omentectomy with or without removal of nodes followed by adjuvant chemotherapy
- Ovarian endometrioma – treatment (medical or surgery)

Sample answer

(a) What clinical features will help you in making a diagnosis? (12 marks)

In the management of this patient, obtaining more information about her presenting complaints is essential. The swelling may be associated with abdominal pain. If the pain is intermittent, then torsion may be a complication of the cyst. The pain may also be constant and increasing in intensity. This will point to the possibility of haemorrhage into an ovarian cyst. Where a cyst has ruptured, the pain tends to be excruciating and of very sudden onset. However, where the pain started intermittently and later became constant, the likely cause will be torsion. Associated symptoms may depend on the size of the ovarian cyst. These will usually be gastrointestinal and include dyspepsia, constipation and bloatedness of the abdomen.

Following this, a clinical examination should be undertaken to identify signs of ovarian pathology. These include the origin and size of the mass, associated ascites, fixity, pleural effusion and cachexia. A pelvic examination will confirm the presence of a pelvic mass, although this may be completely abdominal and thus difficult to feel vaginally. Bilaterality of the tumour, its consistency and fixity to the pelvis may indicate a possible malignancy.

(b) Evaluate the investigations you will perform on her. (4 marks)

Necessary investigations include a serum CA125. This may be raised in ovarian epithelial cancers, endometriosis, other epithelial cell tumours and infections. A high value is therefore not necessarily indicative of malignancy. However, it is important to establish a baseline in case serial monitoring is necessary. An ultrasound scan will define the origin of the cyst more precisely, although this is not always the case. Other features which may be identified on ultrasound scan include bilaterality of the tumour, the characteristics of the cysts, such as the presence of solid areas, irregular walls with excrescencies, papillary growths, bright material within the cyst and the size of the cyst. These features may distinguish a benign from a suspected malignant ovarian cyst.

If the ultrasound scan is inconclusive, MRI or computerised tomography (CT) scan may be necessary. In addition to defining the ovarian cyst and other features suggestive of malignancy, this will exclude secondaries in the liver and enlarged lymph nodes. A very large ovarian cyst may cause ureteric obstruction. This may be identified (by ultrasound or MRI of the kidneys) as hydronephrosis and/or dilation of the ureters. In some cases, ultrasound scan may not be conclusive, especially if the cyst is small; a diagnostic laparoscopy may therefore be better at defining the nature and origin of the pelvic pathology. In addition, definitive treatment may be offered at the time of the laparoscopy.

(c) How will you treat her? (4 marks)

The treatment will depend on the type of cyst, its size and associated complications. Ovarian endometriomata are best treated by oophorectomy, ovarian cystectomy or a combination of ovariotomy and medical therapy. Where the cyst is torted, it must be treated as an emergency. At the time of surgery, whether or not the ovary is saved (i.e. a cystectomy is performed) will depend on the viability of the ovary after it is untwisted. Oophorectomy will be performed if the ovary is not viable. In these situations the Fallopian tube tends to become necrotic with the ovary, and often a salpingo-oophorectomy is the treatment of choice. For an uncomplicated benign cyst, a cystectomy will be performed, either laparoscopically or via laparotomy. Where a malignancy is suspected, the patient should be referred to an oncologist for the most appropriate management, which will consist of a total abdominal hysterectomy, bilateral salpingo-oophorectomy and omentectomy followed by chemotherapy.

If the cyst is an endometrioma, the options will be surgery with or without medical treatment. Deroofing and diathermy or laser to the wall of the endometrioma and cystectomy had in the past been regarded as equally effective. It is now generally agreed that ovarian cystectomy has better results. This will be performed at laparotomy or laparoscopy. This may be followed by medical treatment with a gonadotropin-releasing hormone agonist but this additional treatment will depend on whether the patient is trying for a baby or not. In the absence of any other sites of endometriosis, there may be no need for medical treatment.

Whatever the pathology of the cyst in this patient, her management will only be completed after histological examination of the cyst or ovary.

2. A 27-year-old woman presents with intermittent lower abdominal pain. She has also noticed that she has been putting on weight and her clothes have been getting tighter. On examination, you find an abdominal mass consistent with a 36 weeks' gestation. The origin of the mass is uncertain but you suspect that it is ovarian. (a) Which clinical features will indicate that the cyst is benign? (8 marks) (b) Outline with reasons the investigations you will undertake on her. (8 marks) (c) Justify your subsequent management of the patient. (4 marks)

Common mistakes

- Her management depends on her age, parity and desire for further pregnancy
- Management to be determined by an oncologist
- She has ovarian cancer and therefore should not be managed by an general gynaecologist
- Counselling about family history of breast and colon cancer
- Screening for ovarian cancer – listing all the methods for screening for ovarian cancer
- Failure to justify

A good answer will include some or all of these points

(a) Which clinical features will indicate that the cyst is benign? (8 marks)

- History:
  - Slow growing – insidious onset
  - No associated systemic effects, e.g. weight loss, anorexia
  - No associated complications – constipation, dyspepsia
  - Minimal associated comorbidity
- Clinical findings on examination:
  - Abdomen and pelvis:
    - Absence of ascites
    - Unilateral or bilateral mass
    - Solid or cystic, but not mixed
    - Irregular surface
    - Not fixed in pelvis
  - Secondaries – absence of secondaries in lungs and liver
- Clinical findings at surgery

(b) Outline with reasons the investigations you will undertake on her. (8 marks)

- Ultrasound scan – define the location of the cyst, its characteristics, associated ascites and appearance
- Doppler of the ovarian arteries – increased vascularity indicates possible malignancy

- Biochemical markers – CA125, alpha-fetoprotein (AFP), human chorionic gonadotropin (hCG), etc.
- Full blood count (FBC)
- U&Es and liver function tests (LFTs)
- MRI/CT scan if secondaries suspected

(c) Justify your subsequent management of the patient. (4 marks)

- Will depend on diagnosis or suspected diagnosis:
    - Benign – ovarian cystectomy – laparotomy or laparoscopic – option depends on skill of surgeon and facilities available
    - Malignant – discuss with oncologist who should do surgery
    - Chemotherapy if malignancy and set up approach to multidisciplinary team meetings and planned follow-up

Sample answer

(a) Which clinical features will indicate that the cyst is benign? (8 marks)

These will be classified under history and clinical findings. A swelling of insidious onset is more likely to be benign, rather than one that has grown very rapidly over a short period or time. Associated systemic symptoms such as weight loss and anorexia will support a malignant growth although a large ovarian mass may cause nausea and vomiting and may also cause weight loss. The presence of comorbidities such as chest symptoms suggestive of secondaries will be more in favour of a malignant growth. Other symptoms, including those of pressure (e.g. swelling of the feet and vulva, varicose veins, haemorrhoids) and gastrointestinal symptoms (e.g. dyspepsia and constipation) are common to all types of large ovarian tumours. It may be the rapidity with which these symptoms develop that is crucial with regards to the type of tumour. The absence of these will be suggestive of a benign cyst.

Clinical features suggestive of malignancy will include those of general wasting, pallor and the presence of secondaries in the chest. There may be pedal oedema or vulval varicosities. On abdominal examination, a malignant tumour is likely to have a partly solid and partly cystic mass, an irregular surface and associated ascites. These findings will be confirmed on pelvic examination. In addition, the tumour is likely to be bilateral, and to be fixed to the pelvis and side walls.

At surgery, features suggestive of malignancy include a bloody ascites, bilateral tumours whose capsule has been breached and omental secondaries.

(b) Outline with reasons the investigations you will undertake on her. (8 marks)

The following ancillary investigations will be undertaken. A FBC will provide information about her haemoglobin as she may be anaemic and this will have to be corrected if she is to have surgery. Blood should be grouped and saved as transfusion may be required, either prior to surgery or in the perioperative period, while U&Es would indicate renal involvement in the form of ureteric obstruction. In addition, if the cyst is malignant, the patient will require adjuvant chemotherapy and, for this, renal function needs to be normal. A LFT will be performed for similar reasons – to assess secondary involvement in the liver and whether chemotherapy could be offered. An estimation of carcinoma antigen CA125 is essential. This is raised in epithelial cancers, endometriosis and pelvic inflammatory disease (PID). An ultrasound scan will define the nature of the cyst, associated ascites, liver secondaries and renal tract obstruction. However, these may not be conclusive. In this case, an MRI would be undertaken. This has the added advantage of screening for lymphadenopathy of the para-aortic nodes. Although Doppler scans of the ovarian arteries have been suggested as being helpful in distinguishing benign from malignant ovarian tumours, the results are not very encouraging.

(c) Justify your subsequent management of the patient. (4 marks)

The definitive treatment of this patient is surgery. Although a malignancy is unlikely, it must be considered before surgery is untaken. Discussions with the patient must therefore include the nature of the abdominal incision, which in this case will be vertical. In addition, a gynaecological oncologist should be notified and available if needed. At surgery, the contralateral ovary would be inspected for tumours. Any ascites should be sampled, its colour noted and then sent for histology; if none is present, a saline washout of the pelvis and para-aortic gutters would be performed and sent for histology.

The ovarian tumour should then be characterised, essentially identifying features suggestive of malignancy. These include a breached capsule, secondaries on the liver surface or omentum, enlarged abdominal nodes and further characteristics of the tumour, whether cystic or partly solid and cystic. If there are no features of malignancy, treatment will simply be removal of the cyst, omental biopsy and, where nodes are palpable, biopsy. If a malignancy is suspected, an abdominal hysterectomy, bilateral salpingo-oophorectomy and omentectomy will be performed. The definitive treatment will only be completed after histology.

3. A young girl of 17 years presents as an emergency with intermittent lower abdominal pain of 3 days' duration. The pain is now constant and is mainly on the right side and radiating to her back. Her last menstrual period of a 28-day regular cycle was 1 week ago. (a) Critically discuss the investigations you will undertake to help make a diagnosis. (6 marks) (b) Justify your management of the patient. (8 marks) (c) What advice will you give her before she is discharged from hospital? (6 marks)

Common mistakes

- Screen for ovarian cancer and await results before management
- Ultrasound scan must be performed before surgery
- Uterine fibroids are the likely cause
- An ectopic pregnancy is the first differential until proved otherwise
- Failure to justify and critically discuss

A good answer will include some or all of these points

(a) Critically discuss the investigations you will undertake to help make a diagnosis. (6 marks)

- Investigations:
    - FBC – leucocytosis in torsion or infection
    - Group and save – may require transfusion if offered surgery
    - Ultrasound scan – to define the presence of a pelvic mass and characterise the mass
    - Tumour markers – CA125 raised in epithelial tumours and in various pelvic conditions such as endometriosis and PID; not specific to ovarian malignancies – may be raised in epithelial tumours of bowel or breast origin – these are unlikely in this girl
    - Most likely malignancy will be a germ cell tumour for which the markers are AFP and hCG
    - Diagnostic laparoscopy – useful in making a diagnosis and treatment

(b) Justify your management of the patient. (8 marks)

- The most likely diagnosis is torsion of an ovarian cyst:
    - Dermoid cyst – the most likely type of cyst in this young girl
- It is an emergency, hence no place for conservative management
- Diagnostic laparoscopy if out of hours and no facilities for emergency ultrasound scan
- Surgery – laparoscopic or laparotomy
- Ovarian cystectomy or oophorectomy
- Fixation of the contralateral ovary
- Counselling after treatment
- Differential diagnosis – PID or other pathology – treat accordingly

(c) What advice will you give her before she is discharged from hospital? (6 marks)

- Recovery time – depends on the type of surgery
- Follow-up either at the general practitioner (GP) or hospital for histology and check-up that there are no complications
- Educate on the type of surgery offered
- If torsion, counsel about the early warning signs and encourage to present early as late presentation may result in loss of ovary and possibly tube

Sample answer

(a) Critically discuss the investigations you will undertake to help make a diagnosis. (6 marks)

Essential investigations include a FBC. A raised white cell count is recognised to be associated with a torted ovarian cyst. In addition to this, blood should be grouped and saved. A differential diagnosis in this patient is haemorrhage into an ovarian cyst. The cyst may also have ruptured and severe haemorrhage may require transfusion. An ultrasound scan will confirm the presence of an ovarian cyst but this is unlikely to suggest torsion. It will also characterise the mass (e.g. whether there has been haemorrhage into the cyst or it contains features suggestive of a dermoid or an endometrioma). The disadvantage of waiting for this before proceeding with surgery is that this facility may not be available out of hours. However, if it is available it will provide details about the cyst, the size, and what type it may be. If this facility is unavailable, and the ovarian cyst is not more than 14 weeks' gestation in size, a diagnostic laparoscopy may be performed. This procedure has the advantage of defining the type of ovarian pathology and the complications. Where the expertise exists, an ovarian cystectomy or oophorectomy could be performed laparoscopically.

Other investigations, which may not necessarily influence her immediate management, include tumour markers such as CA125 and AFP. CA125 is non-specific for epithelial tumours, which are uncommon in this young age group but may be raised in PID (which could be a differential in this young girl). A raised AFP will be suggestive of a germ cell tumour. The hCG marker could also be measured, not only to exclude pregnancy but also as a marker for germ cell tumours.

(b) Justify your management of the patient. (8 marks)

The most likely diagnosis is torsion of the ovary and the pathology is likely to be dermoid. Definitive treatment for her is therefore an ovarian cystectomy or oophorectomy, depending on the state of the ovary and adjacent tube at the time of surgery. It is an emergency and there is no place for conservative management as this will ultimately result in avascular necrosis of the ovary and tube.

Surgery can either be by laparoscopy or by laparotomy. If it is an out-of-hours' emergency and there are no facilities for ultrasound scan, a laparoscopy will serve as an investigative and treatment tool. Where there is a mass that is more than 14 weeks' gestation, then laparotomy would be the preferred option. If it is less than 14 weeks' size or the expertise is available, then a laparoscopic procedure will be most appropriate. It is associated with a quicker recovery and less analgesia postoperatively.

At surgery, the viability of the ovary and ipsilateral tube should be assessed before proceeding with the definitive surgery. If the torsion has resulted in gangrene of the ovary (and usually this is with the Fallopian tube), a salpingo-oophorectomy will be the treatment of choice. If the ovary is still viable after untwisting, a cystectomy will be performed. The ovary on the opposite side has to be inspected to ensure that it has no cyst. If it has, the cyst has to be removed, otherwise it could undergo a similar complication. The remnant ovary on the affected side and the unaffected ovary should then be fixed to avoid a recurrence of the torsion.

Other pelvic pathologies such as PID will be treated with systemic broad-spectrum antibiotics covering Gram-positive and Gram-negative organisms, anaerobes and *Chlamydia trachomatis*.

(c) What advice will you give her before she is discharged from hospital? (6 marks)

Prior to her discharge from the hospital, she should be counselled about the type of surgery she had, especially if the tube and or ovary were removed. This will ensure that a diagnosis of an ovarian pathology on the affected side is not entertained when she presents with another emergency. Additionally, armed with this information, she can offer it to others and therefore avoid misdiagnosis and unnecessary interventions.

An important aspect of her postoperative care is counselling about physical activity and when to resume work. This will depend on whether her surgery was done laparoscopically or by laparotomy. The former is associated with a slow recovery, while the latter is associated with a quicker recovery. She needs to take time off work and this will vary from a few weeks to 2–3 months. She will also be offered a follow-up appointment, either with the GP or at the hospital. At this visit, the histology of the tumour will be discussed but, more importantly, she will be examined to ensure that there are no residual complications from the surgery. Finally, she should be educated on the early features of torsion and to present early, especially if she lost her tube and ovary, as failure to do so will be catastrophic.

6

Vulval and vaginal disorders

1. A 19-year-old woman presents with a painful swollen right labium majorum. (a) Discuss your differential diagnoses of this symptom. (10 marks) (b) What investigations will help you in making a diagnosis? (5 marks) (c) Outline your treatment of this patient. (5 marks)

2. Mrs TP is 24 years old. She presented to the gynaecology outpatient department with primary amenorrhoea. Following investigations, a diagnosis of Müllerian agenesis was made. (a) Comment critically on other problems this patient may have. (8 marks) (b) Outline your management plan. (12 marks)

3. What steps will you take in the management of a 76-year-old woman with a diagnosis of carcinoma of the vagina? (20 marks)

4. A 65-year-old woman presents with a rash on her vulva. (a) What in the history will make you suspect it is lichen sclerosus? (4 marks) (b) What signs may you demonstrate on examination? (8 marks) (c) Briefly discuss the treatment options. (8 marks)

1. A 19-year-old woman presents with a painful swollen right labium majorum. (a) Discuss your differential diagnoses of this symptom. (10 marks) (b) What investigations will help you in making a diagnosis? (5 marks) (c) Outline your treatment of this patient. (5 marks)

Common mistakes

- Take a history and do a physical examination – although this is an important part of management it needs to be a targeted history and physical examination. Just stating that you will take a history and do a physical examination is not enough
- Refer her to a genitourinary medicine (GUM) clinic: although the swelling may be secondary to a sexually transmitted infection (STI), referring her to the GUM clinic without making a diagnosis is assuming that all swellings in the vulva are caused by STIs
- Exclude vulval cancer – this is a possibility although it is highly unlikely in this 19-year-old
- Listing all the gynaecological investigations for a vaginal discharge is not appropriate. Although you may need to undertake some of them, they must be related to the symptoms and signs you elicit
- Failing to discuss the differential diagnoses

A good answer will include some or all of these points

(a) Discuss your differential diagnoses of this symptom. (10 marks)

- Inflammatory:
  - Bartholin's abscess
  - Bartholin's cyst
  - Condylomata acuminata
- Non-inflammatory:
  - Lipoma
  - Fibroma
  - Haemagioma
  - Inguinolabial hernia
- Traumatic:
  - Haematoma

(b) What investigations will help you in making a diagnosis? (5 marks)

- Examination
- Virology
- Bacteriology

- Ultrasound scan if appropriate
- Biopsy
- Colcopscopy – vulvoscopy and cervical smear
- Screen for other STIs if a condylomata

(c) Outline your treatment of this patient. (6 marks)

- Depends on the cause
  - Bartholin's – marsupialisation
  - Antibiotics
  - Haematoma – drainage
  - Fibroma/lipoma – excision
  - Fibroids – myomectomy
  - Condylomata – excision – if localised, cryocautery, laser, podophyllotoxin

Sample answer

(a) Discuss your differential diagnoses of this symptom. (10 marks)

The differential diagnoses can be classified into inflammatory and non-inflammatory conditions. The former category includes Bartholin's abscess and condylomata acuminata. The latter category includes Bartholin's cyst, a lipoma, fibroma, haemangioma, lyphmangioma, an inguinolabial hernia, a haematoma and accessory breast.

In this young girl the most likely diagnosis is a Bartholin's abscess. An associated vaginal discharge and the patient's sexual history are of particular relevance in making a diagnosis. A Bartholin's abscess will present with a swelling that is gradually getting worse and is red and tender. In the case of a Bartholin's cyst, there may be no history of discharge or sexual activity. This may result from an obstruction of the Bartholin's duct, resulting in a non-infective accumulation of fluid within the gland. This can be differentiated from an abscess from physical findings – in the abscess, there is associated inflammation but there is usually none with the cyst.

A history of trauma to the vulva will suggest a haematoma and associated with this may be urinary retention or a swelling in the vagina if the haematoma extends into the paravaginal area. Another possible cause is an inguinolabial hernia that has become strangulated or obstructed. However, this is uncommon in this age group. In this case, there may be a long-standing history of a swelling that was reducible initially. The patient may also give a history of the swelling getting worse with coughing and possible associated complications, such as constipation.

Lipomas of the vulva are uncommon and they tend to occur in the older age group. These tend to be painless and located in the anterior portion of the vulva. Condylomata have a typical appearance that will be identified from physical examination.

(b) What investigations will help you in making a diagnosis? (5 marks)

Investigations will include a physical examination which will reveal signs of the possible cause of the swelling. A Bartholin's cyst or abscess is located on the posterior medial aspect of the labium majorum. It will be tense, fluctuant and tender, and it may be inflamed. Associated with this may be a vaginal discharge. If there is a gonococcal infection, a purulent urethral discharge may be identified. Evidence of trauma will confirm the diagnosis of a vulval haematoma, whereas a soft, non-tender swelling located on the anterior vulva may be diagnostic of a lipoma. A bimanual examination is important, as it will reveal associated features such as bilateral adnexal tenderness associated with pelvic inflammatory disease or a paravaginal swelling in the case of trauma causing a haematoma. A thorough examination of the inguinal ring and a negative cough impulse will exclude an inguinal hernia.

Following a physical examination, the following investigations will be essential in making a diagnosis. Swabs should be obtained from the urethra, vagina and the discharge (if any) from the swelling. These should be sent for microbiology, culture and sensitivity and for virology. The organisms to be screened for include *Neisseria gonorrhoea* and *Chlamydia trachomatis*. Viral cultures for human papilloma virus will be indicated where there is a suspicion of condylomata acuminata. Other investigations will depend on the suspected cause of the swelling. These may include a colposcopy and vulvoscopy, cervical cytology and screening for other STIs if the cause is thought to be an STI.

(c) Outline your treatment of this patient. (5 marks)

Once the diagnosis has been made, the most appropriate treatment would be offered. If a Bartholin's abscess or cyst is the cause of the swelling, the treatment of choice is marsupialisation and antibiotic therapy. Antibiotic therapy must cover Gram-negative and Gram-positive organisms and also be effective against *N. gonorrhoea*. A sample of the pus drained from the abscess should be sent for microbiology and needs to be transported in a medium suitable for the culture of *N. gonorrhoea*. If a haematoma is the cause, it has to be drained.

A lipoma will be excised, whereas a hernia will be referred to a general surgeon for repair. If the bowel is strangulated, there may have to be resection during surgery. There are other causes of a vulval swelling but these are rare and the treatment depends to a large extent on the cause. In this young woman, if a Bartholin's abscess is the diagnosis, STIs must be considered and excluded as they may coexist. Condylomata acuminata will be treated by local excision if this is feasible, by laser or by podophyllotoxin applied to the area affected.

2. Mrs TP is 24 years old. She presented to the gynaecology outpatient department with primary amenorrhoea. Following investigations, a diagnosis of Müllerian agenesis was made. (a) Comment critically on other problems this patient may have. (8 marks) (b) Discuss her management options. (12 marks)

Common mistakes

- Take a history and physical examination
- Discussing the causes of primary amenorrhoea
- Investigations of primary amenorrhoea
- Investigations to confirm Müllerian agenesis – the diagnosis has already been made. No need therefore to confirm
- Failure to comment critically
- Discussing karyotypic anomalies and androgen-insensitivity syndrome

A good answer will include some or all of these points

(a) Comment critically on other problems this patient may have. (8 marks)

- Vagina agenesis – partial or complete
- Absent uterus – infertility
- Agenesis – difficulties creating a new vagina – surgery/non-surgical
- Psychological problems associated with infertility, amenorrhoea and apareunia/dyspareunia

(b) Outline your management plan. (12 marks)

- Education/counselling
- Psychological support
- Creating of new vagina
- Fertility advice:
  - Option – adoption, surrogacy with patient's eggs and surrogate mother

Sample answer

(a) Comment critically on other problems this patient may have. (8 marks)

Typical Müllerian agenesis consists of an absent uterus and vagina. Therefore, it is important to establish how severe the agenesis is in this patient. The complete syndrome includes an absent vagina and uterus. In the incomplete variety, there may be partial fusion of the upper portion of the Müllerian system. Vaginal agenesis will result in apareunia or severe superficial dyspareunia if it is of the incomplete variety. An absent uterus invariably means infertility. However, there may be a rudimentary uterus, usually with no vagina. Such a rudiment could eventually become enlarged with blood and present as an abdominal mass and/cyclical pains and obstructive complications, especially on the renal tract.

The psychological effects of this diagnosis will not only be secondary to the abnormality itself but also to its implications (difficulties with sexual intercourse and infertility). Communication about the diagnosis needs to be very tactful and sensitive. Most patients will initially respond by denial and then anger, but will eventually come to terms with it. If available, psychological support from staff with appropriate skills in counselling should be offered. Subsequently, counselling must explain the full implications of the condition to the patient (she will remain amenorrhoeic and will not be able to become pregnant).

(b) Outline your management plan. (12 marks)

The next step will be to discuss the options available to the patient and to determine her needs. It is unlikely that she is sexually active. In fact, she may have experienced apareunia and offering an explanation for this may be very reassuring. The main treatment option is to create a new vagina. This is probably the only treatment that she could be offered.

A neovagina may be created surgically or non-surgically. If it is to be created surgically, the patient would have to be referred to someone with an experience in the creation of a neovagina. This is often successful initially but is commonly followed by adhesions and therefore results may not be as good. A neovagina can also be created by use of vaginal dilators and an Ingram's bicycle seat. This requires the patient to apply dilators of increasing size and length for 30 minutes every day for about 3–6 months. If the patient is well motivated, and can tolerate this, the results are often very good. However, some patients experience a pulling sensation in the vagina after completing the therapy. The disadvantage of this option is that after creation of the neovagina, it must be maintained by frequent dilatation. Often, this is done by sexual intercourse.

The long-term consequence of the diagnosis relating to the patient's inability to become pregnant must be discussed. She needs to be informed that, although she cannot become pregnant, she could have children from her own eggs through surrogacy. Adoption is another option that should be discussed. A diagnosis of Müllerian agenesis requires a team approach to its management. In some cases, a clinical psychologist or a psychotherapist may be necessary.

3. What steps will you take in the management of a 76-year-old woman with a diagnosis of carcinoma of the vagina? (20 marks)

Common mistakes

- Take a history and perform a physical examination
- Discussing the aetiology of vaginal carcinoma
- Symptoms of vaginal carcinoma
- Details of the screening for vaginal intraepithelial neoplasia (VAIN)
- Management of VAIN

A good answer will include some or all of these points

- Carcinoma of the vagina is rare
- Need for a thorough examination under general anaesthesia:
    - Colposcopy at the same time to identify coexisting VAIN
    - Combined rectal and vaginal examination
    - Cystoscopy if anterior spread is suspected
    - Proctosigmoidoscopy if posterior spread is suspected
- More elaborate assessment, depending on the suspected extent of the disease
- Need for a full-thickness biopsy
- Other investigations:
    - Full blood count
    - Chest X-ray (CXR)
    - Intravenous urogram (IVU)/ultrasound of the renal tract
    - Lynphangiography – not recommended by all experts
- Treatment of choice – surgery:
    - Stage I – radical vaginectomy, radical hysterectomy and lymphadenectomy
    - More advanced disease – exenteration is treatment of choice:
        - Anterior spread – anterior exenteration and reimplantation of the ureters in bowel creating an ileal conduit
        - Posterior spread – posterior exenteration with the creation of a colostomy
- Other treatment options:
    - Radiotherapy
    - Combination or both (surgery and/or radiotherapy)
- Follow-up

Sample answer

Carcinoma of the vagina is uncommon and best managed by a gynaecological oncologist, to whom the patient should be referred. It typically presents with postmenopausal bleeding.

Once the diagnosis is made, attempts must be made to define the extent of the disease. This is best done by examination under anaesthesia (EUA). During this procedure, a colposcopy may also be performed to identify coexisting VAIN and also to define the location of the lesion. An EUA is incomplete without a combined rectal and vaginal examination.

If, during EUA, an anterior or posterior spread is suspected, a cystoscopy and/or a proctosigmoidosccopy, respectively, should be performed. A generous, full-thickness biopsy should also be taken for an adequate histological evaluation. Further investigations would be undertaken to exclude distant metastases. A CXR will exclude secondaries in the lungs, whereas an IVU will exclude parametrial spread affecting the ureters. However, an IVU may be avoided if an ultrasound scan of the renal system is performed. Lymphangiography has been recommended by some experts to help map out any nodal involvement but this is not universally available.

The treatment of choice for this patient is surgery. This will depend on the stage of the disease and her suitability for surgery. If she has Stage I disease, the treatment of choice will be a radical hysterectomy, radical vaginectomy and lymphadenectomy. For more advanced disease, an exenteration is the treatment of choice. This will depend on the extension of the disease. For an anterior spread, this will take the form of an anterior exenteration and reimplantation of the ureters in the bowel or creating an ileal conduit. For a posterior spread, a posterior exenteration with the creation of a colostomy will be the surgery of choice. If the spread is both anterior and posterior, a total exenteration will be the treatment of choice. These radical options will only be offered if the patient is fit. Where she is unable to withstand such extensive surgery, radiotherapy should be offered as the treatment of choice. In fact, it is regarded as the treatment of choice in some patients by some oncologists. It is associated with less morbidity and mortality, especially for older patients. This is offered as combined internal and external radiotherapy. Whatever the treatment, regular follow-up is essential to identify recurrences.

4. A 65-year-old woman presents with a rash on her vulva. (a) What in the history will make you suspect it is lichen sclerosus? (4 marks) (b) What signs may you demonstrate on examination? (8 marks) (c) Briefly discuss the treatment options. (8 marks)

Common mistakes

- Repeating the question
- Discussing the aetiological factors considered to be involved in lichen sclerosus
- Discussing the pathology of the condition
- Referring the patient to a gynaecological oncologist for radical vulvectomy
- Counselling on the risks of diabetes mellitus
- Detailing the investigations you will undertake
- Discussing the differential diagnoses and their management/treatment

A good answer will include the following

(a) What in the history will make you suspect it is lichen sclerosus? (4 marks)

- Associated itching
- Chronology of symptoms – itching
- Scratching leading to breakage of the skin with ulceration
- Ensuing scar may result in superficial dyspareunia
- Associated perianal symptoms
- If the urethral meatus is involved with obstruction, voiding may be difficult

(b) What signs may you demonstrate on examination? (8 marks)

- Appearance of the lesions – thin skin, pearly or porcelain white with crinkly plaques
- Slightly raised areas within the lesion
- Lesion may be multiple – involving more than one area
- Appearance of the lesion may be the typical figure-of-eight pattern surrounding the vulva
- There may be shrinkage of the labia minora with coaptation of the labia across the clitoris resulting in the formation of phimosis and narrowing of the introitus
- Ulcerations may be present – usually secondary to scratching
- Areas of ecchymosis and subsequent pigmentation may be identified
- There may be lesions on the trunk or limbs – these are involved in 18 per cent of patients

(c) Briefly discuss the treatment options. (8 marks)

- Topical steroids creams or ointments to treat symptomatic skin lesions

- Treatment should be continued for up to 3 months
- If coexisting fungal infection? Treat
- If failure to respond to treatment? Rule out coexisting malignancy (in approximately 2.5–5 per cent)

Sample answer

(a) What in the history will make you suspect it is lichen sclerosus?(4 marks)

The typical history is usually that of vulval itching. It is most likely that this was the preceding symptom in this patient and scratching resulted in the ulcer. Other symptoms will include perianal itching, superficial dyspareunia and occasionally difficulties voiding if there has been scarring involving the urethral meatus. The patient may also have coexisting lesions on other parts of the body, especially the limbs, and these may be present in up to 18 per cent of cases.

(b) What signs may you demonstrate on examination? (8 marks)

The typical signs that may be demonstrated include the appearance of a thin pearly or porcelain white vulval skin, which may have crinkly plaques. There may be ulcers, some of which could have fungal superinfection. The typical appearance of the figure-of-eight lesion surrounding the labia will be diagnostic. Other signs that may be demonstrated include shrinkage of the labia minora with coaptation of the labia across the introitus making it difficult if not impossible to perform a speculum examination let alone a digital examination because of the coaptation and resulting phimosis. Where there is superinfection, there may be ecchymosis with subsequent pigmentation.

Since the pathology may involve other parts of the body, especially the trunk and limbs (in approximately 18 per cent of cases), the typical whitish lesions may also be demonstrated in the different parts of the body.

(c) Briefly discuss the treatment options. (8 marks)

The most common treatment option is the application of topical steroids and a bland emollient to the affected area. Topical steroids are the most effective treatment option and should be applied nightly for up to 3 months. If she responds to this treatment this should become obvious within a few weeks of commencing it, otherwise differentials should be excluded; e.g. where there has been failure to respond to this treatment, consideration should be given to excluding a malignancy and superinfection. Additionally, a fungal superinfection should be excluded and appropriate antifungal treatment added to the steroids and emollient creams if this were the case. If treatment for this suspected fungal superinfection fails to respond, then a malignancy must be excluded by the appropriate biopsy. Vulval malignancies coexist with lichen sclerosus in 2.5–4 per cent of cases.

Although it is important to improve the introitus for coitus if it is very narrow, there is no evidence that oestrogen creams applied topically are of any benefit.

Further reading

Maclaren A, Dina R (2003) Benign disease of the vulva and the vagina. In: Shaw RW, Soutter WP, Stanton SL (eds) *Gynaecology*, 3rd edn. Edinburgh: Churchill Livingstone, pp. 603–4.

7

Gynaecology, endocrinology

1. A 19-year-old woman with hirsutism has been referred to the gynaecologist by her general practitioner (GP). (a) What important clinical signs will you look for? (6 marks) (b) Justify the investigations you will undertake on her. (6 marks) (c) Evaluate the treatment options for this young woman, if no obvious cause is found after investigating. (8 marks)

2. What advice will you give a 34-year-old, well-educated woman with polycystic ovary syndrome (PCOS) about (a) her fertility (6 marks) and (b) the wider health implications of her condition? (14 marks)

3. Critically appraise the management of a 27-year-old woman presenting with inappropriate galactorrhoea and secondary amenorrhoea. (20 marks)

4. An 18-year-old girl who is *virgo intacta* attended the gynaecology clinic because she is yet to start menstruating. (a) Justify any additional information you will obtain from her to help you make a diagnosis. (8 marks) (b) What investigations will you order on her? (5 marks) (c) How would you manage this patient? (7 marks)

> 1. A 19-year-old woman with hirsutism has been referred to the gynaecologist by her GP. (a) What important clinical signs will you look for? (6 marks) (b) Justify the investigations you will undertake on her. (6 marks) (c) Evaluate the treatment options for this young woman, if no obvious cause is found after investigating. (8 marks)

Common mistakes

- Discussing the pathogenesis of hirsutism
- Listing all the causes of hirsutism
- Detailing the symptoms of PCOS and the physiological bases of hyperandrogenism in PCOS
- Management of infertility and menstrual abnormalities
- Defining hirsutism and the use of Gallwey and Ferriman classification of hirsutism
- Advising the patient to lose weight – not told that she is obese
- Treating all the associated symptoms of PCOS, e.g. menstrual abnormalities, acne, infertility, obesity, etc.
- Use of trade names of very unfamiliar drugs

A good answer will include some or all of these points

(a) What important clinical signs will you look for? (6 marks)

- Body habitus (height, weight):
  - Signs of virilisation, and in some cases features of classic endocrine disorders – Cushing's syndrome or acromegaly
- Breast examination – galactorrhoea (especially if menstrual abnormalities), atrophy
- Thyroid gland – enlargement
- Abdomen and pelvis for masses – adrenal or ovarian
- Acanthosis nigricans – back of neck and vulva
- Hair distribution:
  - Semi-quantitative assessment of degree of hirsutism – Ferriman–Gallwey score
  - Baldness, acne
- Secondary sexual characteristics

(b) Justify the investigations you will undertake on her. (6 marks)

- Blood:
  - Serum testosterone – elevated in only 40 per cent of cases:
    - Mainly to exclude serious disorders of androgen secretion (e.g. congenital adrenal hyperplasia, Cushing's syndrome, adrenal or ovarian tumours)

- - Testosterone levels <3 nm/L in those with idiopathic hirsutism; levels >5 nmol/L are rare in those with PCOS
  - If >5 nmol/L, further test for adrenal function must be undertaken (computerised tomography (CT)/magnetic resonance imaging (MRI))
- Sex-hormone-binding globulin
- Follicle-stimulating hormone (FSH)/luteinising hormone (LH)
- Free androgen index
- Dehydroepiandrostendione sulphate (DHEAS),
- Radiological:
  - Ultrasound scan of the ovaries and adrenals; best performed in the early follicular phase to define ovarian morphology and exclude rare tumours
  - MRI/CT scan if raised testosterone

(c) Evaluate the treatment options for this young woman, if no obvious cause is found after investigating. (8 marks)

- Reassurance – especially if familiar; no treatment needed and patient feels normal
- Mechanical (cosmetic) – waxing, shaving, electrolysis, depilatory creams, bleaching and laser; most are cheap, patient feels normal and that she does not have a disease, not medicalised
- Medical:
  - Antiandrogens:
    - Cyproterone acetate (CPA) alone or in combination with oestrogens (Dianette®)
    - Spironolactone
    - Flutamide
  - Ovarian suppression:
    - Combined oral contraceptive pill
    - Gonadotropin-releasing hormone (GnRH) analogues
  - Eflornithine hydrochroride (Vaniqa®)
  - 5-Alpha-reductase inhibitor:
    - Finasteride

Sample answer

(a) What important clinical signs will you look for? (6 marks)

Physical examination will first determine her weight, height and therefore body mass index and muscle distribution. The aim of this is to identify obesity and if present whether it is central or not. Acanthosis nigricans should be noted. Other features that may be identified on examination include those of virilisation and, in some cases, those of the classical endocrinopathies such a Cushing's syndrome (moon-face appearance). Hair distribution and the type of hair should be noted and scored by the Ferriman–Gallwey method of semi-quantification. Any acne or degree of baldness should also be noted. All secondary sexual characteristics including the Tanner stage of breast development should also be recorded. The breasts should be examined for atrophy and discharge, while the thyroid gland is examined for enlargement and features of thyrotoxicosis. Examination of the abdomen should aim to identify masses such as adrenal and ovarian, while a pelvic examination will confirm the presence of ovarian masses, which may be the source of androgens causing the hirsutism.

(b) Justify the investigations you will undertake on her. (6 marks)

A blood sample should be obtained for a hormone profile (including serum testosterone, FSH and LH, sex-hormone-binding globulin, DHEAS and free androgen index) to exclude or diagnose PCOS. A thyroid function test (free thyroxine (FT4) and thyroid-stimulating hormone (TSH)) should also be undertaken if thyroid dysfunction is suspected. If the testosterone level is <5 nmol/L, then PCOS is a more likely to be a cause but if >5 nmol/L, then an adrenal tumour would look more likely. For a raised testosterone level, an MRI/CT scan of the abdomen should be undertaken as this is more likely to diagnose a tumour.

An ultrasound scan of the pelvis and abdomen will be essential to rule out any tumours within the ovary and adrenals and more importantly to exclude features consistent with PCOS. This scan is best done in the early follicular phase.

(c) Evaluate the treatment options for this young woman, if no obvious cause is found after investigating. (8 marks)

Where no obvious cause is found, it is classified as idiopathic and may well be constitutional. The first approach is reassurance; such reassurance is much better if there is a strong family history of hirsutism.

The next option will be shaving the excessive hair. If this is unacceptable, other mechanical treatments such as plucking or waxing could be considered. Some of these are cheap and effective but require repeated application. The myth that shaving increases hirsutism needs to be dismissed in order to motivate this patient appropriately. Where she objects to this, or has previously tried these methods unsuccessfully, she should be offered bleaching and/or laser treatment. These methods are effective but are more expensive. Electrolysis is thought to be the only permanent way of removing hair and gives the best cosmetic result. This may be offered as an option if the others are unsuccessful or unacceptable. However, it is expensive and needs to be performed by an experienced operator to minimise the risks of scarring or infection.

Medical treatment will be the last option for this young woman. The first will be a combination of CPA (an antiandrogen) and an oestrogen in the form of Dianette®. This offers the added advantage of effective contraception, if required, and also corrects any menstrual abnormalities. It is cheap and effective, but compliance may be a problem as it has to be taken regularly. In a young woman this may be an important consideration. It is important to emphasise that the effects of this treatment are not immediate and it may take up to 4 months for a significant difference to be noticed. More than 70 per cent of women treated with this regimen report a significant improvement in symptoms within 12 months. Side-effects, of which the patient must be warned, include depression, weight gain and breast tenderness.

More recently, eflornithine hydrochloride (Vaniqa®) has been shown to be effective, especially for facial hair, and this may therefore be offered if the patient does not require contraception. Other options to consider include CPA given on its own. Again, motivation is required as it is taken daily. There are side-effects of this treatment, which may be unacceptable to the patient and therefore result in poor compliance. If this is not acceptable, spironolactone (an aldosterone antagonist with androgenic-receptor-blocking activity) or flutamide (a non-steroidal antiandrogen) may be used. Flutamide may also be used in combination with a combined oral contraceptive pill to achieve results comparable to those of spironolactone or CPA. Flutamide has several side-effects and may be poorly tolerated. A comparative trial of spironolactone and CPA did not show any significant difference in response between the two groups, but spironolactone is not the drug of choice because of its side-effects and cost. In addition, when used it must be combined with effective contraception.

Other less-effective options that may be considered include ketoconazole, a synthetic imidazole derivative, which blocks gonadal and adrenal steroidogenesis. Unfortunately, marked side-effects, such as nausea, asthenia and alopecia, necessitate close monitoring during treatment and may also result in poor compliance. Clinical response to this option is also relatively poor.

Ovarian suppression with low-dose contraceptive pills and GnRH analogues are effective in some patients. The former will be suitable in this young woman, but the latter, though effective, will have severe hypo-oestrogenic side-effects, making it less acceptable.

An important aspect of her management is the emphasis on the absence of pathology. Such reassurance and encouraging the patient to have a more positive image of herself may be all that is necessary.

2. What advice will you give a 34-year-old, well-educated woman with PCOS about (a) her fertility (6 marks) and (b) the wider health implications of her condition? (14 marks)

Common mistakes

- Discussing:
  - Infertility in PCOS
  - Irregular periods, and how to manage them
  - Acne and hirsutism, and how to manage them
  - Ovulation induction in women with PCOS
  - The patient did not present with specific symptoms (so do not state that this will depend on her symptoms)
- Do not advise on contraception and other related problems

A good answer will include some or all of these points

(a) What advice will you give a 34-year-old, well-educated woman with PCOS about her fertility? (6 marks)

- Periods – vary from normal to irregular and amenorrhoea
- Anovulation – may struggle to become pregnant; if oligomenorrhoea – may take long to become pregnant
- May require assistance for induction of ovulation – medical/surgical
- Increased risk of miscarriage
- Increased risk of gestational diabetes and, if obese, related complications

(b) What advice will you give a 34-year-old, well-educated woman with PCOS about the wider implications of her condition? (14 marks)

- Insulin resistance, resulting in impaired glucose tolerance and diabetes mellitus
- Need to be aware of early symptoms of diabetes mellitus and make regular check-ups with GP and check urine
- Ischaemic heart disease due to abnormal cholesterol metabolism:
  - General health advice – adequate and regular exercise
  - Dietary – aim to reduce cholesterol levels
  - Early warning signs of heart disease/attacks
- Hypertension – increased risk:
  - Regular blood pressure check
  - Persistent headaches need to be checked

- Malignancies:
  - Endometrial carcinoma:
    - Menstrual disorders – educate on the relevance of this as a symptom of cancer/hyperplasia:
      - Perimenopausal irregular vaginal bleeding
      - Postmenopausal bleeding
  - Breast cancer:
    - Inconclusive evidence; however, obesity, hyperandrogenism and infertility are risk factors for breast cancer. Syndrome *per se* may not be associated with an increase but watchful vigilance is required
    - Regular breast examination and mammography
  - Ovarian cancer:
    - Most likely to be related to ovulation-induction drugs rather than the condition *per se*
    - Those who have had infertility treatment must be followed up with a high index of suspicion since symptoms of ovarian cancer are vague and non-specific
- Excessive weight gain:
  - Dietary control
  - Regular exercises

Sample answer

(a) What advice will you give a 34-year-old, well-educated woman with PCOS about her fertility? (6 marks)

She may conceive spontaneously but because of oligomenorrhoea/amenorrhoea, this may take longer, if it happens at all. Even if she did conceive, there is an increased risk of spontaneous miscarriages, especially in the first trimester. Ovulation induction with different agents, including weight loss and laparoscopic drilling of the ovaries, will significantly improve her fertility. Although the ovulation rate with most of the regimens is high, pregnancy rates are much lower and she will be at an increased risk of multiple pregnancies and ovarian hyper-stimulation syndrome. During pregnancy, she is at risk of developing gestational diabetes and, if obese, the complications thereof.

(b) What advice will you give a 34-year-old, well-educated woman with PCOS about the wider implications of her condition? (14 marks)

She is at increased risk of cardiovascular disorders. These include hypertension and ischaemic heart disease. Abnormal cholesterol metabolism is responsible for this increased risk. Therefore, the advice for the patient will relate to early warning signs of hypertension and ischaemic heart disease. These include headaches, easy fatigability, shortness of breath and precordial chest pain. It is important that she reduces cholesterol in her diet and visits her GP regularly. Her GP must be informed of these increased health risks and monitor the patient's blood pressure and cholesterol levels and examine her cardiovascular system regularly.

She is also at an increased risk of developing insulin resistance. This is due to hyperandrogenism and insulin-like growth factors in PCOS. She must therefore be educated on the early symptoms of diabetes mellitus, such as polyuria, polydypsia and polyphagia. In addition, she must attend her GP clinic regularly for urine testing and occasional blood-glucose estimation.

An important complication of PCOS is the development of endometrial cancer. In educating this patient, it is important to be extremely sensitive and cautious as she could become unnecessarily alarmed. Irregular periods are a recognised symptom of PCOS and may also be a presentation for endometrial cancer; PCOS is one condition in which endometrial cancer may occur before menopause. Therefore, it is important for the patient to visit her GP if any unusual vaginal bleeding occurs and ultrasound scans should be performed and endometrial biopsies taken. Early referral for hysteroscopic assessment of the endometrium would be highly recommended to her GP.

Obesity is an important consequence of this condition. Appropriate dietary and exercise advice should be offered whether or not she is obese. Weight loss will not only reduce the risk of the other wider health issues, such as hypertension and endometrial cancer, but will also reduce the risks of diabetes.

Finally, the advice this patient will be given will need to be reinforced by information she receives from her GP and from information leaflets about the wider health implications of this common endocrine condition.

3. Critically appraise the management of a 27-year-old woman presenting with inappropriate galactorrhoea and secondary amenorrhoea. (20 marks)

Common mistakes

- Assuming that she has a prolactinoma – no definite cause has been provided
- Discussing the treatment of infertility
- Referring the patient to an endocrinologist – indicating that this is the best option and therefore a gynaecologist should not manage her!
- Concentrating on history and physical examination – unnecessary to provide all the details
- Failure to critically appraise your answer

A good answer will include some or all of these points

- There are many causes of galactorrhoea
- A good history to exclude some of these
- Physical examination to exclude disturbances in the visual field; thyroid gland enlargement; breast examination to confirm galactorrhoea
- Investigations to identify the cause of the galactorrhoea: hormone profile – TSH, FT4; FSH, LH, skull X-ray – will only identify gross pathology. Best option is MRI of the skull, especially the pituitary fossa; CT scan if necessary
- Treatment will depend on the cause and the wishes of the patient
- Primary concern amenorrhoea – treat appropriately
- Infertility coexisting – treat accordingly
- May need referral to neurosurgeons for surgery for prolactinomas
- Treatment for prolactinomas: bromocriptine; cabergoline; PCOS; osteoporosis

Sample answer

Inappropriate galactorrhoea is defined as milk production outside lactation. In some cases there may not be an obvious cause, but often it may be due to hyperprolactinaemia. The combination of amenorrhoea and inappropriate galactorrhoea suggests that the patient may be hyperprolactinaemic. In her management, possible causes of galactorrhoea should be excluded before initiating treatment for the amenorrhoea.

Recognised causes of hyperprolactinaemia, such as drugs that inhibit dopamine production or action (e.g. phenothiazides, benzodiazepines, steroids, antihypertensive agents, etc.) may be established from directed questioning of the patient. In addition, symptoms of hypothyroidism, intracranial lesions (headaches, nausea, vomiting, visual field disturbances), chronic renal failure and PCOS or stress may be excluded from the history. Although the history may provide very useful information, it is important to recognise that the most common causes of hyperprolactinaemia are pituitary prolactinomas and idiopathic hypersecretion, both of which are more likely to be asymptomatic. Indeed, the two pathologies may be unrelated and therefore symptoms of other causes of secondary amenorrhoea need to be excluded.

A physical examination may identify signs suggestive of the possible cause of either the inappropriate galactorrhoea or amenorrhoea, or both. These will include visual field disturbances, thyroid enlargement, confirmation of galactorrhoea, features of PCOS (such as hirsutism) and genital tract abnormalities. A series of investigations is essential to diagnose the causes of these problems. A hormone profile (TSH, FT4, FSH, LH and prolactin) will confirm hyperprolactinaemia, if present, or other causes, e.g. hypothyroidism, PCOS, etc. To identify prolactinomas, MRI of the skull, especially of the pituitary fossa, will be required. This offers a better resolution to detect small microprolactinomas, but CT scanning is an equally good alternative and, in the absence of these, an X-ray of the skull would be performed. Although hormone assays may identify causes, normal values do not necessarily exclude them. Similarly, microprolactinomas may not be defined easily from the radiological investigations. X-rays are now considered crude screening methods for gross abnormality of the pituitary fossa or calcification in a craniopharyngioma.

The treatment of this patient will depend on the cause of either the amenorrhoea or the galactorrhoea, or both. Where the causes are unrelated it may not be possible to treat them concurrently, in which case the predominant concern must be treated first. Since most causes of galactorrhoea due to hyperprolactinaemia are idiopathic or of the microprolactinoma varieties, the treatment of choice will initially be for this variety. The treatment of choice will be a dopamine agonist, such as bromocriptine. This is effective in shrinking prolactinomas and reducing prolactin levels in the idiopathic group. Attempts must be made to remove known iatrogenic causes of hyperprolactinaemia, such as drugs, if possible. It is important to counsel the patient on her fertility whilst she is taking bromocriptine. This may not be acceptable to her because of side-effects, such as headaches. In this case, alternatives, such as cabergoline or quinagolides, may be used.

For the macroadenomas, transphenoidal microsurgical excision is the treatment of choice. One of the main consequences of hyperprolactinaemia is osteoporosis. This should be addressed by instituting oestrogen therapy. This may be combined with bromocriptine. The treatment of the patient's amenorrhoea may be the combined oral contraceptive pill, but it must be remembered that this can itself cause hyperprolactinaemia.

4. An 18-year-old girl who is *virgo intacta* attended the gynaecology clinic because she is yet to start menstruating. (a) Justify any additional information you will obtain from her to help you make a diagnosis. (8 marks) (b) What investigations will you order on her? (5 marks) (c) How would you manage this patient? (7 marks)

Common mistakes

- Assuming that she has a chromosomal abnormality and discussing the management of intersexual disorders
- Discussing postpill amenorrhoea and its treatment
- Justifying why she has PCOS and detailing how to manage this
- Investigating her for infertility and offering treatment for this
- Assuming that she has an adrenal problem and discussing its management
- Listing all the causes of primary amenorrhoea in this young girl
- Failure to justify in part (a)

A good answer will include some or all of these points

(a) *Justify any additional information you will obtain from her to help you make a diagnosis. (8 marks)*

- Most likely problem is primary amenorrhoea; history and examination will provide additional information
- Personal:
  - Pubertal milestones – age at thelarche, adrenache
  - Medical history – meningitis, headaches, symptoms of thyroid dysfunction
  - Drug history – drugs, e.g. androgens, and drugs that may cause hyperprolactinaemia (e.g. antidepressants, cimetidine, methyldopa, phenothiazines)
  - Secretions from breast – inappropriate galactorrhoea
  - Associated symptoms, e.g. hirsutism, acne
- Family history:
  - Any female siblings? Age at menarche in sisters and mother
- Physical examination:
  - Height, body mass, secondary sexual characteristics
  - Abdomen for masses
  - *Virgo intacta* – may do a rectal examination otherwise ultrasound scan of pelvis as examination will not provide as much information as an ultrasound scan

(b) *What investigations will you order on her? (5 marks)*

- Hormone profile:
  - FSH, FH, testosterone, oestradiol, prolactin, TSH, free T4

- Radiological:
  - Ultrasound scan of the abdomen and pelvis looking for the uterus, ovaries and adrenals
  - Other radiological investigations to outline the vagina, etc. – vaginography – very specialised investigations
- Karyotype if indicated:
  - If there are external characteristics such as gonads in the groins, abnormal biochemistry, features of Turner's syndrome (short stature, web-necked, etc.)

(c) How would you manage this patient? (7 marks)

- Depends on the cause
- Idiopathic – treatment: reassurance
- Specific cause – treat (e.g. congenital malformation, thyroid dysfunction, drug-induced, etc.)
- If karyotypic abnormality – counselling required not only about amenorrhoea but about implications for fertility

Sample answer

(a) Justify any additional information you will obtain from her to help you make a diagnosis. (8 marks)

The most likely problem in this young girl is primary amenorrhoea, which is defined as failure to start menstruation by the age of 16 years. She is already 18 years but whether this amenorrhoea is pathological or constitutional, as most cases are, will depend on several factors. Therefore, in her management, attempts must be made to exclude pathological causes and then tailor treatment according to the identified cause.

First, it is important to establish the various milestones of puberty. These will include the age at thelarche (the first pubertal secondary sexual characteristic) and pubarche. Where these appeared in the right order and at the right age, primary ovarian function must be considered to be normal.

The age at which her sisters attained menarche should be established. If this was at about her age, all that is necessary is reassurance, as the most likely cause is familiar or constitutional. However, if they attained menarche at an earlier age, pathological causes should be excluded. However, this must not be considered as an obvious indication that there is a cause, as it can still be constitutional. Among important factors that must be excluded from the history are: trauma to the skull, features of an intracranial lesion (such as headaches), visual field abnormalities, galactorrhoea, and features of thyroid dysfunction. Drugs that may induce amenorrhoea should also be excluded, especially those that may interfere with pituitary function, e.g. steroids, antihypertensive agents, etc. Most of these may do so by inducing hyperprolactinaemia.

A physical examination may identify possible causes of the primary amenorrhoea. Initially, the patient's height should be measured. If she is of short stature for her age, it could be an indication of a chromosomal problem, such as Turner's syndrome. Body proportions and secondary sexual characteristics, such as the breasts, pubic and axillary hair, the carrying angle of the arm, location of the nipples and the hair line should also be observed. Palpation of the abdomen and inguinal rings should be undertaken to exclude gonads as in a case of androgen insensitivity syndrome. Since she is *virgo intacta*, a vaginal examination would be inadvisable. However, a rectal examination may be able to palpate the uterus, although this may not be necessary, especially with the ready availability of ultrasound facilities.

(b) What investigations will you order on her? (5 marks)

A series of investigations are essential in helping make a diagnosis and therefore tailoring treatment. A complete hormonal profile is required. This will include serum FSH, LH, TSH, free T4, prolactin, testosterone, sex-hormone-binding globulin and 17-beta-oestradiol. In addition, an ultrasound scan of the pelvis will be performed, which will define the uterus and ovaries. However, it must be recognised that sometimes these radiological investigations fail to reveal pathology. Where there is a suspicion of a chromosomal abnormality, karyotyping should be performed. The best sample for this is peripheral blood where lymphocytes may be harvested.

(c) How would you manage this patient? (7 marks)

The treatment will depend on the cause. Where it is constitutional, reassurance is often adequate. However, if this is unacceptable, the combined oral contraceptive pill may be used to induce menstruation. It must be recognised that when the patient comes off the pill, she may suffer from amenorrhoea and/or irregular periods. Where the cause is PCOS, as defined by an abnormal hormone profile, appropriate treatment could be instituted. This may take the form of the combined oral contraceptive pill or cyclical progestogens. Effectively, the choice is determined by the presence of other symptoms requiring treatment.

If the primary amenorrhoea is secondary to drugs, these should either be discontinued or modified. However, if it is not possible to do this, hormonal therapy should be instituted, provided the hormones do not interfere with the drugs. Other causes, such as hypothyroidism, will be treated accordingly. The more difficult problems to treat are those related to agenesis of the Müllerian system and intersexual disorders. For disorders secondary to agenesis of the Müllerian system, appropriate counselling is required and, if the vagina is not formed, a neo-vagina is created either by surgery or by use of sustained pressure as described by Ingram (Folch *et al.*, 2000).

Counselling about fertility is important in the management of this patient. Where the cause is Turner's syndrome, secondary sexual characteristics will be absent and she could be short. Here, the treatment of choice is oestrogen to stimulate the uterus and induce growth. Once this has been achieved, the patient will start menstruation. However, she may be infertile and require ovum donation. If the cause of the amenorrhoea is androgen-insensitivity syndrome, the gonads need to be removed and the patient offered hormone replacement therapy. Again, appropriate counselling will be required to address the issue of fertility.

Reference

Folch M, Pigem I, Konje JC (2000) Müllerian agenesis: etiology, diagnosis and management. *Obstet Gynecol Surv* **55**: 644–9.

8

Infertility

1. A couple investigated for infertility were categorised as 'unexplained infertility'. (a) What factors will influence the results of treatment offered? (8 marks) (b) Summarise the options available to them. (12 marks)

2. During the course of investigating a couple who attended for secondary infertility of 2 years' duration, you opt to assess tubal function. (a) What radiological options will you consider? (7 marks) (b) Critically appraise the non-radiological options. (7 marks) (c) Outline the complications of these procedures. (6 marks)

3. An obese, 25-year-old woman with polycystic ovary syndrome (PCOS) presents with infertility, which is secondary to anovulation. (a) Critically appraise the non-medical methods by which ovulation can be induced in this patient. (6 marks) (b) Discuss the anti-oestrogens that could be used for ovulation induction. (7 marks) (c) Discuss how you will induce ovulation using gonadotropins. (7 marks)

4. Ovarian hyperstimulation syndrome (OHSS) is an important cause of severe morbidity and mortality in assisted reproduction. (a) Which factors predispose to OHSS? (3 marks) (b) What steps will you take to minimise the risk of OHSS? (8 marks) (c) How will you recognise OHSS? (4 marks) (d) Briefly discuss its management. (5 marks)

5. A couple attending the infertility clinic have been investigated and the husband's semen analysis was described as oligozoospermic. Evaluate the options available to the couple. (20 marks)

1. A couple investigated for infertility were categorised as 'unexplained infertility'. (a) What factors will influence the results of treatment offered? (8 marks) (b) Summarise the options available to them. (12 marks)

Common mistakes

- Discussing the causes of infertility – there is no need to list the causes of infertility as the question explicitly demands summarising options for a particular type of infertility – the unexplained type
- Do not discuss the contributions of every factor involved in infertility
- Taking a history and doing a physical examination is irrelevant. The couple have already been investigated and categorised as unexplained!
- Details of infertility treatment in general, e.g. ovulation induction regimens in women with anovulation, *in vitro* fertilisation with embryo transfer (IVF-ET), etc. These details are irrelevant to this question

A good answer will include some or all of these points

(a) What factors will influence the results of treatment offered? (8 marks)

- Age of the woman – the younger she is, the better the prognosis
- Previous obstetric history – the chances of a successful pregnancy are greater in women who have had previous pregnancies compared to those who have not
- How was the diagnosis made – the extent of the various investigations undertaken, i.e. all subtle causes have been excluded. A more thorough investigation is more likely to have excluded subtle factors, hence the prognosis is more likely to be better
- Period of waiting/expectant management

(b) Summarise the options available to them. (12 marks)

- Counselling – the first important stage – support – success rate – influence of natural conception rates superimposed on infertility
- Assisted reproductive techniques:
  - Induction of ovulation
  - IVF-ET
  - Artificial insemination by husband (AIH), artificial insemination by donor (AID)
  - All these are expensive – complications – psychological problems with failure
- Adoption

Sample answer

(a) What factors will influence the results of treatment offered? (8 marks)

The outcome of unexplained infertility depends on various factors. These include the age of the female patient, and the duration and type of infertility. If the woman is over 35 years, the success of expectant management is poor. Hull *et al.* (1985) showed that the chances of spontaneous conception are closely related to the duration of infertility and whether it is primary or secondary in nature. The outcome is better in those with secondary infertility than those with primary infertility. Where the investigations are more extensive, the pregnancy rates tend to be much higher, hence the facilities available for investigation and labelling the couple 'unexplained' are critical in influencing outcome. The longer the period of expectant management, the better the success rate.

(b) Summarise the options available to them. (12 marks)

The first option for any couple with this diagnosis is counselling and reassurance. The eventual pregnancy rate after 3 years' expectant management is between 60 and 70 per cent (Hull *et al.*, 1985). In this option, sympathetic explanation of the diagnosis and the success rate of expectant management are offered to the couple. A young couple is the most likely to succeed with this option. This option is frustrating at the best of times, not only to the couple but also to the physician. For older women the success rate is lower, simply because age has an important effect on spontaneous conception rates.

The next option for the couple is assisted reproduction techniques for infertility. Options under this category include AIH and IVF-ET. AIH is inexpensive and likely to be acceptable to the couple. With IVF-ET, superovulation is induced and, after harvesting the eggs, fertilisation is facilitated *in vitro* and the fertilised embryo transferred into the uterus. The advantage of this technique is that fertilisation is guaranteed and extra embryos may be stored for further attempts. However, this is a very expensive option and one whose failure may be associated with many psychological problems. This option may be complicated by OHSS, with associated severe morbidity and sometimes mortality and multiple pregnancies.

The last option for the couple is adoption. Adopting may sometimes remove the anxiety associated with attempting to conceive and result in a natural conception. Whatever the case, there is the need to be more proactive in the older than the younger couple. Those with primary infertility have a lower success rate with expectant management than those with secondary infertility. Where the duration of infertility is less than 3 years, expectant management is associated with an 8 per cent success rate.

Reference

Hull MG, Glazener CM, Kelly NJ, Conway DI, Foster PA, Hinton RA, *et al.* (1985) Population study of causes, treatment and outcome of infertility. *BMJ* **291**: 1693–7.

Further reading

McClure N (2003) Investigation of the infertile couple. In: Shaw RW, Soutter WP, Stanton SL (eds) *Gynaecology*, 3rd edn. Edinburgh: Churchill Livingstone, pp. 281–94.

2. During the course of investigating a couple who attended for secondary infertility of 2 years' duration, you opt to assess tubal function. (a) What radiological options will you consider? (7 marks) (b) Critically appraise the non-radiological options. (7 marks) (c) Outline the complications of these procedures. (6 marks)

Common mistakes

- Causes of tubal infertility – the question specifically asks about assessing tubal function
- Although tubal function can be assessed in the male partner, it is unusual for the gynaecologist to assess him
- Listing all the causes of infertility
- History, physical examination and investigations
- Treatment of causes of tubal infertility
- Comparing and contrasting
- Screening for *Chlamydia* antibodies, etc.

A good answer will include some or all of these points

(a) What radiological options will you consider? (7 marks)

- Hysterosalpingography (HSG):
  - Cannula in the cervix
  - Injection of oil-based contrast medium through the uterine cavity and Fallopian tubes under fluoroscopy
  - X-rays taken
  - Outlines uterine cavity and Fallopian tubes
  - Defines site of blockage, intrauterine adhesions
- Hysterosalpingo-contrast-sonography (HyCoSy):
  - HyCoSy injected into the uterine cavity
  - Ultrasound examination during injection
  - Saline HSG. Enables ovarian cysts to be diagnosed. May be useful in the diagnosis of Asherman's syndrome. Requires skilled personnel and equipment. Contrast ultrasound (Echovist®) similar to saline ultrasonography

(b) Critically appraise the non-radiological options. (7 marks)

- Laparoscopy and dye test:
  - Enables diagnosis of tubal adhesions, pelvic pathology such as endometriosis
  - Option of treating the adhesions and endometriosis
  - Unable to define uterine pathology and site of tubal blockage

- Requires general anaesthesia (GA) although could be done under local anaesthesia (LA)
- Falloposcopy and salpingoscopy – useful to assess the internal anatomy of the tubes. Requires GA and a very skilled operator and equipment. Unlikely to be available to all patients
- Salpingoscopy

(c) Outline the complications of these procedures. (6 marks)

- Radiological – flare-up of subclinical pelvic inflammatory disease
- Allergic reaction to dye
- Pain from grasping the cervix leading to vasovagal attacks
- Trauma to the cervix and infections
- Risks of laparoscopy:
  - GA
  - Injury to viscera
  - Infections
  - Embolisation of dye and contrast – Echovist®

Sample answer

(a) What radiological options will you consider? (7 marks)

Tubal function can be assessed by radiological and non-radiological tests. The radiological approaches to tubal function assessment include HSG and HyCoSy or saline.

Hysterosalpingography is an outpatient procedure, usually performed without GA. It involves the administration of a contrast medium (e.g. Urografin®) through the cervical and uterine canals into the Fallopian tubes. This allows visualisation of the course of the tubes, and localisation of any blockage and peritubal adhesions. Where there is tubal blockage, it localises the site of obstruction. It has the added advantage of being able to diagnose cervical weakness (incompetence) and intrauterine adhesions/suspected polyps. In addition, pathognomonic appearances may aid in the diagnosis of pelvic tuberculosis affecting the Fallopian tubes. The major disadvantages of this procedure include flare-up of subclinical chronic PID, vasovagal attacks and trauma to the cervix. In addition, false-positive tubal blockages may be reported because of tubal spasm. Unfortunately, this procedure does not allow for the examination of the rest of the pelvis and therefore the exclusion of other factors associated with infertility, such as endometriosis.

Contrast or saline hysterosonography using ultrasound for tubal patency assessment is an option that is increasingly being applied in most units. These procedures have the same advantages as those of HSG, but tubal function has to be assessed dynamically during the procedure. The main advantage over the latter is the use of ultrasound, which may allow the exclusion of ovarian pathology and intramural fibroids (a possible cause of infertility that laparoscopy may not identify).

(b) Critically appraise the non-radiological options. (7 marks)

The non-radiological methods of assessing tubal function are mainly endoscopic. The first of these and possibly the gold standard is a diagnostic laparoscopy and dye test. Although it can be performed under sedation and LA, it is most commonly performed under GA in the UK. The advantages include its ability to identify abnormal fimbriae and associated pelvic pathologies, such as adhesions and endometriosis. In addition, some of these pathologies may be treated (e.g. adhesiolysis) during the procedure. Unfortunately, it does not define the site of tubal obstruction and cannot exclude uterine pathology, such as synechiae. Skilled clinicians need to perform the procedure, which is more expensive than HSG. Where IVF may be a treatment option for the infertility, it allows for the assessment of the ovaries *vis-à-vis* oocyte retrieval.

Although the above two diagnostic procedures are most common, others, such as falloposcopy (examination of the internal surface of the Fallopian tubes through the uterine canal) and salpingoscopy (examination of the internal surfaces of the Fallopian tubes through the external ostium of the tubes at laparoscopy), are available for the assessment of tubal function; these procedures are quite specialised and therefore are only available in a few units. They require skill and expensive equipment. The advantage of both procedures is their ability to identify intratubal pathologies, which neither of the other two methods will identify. These include thinning of the epithelium and adhesions (synechiae). Again, they are commonly performed under GA, although they can be performed under sedation and LA. These additional assessments may help in the counselling of patients on their suitability for tubal surgery.

(c) Outline the complications of these procedures. (6 marks)

The complications of these procedures for assessing tubal patency depend on the procedure being undertaken. For the radiological procedures, the complications include allergic reaction to the contrast, flaring up of pelvic inflammation, trauma from instrumentation, pain and occasional vasovagal attack from pain. Secondary pelvic infection may result from the introduction of the cannula into the cervix. These complications are similar to those occurring with HyCoSy.

The complications of the various endoscopic procedures include procedure-related complications such as injury to viscera, blood vessels, infections, gas embolism and emphysema and anaesthetic-related complications such as atelectasis and respiratory tract infections.

Further reading

Djahanbakhch O, Saridongan E (2003) Tubal disease. In: Shaw RW, Soutter WP, Stanton SL (eds) *Gynaecology*, 3rd edn. Edinburgh: Churchill Livingstone, pp. 361–70.

3. An obese, 25-year-old woman with PCOS presents with infertility, which is secondary to anovulation. (a) Critically appraise the non-medical methods by which ovulation can be induced in this patient. (6 marks) (b) Discuss the anti-oestrogens that could be used for ovulation induction. (7 marks) (c) Discuss how you will induce ovulation using gonadotropins. (7 marks)

Common mistakes

- Induction of ovulation and treatment for infertility in general
- Discussing options for infertility treatment
- Concentrating on drug therapy only
- Treatment of male infertility
- Details of IVF-ET
- Discussing treatment for non-fertility symptoms of PCOS
- Failure to critically appraise your answer

A good answer will include some or all of these points

(a) Critically appraise the non-medical methods by which ovulation can be induced in this patient. (6 marks)

- Weight loss:
  - Does not require medication
  - Free of side-effects
  - Requires no medication
  - If successful, there is no increased risk of multiple pregnancy, and pregnancy complications related to obesity are reduced
  - If weight loss is successful in inducing ovulation, it will, however, complement other methods of induction ovulation
  - For most patients, this is unlikely to work, mainly because of failure to lose weight
- Ovarian drilling:
  - Either by laparoscopy or laparotomy – most commonly by laparoscopy
  - Using laser or diathermy
  - Associated with a high success rate and minimal risk of multiple pregnancy and OHSS
  - Risk of anaesthesia and difficulties in performing laparoscopy in obese patient
  - Effectiveness is time limited

(b) Discuss the anti-oestrogens that could be used for ovulation induction. (7 marks)

- Clomifene citrate. Induces ovulation in 60–80 per cent of cases, but successful pregnancy in only 40–60 per cent of cases

- Risk of multiple pregnancy (approx. 10 per cent)
- OHSS
- Requires ultrasound scan (USS) to monitor follicular development (ideal)
- Increased risk of ovarian cancer
- Not recommended to be given more than 6 months after ovulation is achieved
- Can be given in escalating doses up to 150 mg on day 2–6 of cycle
- May be combined with other methods, e.g. weight loss and other medications (metformin)
- Other anti-oestrogens include cyclofenil, tamoxifen, and the aromatase inhibitors anastrozole and letrozole

(c) Discuss how you will induce ovulation with gonadotropins. (7 marks)

- Expensive and have to be administered parentally
- Require serial monitoring by USS and serum oestradiol to help reduce the risk of OHSS and time the administration of human chorionic gonadotropin (hCG)
- Given as combined follicle-stimulating hormone (FSH) and luteinising hormone (Metrodin®) or as recombinant FSH. Recombinant FSH is free of protein, hence minimal risk of allergic reaction
- Gonadotropins can be given in three approaches starting on day 2–3 of the cycle:
  - Regular dose step-up
  - Chronic low dose step-up
  - Step-down protocols
- Increased risk of multiple pregnancies and OHSS
- Concomitant use with gonadotropin-releasing hormone (GnRH) agonist not shown to be of any real additional benefit but can be used in women who show premature luteinisation

Sample answer

(a) Critically appraise the non-medical methods by which ovulation can be induced in this patient. (6 marks)

The first non-medical option is weight loss. It does not require medication, is free of side-effects and is inexpensive. In addition, with successful induction of ovulation, pregnancy rates are higher compared to that of other methods. Weight loss does not increase the risk of multiple pregnancies and overweight-related complications of pregnancy are reduced. Additionally, weight loss increases the success rate of other methods of induction ovulation. The main drawback is the need for motivation and the fact that it may take some time to be successful.

The other non-medical method is laparoscopic (although this can be done by laparotomy) laser or diathermy drilling of the ovaries. However, the procedure-related risks are greater in this obese woman. It is expensive and involves hospital care, even if this is only during the time of surgery. The complications of the procedure include visceral injury, gas embolism, infections, adhesion formation and those of GA. In skilled hands, this may be best performed at the time of laparoscopic assessment of tubal function. This option is not associated with an increased risk of multiple pregnancies. Wedge resection of the ovary has generally been superseded by modern techniques, but may still be considered in some developing countries.

(b) *Discuss the anti-oestrogens that could be used for ovulation induction. (7 marks)*

Clomifene citrate is the most commonly used anti-oestrogen, usually administered in the early menstrual phase. It is inexpensive and induces ovulation successfully in about 30–40 per cent of patients with PCOS, although that rate may be as high as 80 per cent in properly selected patients. The 6 months' cumulative conception rate, where ovulation has been successfully induced, is similar to that of normal fertility (60 per cent) with most occurring in the first six ovulatory cycles. It has the added advantage that the multiple pregnancy rate is only 5–10 per cent and significant OHSS is rare compared to after ovulation induction with gonadotropins. Unfortunately, because of the anti-oestrogenic effects, clomifene citrate may induce ovulation but not result in successful pregnancy. Therefore, patients may often have to take multiple courses before pregnancy can be achieved. Clomifene is licensed for 6 months in the UK and if being used beyond this duration, appropriate counselling must be offered.

Where clomifene citrate has been unsuccessful, cyclofenil could be the next option. It has less anti-oestrogenic effects on the cervical mucus. It may theoretically be associated with higher pregnancy rates than clomifene citrate. However, cyclofenil is more expensive and associated with more side-effects when compared to clomifene citrate.

Other anti-oestrogens, such as the aromatase inhibitors anastrozole and letrozole, have been used in a similar way to clomifene citrate and have been shown to improve ovulation induction rates in those who are refractory to clomifene. Although the selective oestrogen receptor modulator tamoxifen has been used only occasionally, it is another option.

(c) *Discuss how you will induce ovulation using gonadotropins. (7 marks)*

Ovulation can be induced with human menopausal gonadotropin (hMG) or pure FSH (Pergonal®, Normagon® or Metrodin®), extracted from the urine of postmenopausal women or recombinant FSH. Recombinant FSH is free of extraneous proteins to which some patients may develop allergic reactions or antibodies. Gonadotropins are effective but more expensive methods of ovulation induction that have to be administered parenterally (usually daily and starting in the menstrual phase). The patient should have follicular tracking and serial oestradiol monitoring to time the administration of hCG, in order to minimise the risk of multiple pregnancies and OHSS.

Although there are several approaches to the use of gonadotropins, three are most common. These are the regular dose step-up, chronic low dose step-up and the step-down protocols. If she is to have the regular dose step-up option, she will be started on FSH 150 IU/day on day 2–3 of her cycle and increased by 75 IU/day every 3–4 days according to ovarian response assessed by serum oestradiol or ultrasound follicular measurement. Once 1–2 dominant follicles reach 18 mm, hCG is administered. It is associated with a higher incidence of multiple pregnancies and OHSS.

The next protocol that she could be offered is the chronic low dose step-up protocol. This is aimed at reaching the FSH threshold gradually and thereby avoiding excessive stimulation and development of multiple follicles. The starting dose is about 37.5–75 IU/day of FSH and continued for 10–14 days followed by increases of 37.5 IU/day every week to a maximum of 225 IU/day. When the dominant follicle reaches 18 mm, hCG is administered. The main disadvantage is that it may take longer to reach the FSH threshold and she will have to be counselled appropriately. This regimen is associated with fewer multiple pregnancies and a lower risk of OHSS compared to the regular dose step-up protocol.

The last option is the step-down protocol whose aim is to mimic the physiological changes of a normal menstrual cycle. She would be given FSH starting with 150 IU/day on day 2–3 of cycle and follicular tracking monitored every 2–3 days. Once the dominant follicle is at least 10 mm, the dose is reduced to 112.5/day followed by a further decrease to 75 IU/day after 3 days. This is continued until hCG administration, the timing of which is determined by the size of the dominant follicle.

Combining gonadotropins with GnRH agonist has not been shown to confer any additional benefits in women with PCOS and is therefore only appropriate in women with premature luteinisation.

Further reading

Balen A (2003) The polycystic ovary syndrome. In: Shaw RW, Soutter WP, Stanton SL (eds) *Gynaecology*, 3rd edn. Edinburgh: Churchill Livingstone, pp. 259–70.
Ng EHY, Ho PC (2003) Ovulation induction. In: Shaw RW, Soutter WP, Stanton SL (eds) *Gynaecology*, 3rd edn. Edinburgh: Churchill Livingstone, pp. 252–3.

4. Ovarian hyperstimulation syndrome is an important cause of severe morbidity and mortality in assisted reproduction. (a) Which factors predispose to OHSS? (3 marks) (b) What steps will you take to minimise the risk of OHSS? (8 marks) (c) How will you recognise OHSS? (4 marks) (d) Briefly discuss its management. (5 marks)

Common mistakes

- Classification and details of OHSS
- Treatment and management of the causes of OHSS
- Mentioning irrelevant points, e.g. OHSS does not occur with GnRH analogues (this is not true and if you are uncertain do not mention it) – OHSS occurs in natural cycles!
- Vaginal examination is contraindicated in OHSS
- Scanning before induction of ovulation to determine suitability for induction. Listing investigations for OHSS
- Inaccurate facts, e.g. features of OHSS include hirsutism, irregular periods and vaginal bleeding
- Use of clomifene for more than 6 months inadvisable because of OHSS
- Stating that it only occurs in PCOS patients in whom injudicious use of gonadotropins has occurred
- Defining the features of OHSS (enlarged ovaries, abdominal distension, nausea, vomiting, diarrhoea, and, in severe forms, ascites, pleural effusions, hypovolaemia, hypotension and polycythaemia)

A good answer will include some or all of these points

(a) Which factors predispose to OHSS? (3 marks)

- Predisposing factors:
  - Large number of follicles (especially induced by gonadotropins and βhCG)
  - βhCG administration
  - Younger patients
  - Pregnancy – four times higher incidence in conception cycles. Pregnancy is three times more likely in OHSS cycles
  - Low body mass index (weight) (BMI <19)
  - PCOS

(b) What steps will you take to minimise the risk of OHSS? (8 marks)

- Serial follicular tracking to ensure no hCG administration for more follicles
- Oestradiol levels >6000 pmol, do not administer βhCG
- Advice against sexual intercourse if oestradiol levels high or large number of follicles

- Progestogens rather than βhCG to support pregnancy
- Ovarian drilling/diathermy for PCOS
- Clomid® rather than gonadotropins
- hMG + GnRH agonists decrease the risk of OHSS compared to gonadotropins alone

(c) How will you recognise OHSS? (4 marks)

- Symptoms – mild, moderate or severe (abdominal pain, vomiting, chest pain, enlarged abdomen)
- Ultrasound – follicles, ascites
- Biochemistry – deranged urea and electrolytes (U&Es), hypovolaemia, low urine output, pleural effusion – chest X-ray (CXR)

(d) Briefly discuss its management. (5 marks)

- Should be protocol driven:
  - Mild cases may be managed at home – moderate to severe cases to be admitted
- Divided into several aspects:
  - Symptom control:
    - Pain relief – avoid non-steroidal anti-inflammatory drugs (NSAIDs) as these may precipitate renal failure
    - Nausea and vomiting – metoclopramide/prochlorperazine
  - Fluid replacement – most of the fluid is in the extravascular compartment, hence the intravascular volume is constricted and needs replacing:
    - Oral if mild and no vomiting/nausea
    - Intravenous – if moderate to severe and/or there is nausea and vomiting – colloids preferred to crystalloids
  - Fluid accumulation:
    - Drainage if necessary – ascites or hydrothorax
  - Thromboprophylaxis:
    - Thromboembolic deterrent (TED) stocking
    - Low-molecular-weight heparin (Fragmin®)

Sample answer

(a) Which factors predispose to OHSS? (3 marks)

The factors predisposing to OHSS include the age of the patient (the younger the patient, the greater the risk), PCOS, low body mass index (BMI <19), βhCG administration, high serum oestradiol levels during ovulation induction, and a larger number of follicles (>18–20 mm in diameter) during ovulation and pregnancy. Pregnancy is three times more likely in OHSS cycles.

(b) What steps will you take to minimise the risk of OHSS? (8 marks)

Minimising the risk of OHSS must involve reducing the predisposing factors. First, ovulation induction is best undertaken by drugs that are least likely to induce the condition, e.g. use anti-oestrogen agents such as clomifene citrate instead of gonadotropins. However, this may not necessarily be the case, as these drugs may be ineffective. Therefore, alternatives to gonadotropins, such as ovarian drilling, must also be considered. Where gonadotropins are employed, the ovulation induction process must be monitored closely. This will include follicular tracking with ultrasound to ensure that there are not too many follicles ready to rupture. This can be complemented with serum oestradiol estimations. If the number of follicles above 12 mm in diameter is more than 15, or serum oestradiol levels are above 2000 pg/mL, then βhCG should be withheld. This will delay, or prevent, release of the ova from the follicles. In some cases, it has been suggested that delaying rather than omitting the βhCG may also minimise the risk of OHSS.

Where ovulation induction is for a natural conception, advising against sexual intercourse will minimise the risk of OHSS. This will prevent pregnancy and therefore reduce the chances of OHSS developing. If pregnancy does occur, the use of progestogens rather than βhCG to support the early phase of pregnancy will significantly minimise the risk of OHSS.

Ovulation induction with GnRH agonists with βhCG or hMG is associated with a lower risk of OHSS compared to the use of hMG and hCG. Used in a pulsatile fashion, this has been shown to result in successful pregnancy without the risk of developing the condition. In patients who have raised oestradiol levels, GnRH agonists with βhCG or hMG may be used during induction of ovulation with gonadotropins. Imoedemhe *et al.* (1991) used 8-hourly intranasal buserelin in patients with >4000 pg/mL oestradiol levels and achieved a 22 per cent pregnancy rate with no case of OHSS. Alternatively, follicular aspiration may be used. Pregnancies after IVF are rarely complicated by OHSS, because of aspiration of the follicles. Therefore, where there are many follicles above the threshold diameter, repeated aspiration will minimise the risk of OHSS.

Although other methods of minimising the risk of OHSS have been employed, e.g. intravenous administration of albumin and also corticosteroids, these are not commonly used. The most effective method of minimising this complication of superovulation is to monitor the patient closely and to offer interventions that will minimise it. It is also important to identify early symptoms and signs of OHSS and to take the steps necessary to prevent progression.

(c) How will you recognise OHSS? (4 marks)

Ovarian hyperstimulation syndrome consists of ovarian enlargement, abdominal distension, ascites, nausea, vomiting and diarrhoea, and, in severe forms, pleural effusion, hypovolaemia, hypotension and polycythaemia. If improperly managed, it could be fatal. Recognition should start with a high index of suspicion and then the clinical features enumerated above. This can be confirmed by ancillary investigations which must include USS for ascites, U&Es, liver function tests and, if indicated, a CXR.

(d) Briefly discuss its management. (5 marks)

Treatment should be protocol driven and intensive as this is a recognised cause of mortality. Mild cases may be managed at home but moderate and severe cases should be admitted into hospital. Treatment should be directed at the control of symptoms, fluid replacement, removal of accumulated fluids and thromboprophylaxis. With regards to symptoms, pain should be treated with simple analgesics (avoiding NSAIDs) and nausea and vomiting treated with antiemetics such a metoclopramide and prochlorperazine. Occasionally, something stronger may have to be administered. In OHSS there is constriction of the intravascular compartment, hence plasma expanders should be considered. If there is no nausea/vomiting and it is mild, oral fluids should be prescribed. Where there is nausea and vomiting or if it is more than mild, intravenous plasma expanders such as colloids may be offered. Drainage of extracellular fluid, especially that which affects the woman's health, should be considered (e.g. drainage of a pleural effusion).

An important cause of mortality in these patients, especially those with severe disease, is venous thromboembolism. Prophylaxis in the form of TED stockings, appropriate mobilisation and prophylactic low-molecular-weight heparin should be offered.

Reference

Imoedemhe DAG, Chan RCW, Signe AB, Papaco ELA, Olaza AB (1991) A new approach to the management of patients at risk of ovarian hyperstimulation in an *in vitro* fertilization programme. *Hum Reprod* **6**: 1088–91.

Further reading

RCOG (2006). *Green-top Guideline No 5. The Management of Ovarian Hyperstimulation Syndrome.* September 2006. London: Royal College of Obstetricians and Gynaecologists.
Rizk B (1994) Ovarian hyperstimulation syndrome. In: Studd J (ed.) *Progress in Obstetrics and Gynaecology*, vol. 12. London: Churchill Livingstone, pp. 311–49.

5. A couple attending the infertility clinic have been investigated and the husband's semen analysis was described as oligozoospermic. Evaluate the options available to the couple. (20 marks)

Common mistakes

- Taking a history and doing a physical examination – this would have been done before the investigations
- Details of investigations for infertility are irrelevant
- Discussing treatment of zoospermia
- Offer a procedure and then state that it is most unlikely to succeed – if so, why offer it in the first place? If you were the patient, would you accept it?
- You have been asked to evaluate the options and not to outline how to investigate the infertile couple
- Failure to evaluate the treatment options

A good answer will include some or all of these points

- Assumption – repeat semen analysis remains abnormal and female investigations are normal
- Options – four main ones:
  - Identify cause of oligozoospermia and correct if treatable. This is the most cost effective option and there is no need for invasive procedures, which may be associated with higher pregnancy rates. May need referral to a urologist. Modification of lifestyle to remove risk factors
  - Assisted conception techniques: artificial insemination with husband's sperm (AIH) or donor sperm (AID) and intrauterine insemination – sperm preparation and concentration. Only extra requirement is sperm preparation. Success rate may be improved by induction of ovulation. Use of husband's sperm, therefore biological father – more acceptable; AID – least likely to be accepted at the outset (as first suggestion); AIH and AID cheaper than IVF
  - Advanced assisted conception techniques:
    - IVF – expensive and low success rate; may still need donor sperm
    - Gamete intrafallopian transfer – cheapest of the three; may still need donor sperm;
    - Intracytoplasmic sperm injection (ICSI) – if sperm cannot fertilise or are morphologically abnormal; expensive and associated with the complications of superovulation and OHSS
  - Adoption: child not biological offspring of parents

Sample answer

It is to be assumed that the semen analysis was performed at least twice in this couple and that the results were basically similar. Therefore, there is no need to repeat the semen analysis. In the first instance, the cause of the oligozoospermia should be identified if possible. If treatable, this will be the most suitable option to be offered. However, in most cases the cause is difficult to identify and treatment is neither a logical nor a satisfactory option. If there is no known cause, the husband should be referred to a urologist for further evaluation and management if necessary. Sometimes a simple modification of lifestyle, such as working habits, smoking, drugs, etc., may be all that is necessary to improve the quality of the semen. Therefore, before referral, information about lifestyle factors that could influence semen analysis should be elicited and appropriate counselling offered.

The second option is AIH. In this case, the sperm have to be prepared so that only normal ones are present and, in addition, the concentration is significantly improved. This may go in tandem with ovulation induction in order to improve the success rate. For this option, the only requirements are facilities for sperm preparation and introduction into the cervical canal. The main advantage is involvement of both partners and the offspring will be genetically from both parents. However, AID may be another alternative. In this case, the biological father is a donor. Psychologically, this may be more difficult for the couple to accept.

Advanced assisted conception techniques may be offered in two different ways. The first is IVF where ovulation induction is undertaken followed by fertilisation with the husband's sperm (specially prepared) if they are morphologically normal, or by ICSI using spermatids aspirated from the testis. This option is expensive and some couples may not be able to afford it, especially where it is only available privately. Also, ICSI is likely to be an option only in highly specialised tertiary centres or private units. Complications with these advanced techniques may negate their availability.

The last option for the couple is adoption. This is complex, time consuming and very lengthy, which make it a very frustrating option for the couple. In addition, the couple are not the biological parents of the adopted child and may be apprehensive about this. Oligozoospermia is a complication that must be handled with sensitivity and adequate empathy. The treatment options are many but the couple have to be comfortable with the one they eventually choose.

Further reading

Anderson RA, Irvine S (2003) Disorders of male reproduction. In: Shaw RW, Soutter WP, Stanton SL (eds) *Gynaecology*, 3rd edn. Edinburgh: Churchill Livingstone, pp. 295–315.

9

Family planning

1. A 31-year-old woman has attended the clinic requesting reversal of sterilisation. (a) What principles will underpin your management? (16 marks) (b) How will you counsel her after the procedure? (4 marks)

2. Briefly outline the non-contraceptive uses of the combined oral contraceptive pill (COCP). (20 marks)

3. A 30-year-old woman wishes to have the levonorgestrel intrauterine system (Mirena®) for contraception. (a) Discuss the unwanted side-effects of this method of contraception. (8 marks) (b) What are the additional benefits of Mirena®? (5 marks) (c) What advice will you give her after inserting the device? (7 marks)

4. A 46-year-old woman attends the Well Women Clinic asking for advice on contraception. (a) Evaluate her contraceptive options. (12 marks) (b) How will her age influence your recommended method? (4 marks) (c) What advice will you give about contraception and HRT? (4 marks)

1. A 31-year-old woman has attended the clinic requesting reversal of sterilisation. (a) What principles will underpin your management? (16 marks) (b) How will you counsel her after the procedure? (4 marks)

Common mistakes

- Illogical in management – not following a logical order
- Describing the details of reversal of sterilisation – microsurgical or macrosurgical techniques; describing these in detail, etc.
- It is not offered in the National Health Service, hence she should be offered *in vitro* fertilisation (IVF)!
- Refer to the private sector for reversal
- Discussing the causes of tubal damage and how these can be prevented to avoid reversal of sterilisation
- Commenting on the regret rate following sterilisation and discussing how this can be minimised with appropriate counselling
- Listing the reasons why a reversal should be performed
- Highlighting the cost of reversal

A good answer will include some or all of these points

(a) What principles will underpin your management? (16 marks)

- The request needs to be justified (this is not a scientific concept)
- Information about the type of sterilisation (from history or from gynaecology notes if patient cannot remember). If notes are not available, request them – diathermy poor success rate; clips or rings – good success rate
- Ovulating or not – investigate
- Semen analysis – normal?
- Assess Fallopian tubes at laparoscopy – what will be the length of Fallopian tube left after reversal?
- If residual Fallopian tube is less than 4 cm, success rate is poor
- Type of reversal – microscopic or macroscopic
- Complications
- Alternatives to reversal of sterilisation if unaccepted

(b) How will you counsel her after the procedure? (4 marks)

- Pregnancy rates highest within the first 12 months of the procedure
- Increased risk of ectopic pregnancy – therefore to report if period missed or at the earliest positive pregnancy test
- Avoid the intrauterine contraceptive device (IUD) as a form of contraceptive for the future

Sample answer

(a) What principles will underpin your management? (16 marks)

A request for reversal of sterilisation is not uncommon, especially as approximately 10 per cent of women in the UK regret the decision to undergo sterilisation. In the first instance, this request needs to be assessed to determine whether it is justified. For most units, there are strict criteria that have to be fulfilled before a reversal can be allowed.

Following justification of the procedure, additional information is required about the type of sterilisation the patient had. A laparoscopic sterilisation with clips offers the best success rate of reversal, followed by sterilisation by rings. Open sterilisation, where portions of the Fallopian tubes were excised, and diathermy sterilisation have poorer reversal success rates. If she had diathermy sterilisation, the success rate is so poor that it might not even be advisable to offer her a reversal.

Factors that could potentially affect the success rate of a reversal must be excluded. These include ovulation and good quality semen. If any of these is abnormal, attempts have to be made to identify the cause and to correct them before the reversal. Assessment of ovulation is best done by serial luteal-phase progesterone assays, whereas a semen analysis will identify any abnormal male factor.

If the decision is to offer a reversal, the next principle will be to determine how much residual Fallopian tube will be left after the procedure. This may be assessed at the time of the reversal or as a separate procedure. The advantage of making such an assessment as a separate procedure is the opportunity it provides for the assessment of the pelvis for coexisting factors, such as endometriosis or pelvic adhesions, which could affect fertility if not rectified. Some surgeons believe that such a separate procedure exposes the patient to an unnecessary risk of repeated general anaesthesia. However, there are others who believe that this separate assessment is important as it provides an opportunity for a prognostic assessment before surgery. If the residual Fallopian tube is judged to be considerably less than 4 cm, it may not be worth undertaking the procedure.

Where the patient is suitable for reversal, the success of the procedure will depend on the type of reversal and the expertise of the operator. Microscopic reversal has a higher success rate than macroscopic reversal. In addition, when performed by a skilled operator the procedure has a better success rate. In good hands, and by use of microsurgical techniques, the success rate is in the order of 70–80 per cent. Any complications (especially infections) arising after the procedure will influence success. Attempts must therefore be made to maintain meticulous asepsis and also to offer prophylactic antibiotics to minimise the risk of infection.

Where the request is unacceptable or is considered unsuitable, alternatives such as IVF with embryo transfer should be discussed and offered if available.

(b) How will you counsel her after the procedure? (4 marks)

The success rate will also be influenced by the interval between the reversal and pregnancy. It is highest within the first 12 months of surgery. This should be emphasised during the counselling offered before the reversal, as there is no benefit in undertaking the procedure if the patient is uncertain about trying for a baby for at least 12 months. The risk of ectopic pregnancy is increased and the patient should be educated not only on the early warning symptoms but also on the importance of seeking medical advice early following a missed period or an early pregnancy test. The IUD is not advisable even when she has completed her family, as the risk of ectopic pregnancy is also higher.

2. Briefly outline the non-contraceptive uses of the COCP. (20 marks)

Common mistakes

- Listing the indications for the COCP
- Advantages and disadvantages of the COCP
- Different types of the COCP
- Complications of the COCP
- Discussing how the oral contraceptive works
- Discussing the contraindications to the use of the COCP

A good answer will include some or all of these points

- Control of menstrual problems – most common:
  - Regulation of menstruation
  - Treatment of amenorrhoea
  - Premenstrual syndrome (PMS)
- Stimulation of the uterus in Asherman's syndrome
- Control of menopausal symptoms
- Control of dysmenorrhoea
- Treatment of endometriosis
- Hirsutism and acne in polycystic ovary syndrome (PCOS)

Sample answer

The most common application of the COCP is in the control of menstrual problems. It may be used in the treatment of menorrhagia, irregular vaginal bleeding and dysmenorrhoea. In the treatment of these menstrual dysfunctions, it is administered in a similar way to its use as a contraceptive. In most of these situations, it provides a dual role of contraception and of menstrual dysfunction control. It is effective in perimenarchal girls with heavy and painful periods; however, caution must be exercised when prescribing for this group of patients as the oestrogen component may affect the ultimate height of the young patient.

Another application is in the treatment of endometriosis. This is offered continuously without the pill-free interval. When the COCP is used as a contraception, it has also been shown to be effective, although less than when used continuously. The duration of treatment is commonly 6 months. The major drawback is breakthrough bleeding. Its use in the treatment of adenomyosis has not been shown to be as effective as that in endometriosis.

The COCP may be used in PMS, although there is no strong evidence to support the effectiveness of this treatment. However, in some patients, this treatment may make the symptoms worse. Other non-contraceptive uses of the COCP include the control of menopausal symptoms and treatment of amenorrhoea where the cause is secondary to oestrogen deficiency. In

PCOS, where there is oligomenorrhoea or irregular vaginal bleeding, the less androgenic COCP may be used to regulate the menstrual cycle. Some patients with PCOS and hirsutism may also be treated with a less androgenic COCP or one containing cyproterone acetate (Dianette®) or Yasmin® (which contains the progestogen drospirenone).

Another uncommon use of the COCP includes the treatment of patients with Asherman's syndrome. High doses of oestrogens in the COCP may be offered to induce proliferation of the epithelium of the deep glands following separation of adhesions. However, the COCP is less effective than oestrogens alone in this regard.

3. A 30-year-old woman wishes to have the levonorgestrel intrauterine system (Mirena®) for contraception. (a) Discuss the unwanted side-effects of this method of contraception. (8 marks) (b) What are the additional benefits of Mirena®? (5 marks) (c) What advice will you give her after inserting the device? (7 marks)

Common mistakes

- Discussing how Mirena® works
- The pros and cons of Mirena®
- Discussing data on its efficacy in menorrhagia
- Cost of Mirena® compared to other forms of contraception
- Expulsion rates and continuation rates of Mirena®
- Discussing the treatment of irregular bleeding

A good answer will include some or all of these points

(a) Discuss the unwanted side-effects of this method of contraception. (8 marks)

- Irregular vaginal bleeding worse over the first 3–4 months
- Localised uterine pain
- Acne, oily skin, fluid retention
- Breast tenderness
- Depression
- Weight gain
- Functional ovarian cysts (10–15 per cent of cases)

(b) What are the additional benefits of Mirena®? (5 marks)

- Menorrhagia – treatment may result in amenorrhoea or hypomenorrhoea
- Dysmenorrhoea
- Fibroids
- Adenomyosis – reduces the size of the adenomyosis
- Endometriosis
- PMS – whether this is the placebo effect is uncertain

(c) What advice will you give her after inserting the device? (7 marks)

- Irregular periods/bleeding – worse over the first 3–6 months
- Most likely to settle into amenorrhoea or hypomenorrhoea or oligoamenorrhoea
- Feel string after each period

- Counsel about side-effects
- If planning on a pregnancy, report for removal, otherwise give date for removal (after 5 years)
- Avoid multiple sexual partners – although may decrease the risk of pelvic inflammatory disease (PID)
- If pregnant, need to exclude an ectopic pregnancy

Sample answer

(a) Discuss the unwanted side-effects of this method of contraception. (8 marks)

The levonorgestrel intrauterine system delivers the progestogen levonorgestrel at a steady rate of 20 μg/day for 5 years. Although this is mainly into the uterine cavity, some of it is absorbed and causes systemic progestogenic side-effects. However, most of the severe side-effects of Mirena® are related to the local effects of the progestogens.

The most common unwanted side-effect is irregular vaginal bleeding. This is unpredictable and is worse over the first 3–4 months. For most women, this is the reason for discontinuation. The systemic side-effects include acne, oily skin, fluid retention (manifesting as weight gain, depression and breast tenderness). The Mirena® is associated with functional ovarian cysts which may present with localised abdominal pain. These cysts occur in approximately 10–15 per cent of cases. Most of them are asymptomatic and do not require treatment. Although rare, some women complain of localised discomfort over the uterus; this is related to the positioning of the Mirena®.

(b) What are the additional benefits of Mirena®? (5 marks)

Mirena® has several non-contraceptive benefits. It is very effective in the treatment of menorrhagia where it has been reported to reduce bleeding by approximately 70–80 per cent in approximately 70 per cent of patients who are placed on the device. It is now a recommended method of treatment for menorrhagia, especially the idiopathic type.

It is effective in other gynaecological conditions, e.g. endometriosis, adenomyosis and fibroids. In women with minimal to moderate endometriosis, it has been shown to be effective with a reduction in pain reported in 70 per cent of patients after 3 years. Although a small cohort of women with adenomyosis has been shown to benefit from Mirena® there are no large studies to confirm this. It has been reported to be beneficial in those with fibroids and PMS. Whether it is the placebo effect in the PMS group is uncertain. What is clear is the fact that it may make the symptoms of PMS worse.

(c) What advice will you give her after inserting the device? (7 marks)

The most important advice to be offered to anyone after insertion of the Mirena® is with regards to irregular vaginal bleeding. This bleeding is unpredictable and could be heavy in some cases. However, it does get better and for most women this tends to be replaced by hypomenorrhoea. Since irregular bleeding is the most common reason for discontinuation, anticipatory counselling will result in better compliance. Several approaches have been tried to reduce this but the most appropriate is counselling.

The device is best inserted during menstruation as it guarantees that the patient is not pregnant. In addition, the insertion is easier. Following insertion, the woman must be advised to feel for the strings of the device especially after the first few periods if they are heavy. If she is planning another pregnancy, the device should be removed; otherwise a date for removal should be given and documented in her notes (usually 5 years from the date of insertion) and the card given to her. Multiple sexual partners should be avoided and she should report early whenever she becomes pregnant to ensure that an ectopic pregnancy is excluded.

4. A 46-year-old woman attends the Well Women Clinic asking for advice on contraception. (a) Evaluate her contraceptive options. (12 marks) (b) How will her age influence your recommended method? (4 marks) (c) What factors in her history will be against her use of LARCs? (4 marks)

Common mistakes

- Details of hormone replacement therapy (HRT) in a perimenopausal woman
- Advantages of HRT
- Diagnosis of menopause
- Contraindications to HRT
- Screening for cervical/endometrial cancer
- Contraception in a perimenopausal woman in general
- Measuring cholesterol levels and discussing their importance

A good answer will include some or all of these points

(a) Evaluate her contraceptive options. (12 marks)

- Sterilisation – consider permanent, one-off procedure, complications of surgery and anaesthesia; risk of ectopic if failure, failure rate = 1:200 cf. vasectomy 1:2000
- LARCs – Mirena®, IUDs, Depo-Provera®, Implanon® – reduced dependence on patient compliance:
  - More effective at the end of reproductive life
  - Need to exclude contraindications
- COCP:
  - If non-smoker and not obese
  - No contraindications
  - Could provide additional benefits as HRT
  - Increase risk of venous thromboembolism (VTE)

(b) How will her age influence your recommended method? (4 marks)

- Older therefore fertility lower and efficacy of all methods better
- More likely to have medical problem which will be a relative contraindication to some of the methods
- More likely to be in a stable relationship, hence reduced risk of PID
- More like to accept sterilisation
- Periods more likely to be irregular, hence contraceptive that may help this likely to be acceptable
- Perimenopausal, hence contraception may act as HRT

(c) What advice will you give about contraception and HRT? (4 marks)

- Contraception important as pregnancy can occur – hormone levels do not exclude the risk of pregnancy
- Age <50 – contraception for 2 years after age 50
- Age >50 contraception for 1 year
- On HRT before menopause – stop and wait for 6 months, then check hormone levels/remains amenorrhoeic
- IUD, surgical sterilisation, COCP

Sample answer

(a) Evaluate her contraceptive options. (12 marks)

The options include tubal ligation (sterilisation), the COCP, the mini-pill and LARCs such as the IUD, Depo-Provera®, Mirena® and Implanon®.

Tubal ligation (sterilisation) is an ideal method for any age group. In the perimenopausal woman, this is even more ideal and it is unlikely that she will return requesting for reversal. However, during counselling, the frequent occurrence of irregular periods in this age group must be emphasized, as some women may blame the irregularity of their periods on the sterilisation. The failure rate of female tubal ligation is 1:200 compared to 1:2000 for vasectomy. The latter is easier to perform and has fewer side-effects and complications. It can also be performed under local anaesthesia.

The COCP is another option. The low-dose oestrogen COCP will be more suitable in this age group. However, since this is associated with an increased risk of VTE, the risk factors for this complication, such as smoking, obesity, hypertension, family history and thrombophilia, must be excluded. Again, this is more effective in this age group. It may provide the added benefit of counteracting perimenopausal symptoms, which may require HRT. The mini-pill is an effective form of contraception; however, the complication of irregular vaginal bleeding may cause unnecessary anxiety derived from the need to exclude hyperplasia or endometrial carcinoma. However, the mini-pill may offer relative protection against oestrogen-induced endometrial hyperplasia. For this option, compliance is an important factor.

The LARCs, just like all forms of contraception, are more effective in this age group compared to younger women. However, they must be acceptable to the patient. The first in this group are the IUDs (copper medicated or the Mirena®). The complication of irregular vaginal bleeding, especially during the early months after administration, may result in early discontinuation, especially with Mirena®. For most women, adequate counselling will result in a high continuation rate. Since the duration of this form of contraception depends on the type of LARC, the choice could be such that, once administered it potentially covers the rest of the reproductive life of the woman. The irregular vaginal bleeding with this method may require investigating and therefore generate significant anxiety. For women who also need HRT, the Mirena® may be combined with HRT to offer endometrial protection.

(b) How will her age influence your recommended method? (4 marks)

The efficacy of any chosen method of contraception is higher in the older woman as fertility declines. The permanent form of contraception is more acceptable to older women, who are more likely to have medical problems such a diabetes mellitus and hypertension which may be considered relative contraindications to some forms of contraception. The older woman is at risk of VTE and added risk factors such as smoking will limit the choice of method. Advancing age is associated with irregular periods which are themselves a relative contraindication to some forms of contraception. However, having said that, the older woman is more likely to accept irregular vaginal bleeding and other side-effects of contraceptives. The chosen methods may also induce amenorrhoea more easily in these women. Finally, the timing of replacements of various options may differ significantly because of reduced fertility.

(c) What advice will you give about contraception and HRT? (4 marks)

Contraceptive advice is extremely important in the woman who is on cyclical HRT or is about to start HRT and is perimenopausal. She should continue with an adequate form of contraception for up to 2 years after the presumed age of menopause. As this is difficult to ascertain, it may be advisable for the woman to stop HRT and contraception for 6 months and see whether her periods resume, or measure hormone levels and ascertain that ovulation does not occur. Stopping contraception in these women could be extremely difficult. In those who are under 50 years of age, it is advisable to continue contraception for 2 years after the age of 50 before stopping, and for those over the age of 50, continuation should be for 1 year.

10

Pelvic infections, pelvic pain, chronic vaginal discharge

1. (a) What principles will you follow in the management of a patient who has been suffering from chronic pelvic pain (CPP) for the past 3 years? (10 marks) (b) How will your treatment differ if no cause is found for the pain? (10 marks)

2. A 30-year-old woman presented with lower abdominal pain, low-grade pyrexia and a history of chronic vaginal discharge. On examination, she was found to have a lower abdominal mass, which was tender but there was no ascites. An ultrasound scan showed a multiloculated cystic mass in the pouch of Douglas but no free fluid. A CA125 was slightly raised. You suspect she has a large tubo-ovarian abscess. Critically appraise your management of the patient. (20 marks)

3. During a routine gynaecology consultation, you see a 27-year-old woman presenting with chronic vaginal discharge. (a) What additional information will you obtain from her? (6 marks) (b) Justify the investigations you will undertake on her. (8 marks) (c) How will you manage her? (6 marks)

4. Critically appraise the measures you will undertake to reduce the prevalence of *Chlamydia trachomatis* genital infections. (20 marks)

1. (a) What principles will you follow in the management of a patient who has been suffering from CPP for the past 3 years? (10 marks) (b) How will your treatment differ if no cause is found for the pain? (10 marks)

Common mistakes

- Discussing the management of pelvic inflammatory disease (PID)
- Cause of pain is psychological – it is not possible to make this assumption on the basis of the information provided. However, it is recognised that this is a possible, but not very likely, scenario
- Treat with psychotherapy – this cannot be the only method of treating this patient – has to be combined with another treatment modality
- Offer treatment for infertility after investigating the patient and her partner. This is completely irrelevant. You are not expected to even broach the subject of fertility
- Exclude human immunodeficiency virus (HIV) – on what basis? HIV does not cause pelvic pain
- Assume she has endometriosis and treat – this diagnosis should only be one of the differential diagnoses rather than the sole cause

A good answer will include some or all of these points

(a) What principles will you follow in the management of a patient who has been suffering from CPP for the past 3 years? (10 marks)

- This is a common symptom that could be due to many causes – the most important principle in the treatment is to identify a cause if possible – recognising that the cause may not be identifiable in some cases
- A good history will be required to identify some of the common causes – this needs to be focused and directed
- Physical examination may be useful, but often not
- Investigations – most important – diagnostic laparoscopy
- Treatment – depends on the cause
- Medical: combined oral contraceptive pill; progestogens; gonadotropin-releasing hormone (GnRH) analogues; analgesics
- Surgery: bilateral salpingo-oophorectomy; total abdominal hysterectomy + bilateral salpingo-oophorectomy; laparoscopic uterosacral nerve ablation (LUNA), etc.
- Psychotherapy

(b) How will your treatment differ if no cause is found for the pain? (10 marks)

- Characterise the pain
- Exploration of factors that may be associated with the pain (e.g. sexual dysfunction, physical abuse, other social problems)

- Multidisciplinary team – pain physician (usually an anaesthetist), clinical psychologist, social support worker and gynaecologist with an interest in CPP
- Treatment will depend on type of pain:
  - Cyclical pain:
    - Combined oral contraceptive pill, GnRH agonist (monthly or 3 monthly, Mirena®)
    - Progestogens – norethisterone/Depo-Provera®
    - Diagnostic laparoscopy – diagnostic and therapeutic
    - Analgesics – non-steroidal anti-inflammatory drugs (NSAIDs) and opiates
  - Non-cyclical:
    - Analgesics
    - Injections of trigger spots
  - Associated with other factors:
    - Counselling and appropriate treatment to eliminate the precipitating factor (most patients will deny a causal association with these factors)
    - Clinical psychologist should be involved
  - Other forms of treatment:
    - Acupuncture
    - Transcutaneous electrical nerve stimulation (TENS)
    - Hypnosis
    - Other non-traditional approaches

Sample answer

(a) What principles will you follow in the management of a patient who has been suffering from CPP for the past 3 years? (10 marks)

Chronic pelvic pain is a common symptom and may be due to a variety of gynaecological and non-gynaecological causes. In the management of this patient, fundamental principles that have to be followed include establishing the cause of the pain and directing treatment to this cause. This can only be achieved through a thorough history, physical examination and appropriate investigations.

The relationship of this patient's symptoms to her menstrual cycle must be established. In addition, other associated symptoms, such as vaginal discharge, infertility and deep dyspareunia need to be excluded. A physical examination to identify associated signs, such as vaginal discharge, cervical excitation tenderness and adnexal masses, is the next important step in her management.

Investigations that have to be performed include endocervical and high vaginal swabs. It is unlikely that these will provide any additional information for the diagnosis. However, for completeness, these have to be performed to exclude associated infections. The most important diagnostic investigation is a laparoscopy. This will exclude endometriosis and chronic PID. It is unlikely to exclude irritable bowel syndrome and other non-gynaecological causes of the CPP.

The treatment of choice will depend on the identified cause. If it is endometriosis, treatment options will include the combined oral contraceptive pill, progestogen-only pill or GnRH analogues. The most effective treatment will be GnRH analogues. However, the complications of these drugs must be considered during counselling before treatment.

If chronic PID is the diagnosis, treatment has to be tailored to this. There are no randomised controlled trials of the efficacy of antibiotics in the treatment of chronic PID but in this patient an antibiotic covering *Chlamydia trachomatis*, Gram-negative and Gram-positive organisms, and anaerobes may be offered. Subsequent supportive treatment will be tailored to the patient's symptoms. These will include psychotherapy, surgery and steroids.

Surgical options include total abdominal hysterectomy and bilateral salpingo-oophorectomy, bilateral salpingo-oophorectomy alone and LUNA. In those with pelvic pain of no definite cause, a total abdominal hysterectomy will only eliminate menstrual problems, whereas oophorectomy will alleviate cyclical symptoms related to the ovarian cycle. There is need to counsel the patient about possible failings of these radical treatment options.

(b) How will your treatment differ if no cause is found for the pain? (10 marks)

Where no cause for the pelvic pain is found, treatment will depend on several factors. Initially, the pain should be characterised, e.g. is the pain cyclical or constant? Is there any association with sexual intercourse or bowel habits? Factors such as sexual dysfunction (rape, anorgasmia, dyspareunia), physical abuse or other social problems should be excluded through a sensitive and tactful questioning. Treatment should be multidisciplinary, including a clinical psychologist, an anaesthetist and a gynaecologist with an interest in CPP. A diagnostic laparoscopy alone may be adequate reassurance to some of these patients.

Where the pain is cyclical, treatment options include the combined oral contraceptive pill, GnRH agonists, and the Mirena® intrauterine contraceptive device (IUD). Progestogens have been shown to improve the pain in those with pelvic varicosities (diagnosed by pelvic venography – an investigation rarely undertaken today). Adding NSAIDs and opiates to the treatment would increase the chances of reducing the severity of the symptoms.

For non-cyclical pain, the treatment approach will include simple analgesics, NSAIDs and injections of trigger points.

Whatever the type of pain, attempts must be made to eliminate or reduce the associated factors. Appropriate counselling and treatment to eliminate precipitating factors has been shown to be extremely helpful in these patients.

Finally non-conventional treatment options such as hydrotherapy, acupuncture, TENS and hypnosis must be considered. These may be offered in non-clinical set-ups but increasingly, these alternatives are becoming available within the National Health Service.

Further reading

Sundarapandian V, Shankar M, Konje JC. Chronic pelvic pain: the enigma of gynaecological practice. *Br J Hosp Med* 2006; **67**: 192–6.

2. A 30-year-old woman presented with lower abdominal pain, low-grade pyrexia and a history of chronic vaginal discharge. On examination, she was found to have a lower abdominal mass, which was tender but there was no ascites. An ultrasound scan showed a multiloculated cystic mass in the pouch of Douglas but no free fluid. A CA125 was slightly raised. You suspect she has a large tubo-ovarian abscess. Critically appraise your management of the patient. (20 marks)

Common mistakes

- Take a history and do a physical examination
- Diagnostic laparoscopy to confirm the diagnosis
- Take a sexual history
- Investigate for infertility
- Hormone profile

A good answer will include some or all of these points

- The most likely cause of this patient's symptoms is a sexually transmitted infection (STI)
- The organism responsible must be identified:
  - *Chlamydia trachomatis* testing – antigen from the blood, antibodies (IgM and IgG)
- Definitive treatment – surgery
- Antibiotics before surgery:
  - Broad-spectrum to cover Gram-negative and Gram-positive bacteria and anaerobes
  - *C. trachomatis* antibiotics:
    - Cephalosporins, metronidazole and tetracycline derivatives or azithromycin
- Adequate counselling prior to surgery
- Options at surgery: drainage of the abscess; removal of the Fallopian tubes if necessary; complete antibiotic therapy
- Appropriate counselling after surgery regarding fertility and ectopic pregnancy
- Refer to genitourinary medicine (GUM) clinic if necessary for contact tracing and screening for other STIs
- Laparoscopic surgery
- Counselling:
  - Contraception – IUD contraindicated
  - Fertility may be impaired and is likely to have *in vitro* fertilisation with embryo transfer (IVF-ET)

Sample answer

The cause of this patient's tubo-ovarian abscess is likely to be sexually transmitted. This may be difficult to identify unless samples can be obtained for microscopy culture and sensitivity.

However, a sexual history and associated symptoms, such as vaginal discharge and dysuria, are important. Since *C. trachomatis* is the most common STI associated with pelvic inflammation, attempts must be made to confirm or exclude this diagnosis. A blood sample should therefore be obtained from the patient for chlamydia antigen testing. The presence of IgG antibodies against chlamydia will not suggest recent infection; however, the presence of IgM antibodies will indicate recent infection.

The mainstay of treatment is antibiotics and surgery. In the first instance, she will be offered broad-spectrum parenteral antibiotics. These should cover Gram-negative, Gram-positive and anaerobic organisms, and *C. trachomatis*. The most popular combination will be a cephalosporin, metronidazole and a tetracycline derivative or azithromycin. These will be modified, depending on the sensitivity of the organisms identified from the cultures and sensitivity test.

Laparotomy is essential to drain the abscess. Although the abscess could be managed laparascopically or with ultrasound-guided aspiration, the best approach is laparotomy. At laparotomy, the definitive treatment will depend on the findings. The most likely scenario is a severely damaged Fallopian tube with the ovary stuck to the tube. In such cases, the best option may be to remove the Fallopian tube; swabs must also be obtained for microscopy, culture and sensitivity. After surgery, the course of antibiotics should be completed. Laparoscopic drainage of the abscess is an alternative to laparotomy. Although the morbidity associated with this procedure is lower than that after laparotomy, it requires expertise and special instruments. In addition, the risk of visceral injury may be considerable in view of the adhesions, which tend to coexist as a result of the infection. This procedure should therefore be limited to very skilled clinicians.

An important aspect of the management is counselling after surgery. The counselling needs to emphasise the fertility problems associated with such complications. She needs to be told that pregnancy is unlikely in view of the consequences of the infection on her fertility, and that she may need IVF in future. If the cause of her infection is chlamydia or another STI, contact tracing should be initiated and the patient referred to the GUM clinic where she will be screened for other STIs and the appropriate steps taken. With regards to contraception, she should avoid the IUD.

3. During a routine gynaecology consultation, you see a 27-year-old woman present-ing with chronic vaginal discharge. (a) What additional information will you obtain from her? (6 marks) (b) Justify the investigations you will undertake on her. (8 marks) (c) How will you manage her? (6 marks)

Common mistakes

- Stating that she has an STI and therefore focusing the rest of your answer on managing this
- Screening for HIV – this is unlikely to be applicable unless you can demonstrate that she is at risk. In contemporary practice in the UK, this is not justified. It may be the case in the near future
- History of alcohol and drug abuse – what is the relevance of this to the question?
- Diagnostic laparoscopy – why? Ensure that you justify all your answer – why are you subjecting the patient to any investigation or treatment?

A good answer will include some or all of these points

(a) What additional information will you obtain from her? (6 marks)

- History:
  - Exclude associated symptoms, e.g. irritation, pruritus, bloody discharge – colour of discharge
  - Predisposing factors, e.g. STIs or other infections, e.g. threadworms; contraceptives – oral contraceptive pill, IUD
  - Allergy – soaps, underwear, powders, etc.
  - Drug-induced
  - Systemic diseases
  - Previous treatment of any discharge
  - Last cervical smear
- Examination: systemic; localised pelvic – vulva, vagina; colour of discharge; bimanual

(b) Justify the investigations you will undertake on her. (8 marks)

- Most important – swabs – urethral, high vaginal, rectal, endocervical:
  - Wet film and microscopy, culture and sensitivity
  - Gram stain, *C. trachomatis* specific test (polymerase chain reaction (PCR))
  - Urine for chlamydia PCR
- Stool for threadworms

(c) How will you manage her? (6 marks)

- Treatment: hygiene/remove allergen if known; specific treatment – *Trichomonas vaginalis*/bacterial vaginosis – metronidazole; other specific treatments – cryotherapy; contact tracing if STI; reassurance – oral contraceptive pill and leucorrhoea
- Refer to GUM clinic if STI identified
- Screen for HIV and offer counselling about STI
- Counsel about contraception and sexual behaviour – barrier methods most appropriate

Sample answer

(a) What additional information will you obtain from her? (6 marks)

The first stage in her management is to identify other associated symptoms with the discharge. These include pruritus, superficial dyspareunia and predisposing factors of the discharge, such as STIs, allergy, drug-induced or systemic diseases. The use of the contraceptive pill or an IUD may provide a clue to the cause of the discharge. The nature of the discharge, its colour, associated bleeding and dysuria are important. The time of the patient's last cervical smear must be ascertained.

A general examination will identify systemic diseases that may cause chronic vaginal discharge. During a pelvic examination, swabs should be taken from the high vagina, the endocervix, urethra and rectum. Careful attention must be paid to the character of the discharge, the appearance of the vagina, tenderness in the adnexa and adnexal masses.

(b) Justify the investigations you will undertake on her. (8 marks)

The most important investigation is swabs from various sites for a wet film, Gram stain, microscopy, culture and sensitivity and specialised tests such as *C. trachomatis* PCR. The swabs obtained should be sent for the following investigations: *C. trachomatis*, *Neisseria gonorrhoea*, *Candida albicans* and for bacterial vaginosis. Threadworms should be excluded from the vagina and from stool examination, especially if there is associated pruritus. If potassium hydroxide is applied to a wet preparation from the high vaginal swab, a fishy smell or the presence of clue cells on the slide will confirm *Gardnerella vaginalis* infection.

Chronic vaginal discharge is a devastating symptom and one that can also be extremely difficult to treat. In this young woman, a systematic approach to diagnose the cause of the discharge, followed by tailored therapy, is essential.

(c) How will you manage her? (6 marks)

The treatment will depend on the causes identified. Simple measures, such as hygiene, to remove possible causes and allergens should be offered if applicable. For specific infections (such as *C. albicans*, *T. vaginalis*, *G. vaginalis*, chlamydia and *N. gonorrhoea*) the most appropriate treatment should be instituted. *Trichomonas vaginalis* infection or bacterial vaginosis should be treated with metronidazole, chlamydia with a tetracycline derivative or azithromycin, and *N. gonorrhoea* with a cephalosporin. For some patients, there may be an obvious cervical erosion that is responsible for the discharge. This may be treated with cryocautery or diathermy. Where the identified cause is an STI, attempts must be made to trace all contacts and offer appropriate treatment and screening for HIV. The patient should be screened for other STIs. The GUM clinic should be involved in this aspect of her treatment. However, if there is any associated systemic disease such as diabetes mellitus, then appropriate referral and treatment would be offered.

In most cases, no cause for the discharge will be identified. It could therefore be explained as leucorrhoea, which is normal in some patients. In such cases, adequate counselling and education may be adequate. The use of Betadine® douches has been shown to be helpful in some women. Simple sanitation methods, such as changing of pads and avoiding the use of tampons, may also be all that is required.

4. Critically appraise the measures you will undertake to reduce the prevalence of *C. trachomatis* genital infections. (20 marks)

Common mistakes

- Discussing treatment for *C. trachomatis* in general
- Listing the various methods of diagnosing *C. trachomatis*
- Being too general
- Failing to critically appraise
- History and examination
- Discussing the different types of *C. trachomatis* infection and how they can be acquired

A good answer will include some or all of these points

- *C. trachomatis* infection is one of the most common STIs and causes tubal infertility and chronic PID
- Reducing the prevalence must start with identifying the at-risk groups:
  - Those aged <25 years having at least two partners within 12 months
  - Single women from low socioeconomic class who smoke
  - Women with other STIs
  - Those undergoing termination of pregnancy
  - Partners of those who have been infected
  - Previous or ectopic pregnancy
- Reduction of prevalence:
  - Reduce the infection rate – public health education (mass media, schools, etc. – expensive and no guarantee that it will reach target population)
  - Universal screening or targeted screening? Advantages and disadvantages? Screening all at-risk groups when the opportunity arises?
  - Termination of pregnancy, family planning – especially emergency contraception. Insertion of IUD
  - Prophylactic antibiotics to all at-risk groups? Disadvantages – expensive, increases the risk of causing drug-resistant strains
- Limitation of spread from infected patients: appropriate treatment; contact tracing; leaflets; infertility clinics/ectopic pregnancy; diagnosis procedure – how reliable?
- Improving screening techniques – urethral and endocervical swabs for *C. trachomatis* PCR or urine PCR

Sample answer

Chlamydia trachomatis infection is a common STI in the UK. It is the most common cause of tubal infertility and PID. To reduce the prevalence of this infection, at-risk groups must be identified and targeted measures taken to reduce the risk of transmission. In addition, once the diagnosis is made, institution of the most appropriate treatment and contact tracing will help to minimise the prevalence of the condition. There must be a concerted effort by general practitioners, other clinicians and the media to educate the public at large and, in particular, those at risk of the early symptoms and sequelae of this infection and the benefits of barrier contraception. This could be offered through the mass media and school classrooms. Such programmes may be directed specifically at at-risk groups or at the general population. They are expensive and may be seen as encouraging promiscuity if not managed properly.

Those most at risk are women under the age of 25 years who have had more than two sexual partners, those from a low socioeconomic class, those with other STIs, those undergoing termination of pregnancy or those who have had an ectopic pregnancy. In these at-risk groups, screening for the infection is important. It will identify those with the infection, offer treatment and also allow for contact tracing and treatment. Targeting this at-risk population is thought to be more cost effective than universal screening, but it will invariably result in some cases being missed within the low-risk population.

The second approach is to screen all sexually active women for *C. trachomatis*. This approach ensures that all those at risk are screened. However, such universal screening is not cost effective, especially in areas where the population is low risk. A disadvantage of such targeted screening is that of labelling a defined population as high risk. This may discourage others from seeking services that will immediately label them as high risk.

Instead of targeted screening, prophylaxis has been proposed as a means of reducing the prevalence of *C. trachomatis* in the high-risk population. In this approach, antibiotics sensitive to *C. trachomatis* are offered to all women undergoing termination of pregnancy, or an IUD inserted. Such an approach will ensure that all cases are treated but the major disadvantage is that, without screening, those who are chlamydia positive will not be identified and therefore their sexual contacts will also not be identified and treated. Such an approach runs the risk of minimising the infection temporarily, but repeated infection and its consequences are more likely.

Once the infection has been identified, institution of appropriate treatment, not only to the patient but also to her contact(s), will significantly minimise the prevalence of this infection. Education of those with the infection and/or those at risk about the symptoms and the consequences of the disease is important in prevention. It is essential that screening should employ modern and reliable techniques. Such screening should be available in various clinics, such as infertility units, and other areas attended by at-risk groups. Where patients present with features suggestive of PID, chlamydia screening should be considered. Such an approach will reduce the prevalence, and therefore the spread, of the disease.

An important step in reducing the incidence of *C. trachomatis* infection is improving the detection rate. This can be achieved by obtaining swabs from the urethra and endocervical region when the infection is suspected for *C. trachomatis* PCR. This will improve detection and false-negative tests.

11

Menopause

1. A 45-year-old business executive has been suffering from menopausal symptoms. She wishes to go on hormone replacement therapy (HRT). (a) Briefly discuss the benefits and side effects of HRT for this patient. (10 marks) (b) How will you counsel her? (6 marks) (c) How would this advice differ if she were 54 years old? (4 marks)

2. Pipelle/Vibra aspirators are useful tools in the outpatient investigation of postmenopausal women with irregular vaginal bleeding. (a) Discuss the advantages and disadvantages of using these devices. (10 marks) (b) Discuss the options you will have in managing a 60-year-old woman who is not fit for surgery and has atypical endometrial hyperplasia. (6 marks) (c) How will you manage a fit patient who continues to bleed despite a negative Pipelle? (4 marks)

3. Critically appraise your management of a 72-year-old patient presenting with postmenopausal bleeding. (20 marks)

4. The use of outpatient hysteroscopy has negated the role of ultrasound in the management of women with postmenopausal bleeding. Do you agree with this statement? (20 marks)

5. A 55-year-old woman is anxious about osteoporosis as she is not on HRT. (a) What are the risk factors for osteoporosis that you will want to exclude? (13 marks) (b) How will you screen her for this condition? (3 marks) (c) What advice will you give her with regards to reducing her risk of osteoporosis? (4 marks)

1. A 45-year-old business executive has been suffering from menopausal symptoms. She wishes to go on HRT. (a) Briefly discuss the benefits and side-effects of HRT for this patient. (10 marks) (b) How will you counsel her? (6 marks) (c) How would this advice differ if she were 54 years old? (4 marks)

Common mistakes

- Discussion of HRT in general
- Advantages
- Types
- How to administer
- Complications
- Contraindications
- Cardiovascular disease is the most common cause of female mortality
- Telling patient about low- and high-density lipoproteins and apolipoprotein a
- Check follicle-stimulating hormone (FSH) and FSH and luteinising hormone
- Determine her gravidity and parity – why?

A good answer will include some or all of these points

(a) Briefly discuss the benefits and side-effects of HRT for this patient. (10 marks)

- Symptom relief – vasomotor symptoms such as hot flushes, night sweats, irritability, inability to concentrate
- Genital tract integrity – reduces risk of prolapse and urinary tract infections
- Cardioprotective – when used before the age of menopause or in the perimenopausal period (all the studies indicate that the risk of cardiovascular diseases rises when used by women over 60 years)
- Osteoporosis – protects
- Reduces the risk of bowel cancer and Alzheimer's disease
- Breast tenderness and lumps in breast
- Makes mammography difficult to interpret
- Increased arterial stroke
- Increased risk of breast cancer
- Increased risk of venous thromboembolism (VTE)

(b) How will you counsel her? (6 marks)

- What specific symptoms does she have?
- Contraindications – does she have any – relative or absolute? Identifying some may require a physical examination and screening, e.g. blood pressure (BP)

- Is the uterus intact or not?
- Is she still menstruating and, if still menstruating, does she need contraception?
- These will help determine the type of HRT and, therefore, the route of administration (contraception is important)
- Side-effects – breast cancer (after 10 years' use)
- Need for monitoring – BP, breast and watching for early signs of VTE
- Check contraceptive needs and tailor HRT accordingly
- Selective oestrogen-receptor modulators (SERMs)

(c) How would this advice differ if she were 54 years old? (4 marks)

- Hopefully postmenopausal – natural age at menopause in the UK approx. 51 years
- If menopausal, recommendation are:
  - Instead of HRT, treat symptoms with other options, e.g. phytoestrogens
  - Advice on osteoporosis – exercise, diet and bisphosphonates
  - Only consider HRT for a short time because of risks of cardiovascular disease, VTE and breast cancer

Sample answer

(a) Briefly discuss the benefits and side-effects of HRT for this patient. (10 marks)

The benefits of HRT can be classified under relief of vasomotor symptoms, genital tract effects and systemic effects. Vasomotor symptoms that may be relieved by HRT include hot flushes, night sweats, poor/disturbed sleep, irritability and lack of concentration. The sense of well-being which HRT induces in women improves the quality of their lives and libido. HRT improves the integrity of the urogenital tract, reducing the risk of genital prolapse, recurrent urinary tract infections and atrophic vaginitis, trigonitis and endometritis. Systemic benefits vary with the age of the woman. In this 45-year-old woman, this will offer some cardioprotection, reduce the age at which osteoporosis develops and also reduce the risk of bowel cancer and Alzheimer's disease.

The risks of HRT vary with the type of HRT, the duration of use and the age of the woman when she goes on HRT. For most women the side-effects include breast tenderness, and lumps which may make mammography difficult. There is an increased risk of arterial disease, especially when used in those over the age of 60 years, breast cancer (which is increased after at least 10 years' use), and VTE.

(b) How will you counsel her? (6 marks)

First, it must be established whether the patient does need HRT. This will be determined by her symptoms. In addition, it is important to establish whether or not she has had a hysterectomy, as this will influence the type of HRT offered. If she has not had a hysterectomy, it is important to know whether or not she is still menstruating. Having established her symptoms and physical status, the next step will be to ensure that she does not have any contraindications to HRT.

Contraindications are absolute and relative. Absolute contraindications include active cancer of the uterus and breast, active VTE and active liver disease. Relative contraindications include previous VTE, previous breast cancer and hypertension.

The choice of HRT for this patient also depends on her needs. If she has an intact uterus and no absolute contraindications, she will need combined HRT to minimise the risk of endometrial cancer. If she has had a hysterectomy, she could have oestrogens only. These may be administered in the form of tablets, patches or implants. The disadvantage of implants is mainly that of tachyphylaxis. Before commencing HRT, the patient should be examined to ensure that her BP is normal and that there are no breast masses. Counselling about the side-effects of HRT, such as breast tenderness, premenstrual symptoms, depression, weight gain and breast cancer after more than 10 years' therapy, must also be offered. The ultimate choice of HRT will depend on any contraindications. Lastly, the patient's contraceptive needs must be considered before HRT is offered. It may be that she still requires contraception, in which case this may be combined with HRT.

Where there are contraindications, other forms of HRT, such as SERMs, progestogens and phytoestrogens, should be considered.

(c) How would this advice differ if she were 54 years old? (4 marks)

At 54 years, she would be expected to be postmenopausal, since the natural age at menopause in the UK is 51 years. The advice she will be offered will therefore depend on whether she is postmenopausal or not. If she is postmenopausal, then hormonal HRT will not be recommended unless she has severe menopausal symptoms that have failed to respond to other remedies. The advice will therefore be to treat the various symptoms with other options including anxiolytics, and phytoestrogens. It may be necessary to give her a short course of HRT for severe vasomotor symptoms. This will have to be in the form of combined HRT, in which case she should be counselled about return of menstruation. If she is at risk of osteoporosis, appropriate counselling about exercise, diet and bisphosphonates will be offered. In postmenopausal women, HRT is not recommended for prevention or treatment of osteoporosis.

2. Pipelle/Vibra aspirators are useful tools in the outpatient investigation of post-menopausal women with irregular vaginal bleeding. (a) Discuss the advantages and disadvantages of using these devices. (10 marks) (b) Discuss the options you will have in managing a 60-year-old woman who is not fit for surgery and has atypical endometrial hyperplasia (6 marks) (c) How will you manage a fit patient who continues to bleed despite a negative Pipelle? (4 marks)

Common mistakes

- Discussing the use of Pipelle or Vibra aspirators – indications and how to apply them
- Describing the management of postmenopausal bleeding – ultrasound scan, etc.
- Listing the advantages of hysteroscopy and the management of postmenopausal bleeding
- Detailing the causes of postmenopausal bleeding

A good answer will include some or all of these points

(a) Discuss the advantages and disadvantages of using these devices. (10 marks)

- Advantages:
  - Biopsy at the time of consultation – no need to come back for a diagnostic procedure outpatient/inpatient)
  - No need for anaesthesia – most are done without (in some cases of cervical stenosis, this may be impossible)
  - Accuracy = 70–80 per cent
- Disadvantages:
  - Impossible with stenosed cervix and difficult and painful in nulligravid women
  - Sampling mainly from the fundus of the uterus and therefore could miss pathology originating from the cornual ends
  - A negative biopsy does not exclude a malignancy or potential malignancy

(b) Discuss the options you will have in managing a 60-year-old woman who is not fit for surgery and has atypical endometrial hyperplasia. (6 marks)

- Progestogens – oral or Depo-Provera®. It may result in irregular vaginal bleeding, which will further compound follow-up. Requires follow-up biopsies after 6 months of treatment
- Mirena®
- Radiotherapy, if she is really unfit

(c) How will you manage a fit patient who continues to bleed despite a negative Pipelle? (4 marks)

- Since reliability is only 70–80 per cent and most of the sampling is from the fundus, a hysteroscopy with directed biopsy is essential
- Ultrasound scan for endometrial thickness will only identify those with thickness of >5 mm; however, this could be used as the first step and if thickness if <5 mm and uniform the patient could be observed and only subjected to hysteroscopy if bleeding continues

Sample answer

(a) Discuss the advantages and disadvantages of using these devices. (10 marks)

Postmenopausal bleeding is a common gynaecological problem. The aim of investigating patients presenting with this complaint is to exclude endometrial carcinoma. This is best achieved from histological examination. An endometrial sample is therefore essential for this examination. This can be obtained either as an outpatient procedure with or without local analgesia or under general anaesthesia (GA). The availability of the Pipelle or Vibra aspirators has been responsible for the ease with which these biopsies can be taken on an outpatient basis. However, they do have disadvantages, which must be recognised when using them in clinical practice.

In most cases, there is no need for anaesthesia and the devices are commonly used during routine pelvic examination at gynaecological consultations. They are also commonly used with outpatient hysteroscopy for biopsies. The advantages of these devices are therefore the avoidance of GA and of cervical dilatation, which may be very painful. Tissues are obtained after consultation and patients do not have to go on long waiting lists for hysteroscopy, where this is offered on outpatient basis.

Despite these advantages, application of the devices is blind. Directed biopsies are therefore not obtained. There is a tendency for tissues to be taken mainly from the body of the uterus and pathology limited to the cornual regions of the uterus may thus be missed. The accuracy of these devices in identifying endometrial cancer is thought to be approximately 75–80 per cent. Another disadvantage is their inability to exclude other causes of postmenopausal bleeding, such as endometrial polyps. Failure to obtain tissue does not reliably exclude all the cause of postmenopausal bleeding. Combining the use of these devices with ultrasound or saline sonography is thought to be more effective. In women with fibrotic lesions, such as those taking tamoxifen, the use of these devices to sample the endometrium is ineffective.

The success of obtaining endometrial biopsies depends of the ability of these devices to pass through the cervix. In patients with a very stenosed cervix this may be difficult and persisting with the attempt to pass them may be associated with vasovagal attacks. In addition, there is the added complication of infections and perforation of the uterus. Ideally, therefore, these devices should be used in conjunction with ultrasound or outpatient hysteroscopy to allow for a more effective means of diagnosis. The use of ultrasound and or hysteroscopy will exclude other causes of postmenopausal bleeding and will direct the clinician to a specific focus from which the endometrial biopsy should be taken. In the absence of a thickened endometrium, the use of these devices may not be necessary.

Overall, these devices are now routinely available in all gynaecological outpatient departments in the UK. Their use will therefore continue. Clinicians must be aware of their shortfalls and recognise that where they have produced tissue that excludes a malignancy, and yet the symptoms persist, further investigations must be performed. As long as these drawbacks are appreciated, the use of the Pipelle or the Vibra aspirator to investigate postmenopausal women with abnormal bleeding will remain an acceptable practice.

(b) Discuss the options you will have in managing a 60-year-old woman who is not fit for surgery and has atypical endometrial hyperplasia (6 marks)

Atypical hyperplasia requires treatment, as the risk of progression to malignancy is of the order of 30–40 per cent. In a surgically fit woman, the option of choice is a hysterectomy and bilateral salpingo-oophorectomy. In this surgically unfit patient, the first option will be progestogen therapy. This can be administered in the form of tablets (norethisterone acetate or medroxyprogesterone acetate) in high doses. This will be taken for 6 months followed by ultrasound scan for endometrial thickness and biopsy. This treatment may be associated with irregular vaginal bleeding which may further frighten the patient and make follow-up complicated. The other option is the Mirena® intrauterine system which delivers the progestogen levonorgestrel locally at a steady rate. Again, this may be associated with irregular vaginal bleeding. With this device *in situ*, measuring the endometrium with ultrasound may be difficult, but not impossible.

Radiotherapy is the last option but this should only be considered if none of the above options is suitable. This is because of the side-effects of radiotherapy and the fact that if there is radiation-induced stenosis, follow-up will be difficult.

(c) How will you manage a fit patient who continues to bleed, despite a negative Pipelle? (4 marks)

Pipelle or Vibra aspirations are only reliable in 70–80 per cent of cases. The two approaches to the management of this patient are ultrasound surveillance and hysteroscopy and directed endometrial biopsy. An ultrasound scan will screen for polyps and endometrial thickness. Where this is less than 5 mm, the risk of malignancy is low, and if it is high then a hysteroscopy would be mandatory. Although hysteroscopy and directed biopsy is the gold standard, if this is negative and she continues to bleed, a hysterectomy should be considered as there may well be a pathology that is not readily accessible to the hysteroscope or biopsy.

3. Critically appraise your management of a 72-year-old patient presenting with post-menopausal bleeding. (20 marks)

Common mistakes

- Take a history and perform a physical examination – not being critical
- Listing all the steps in the management of the patient
- Assuming that she has endometrial cancer and discussing the management of endometrial cancer
- Discussing the uses of endometrial biopsies and outpatient hysteroscopy

A good answer will include some or all of these points

- The primary aim is to exclude endometrial cancer and then to identify other causes, which could be treated
- Discuss the importance of a good history; elaborate on the limitations of this
- Physical examination – benefits and limitations
- Investigations: outpatient endometrial biopsy – Pipelle/Vibra aspirator; hysteroscopy; ultrasound scan
- Treatment – no need to go into the details of the pathologies that could cause post-menopausal bleeding

Sample answer

In this 72-year-old patient, the most important diagnosis that must be excluded is endometrial cancer. An appropriate method of excluding this is histological examination of a biopsy of the endometrium. However, prior to doing this it is necessary to identify possible factors for endometrial cancer or other causes of her postmenopausal bleeding. Her risk of endometrial cancer is greater if she is nulliparous or of low parity, suffers from diabetes mellitus or hypertension, or has been on oestrogen-only HRT. In addition, a history of polycystic ovary syndrome (PCOS), or infertility associated with irregular periods, during her reproductive years may also increase the risk of her developing endometrial cancer. If she is taking tamoxifen for breast cancer, the risk of endometrial malignancy is considerably higher. Although a good history may shed some light on the possible causes of the postmenopausal bleeding, it should be recognised that, in most cases, there are no risk factors in the patient's history. However, there may be other factors, such as medical disorders and drug therapy, which may influence the type of treatment that the patient may receive.

Following the history, a physical examination has to be performed. The most important part of this examination will be the abdomen and the pelvis. However, other systemic features, such as hypertension, cardiac and respiratory signs, must be excluded. The presence of all these may influence treatment, e.g. the patient's suitability for surgery. Essential findings on abdominal examination will include an abdominopelvic mass. The presence of such a mass may suggest endometrial carcinoma, although classically patients with endometrial carcinoma do not have an abdominally palpable uterus. However, the presence of ovarian masses may suggest the possibility of a functioning ovarian tumour. A pelvic examination may identify atrophic vaginitis and cervicitis, and a bulky uterus or adnexal masses. In most women with postmenopausal bleeding, these examinations are negative but do not exclude pathology. So, although a pelvic examination may identify possible causes of postmenopausal bleeding, it has significant limitations, as endometrial pathology cannot be excluded by these means.

To exclude endometrial pathology, therefore, an endometrial biopsy is needed. This can be done at the time of the pelvic examination in the clinic by use of a Pipelle or a Vibra aspirator. However, the success of this procedure will depend on the ease with which these instruments can be inserted through the cervix. In addition, a negative biopsy does not completely exclude pathology as it does not identify polyps and is only reliable in approximately 70–80 per cent of cases. Hysteroscopy performed at the time of the biopsy may improve the accuracy of this biopsy. It will also diagnose polyps. The only disadvantage is that this is unlikely to be performed at the outpatient visit. There are patients who may not tolerate these rather invasive procedures, hence they may have to be abandoned. An alternative to an endometrial biopsy or hysteroscopy is an ultrasound scan to assess endometrial thickness. This will identify the thickness of the endometrium and adnexal pathology, which the other diagnostic methods will not do. If the endometrium is more than 4 mm thick, the patient could be offered a biopsy.

Having made the diagnosis, treatment will depend on the cause. If the patient has atrophic vaginitis or cervicitis, oestrogen creams administered sparingly will be adequate. It must be recognised that their prolonged administration can lead to endometrial cancer. If the patient has polyps, these could be removed at hysteroscopy. For endometrial cancer, the treatment of choice will be an abdominal hysterectomy, bilateral salpingo-oophorectomy and node dissection, if appropriate. Adjuvant chemotherapy or radiotherapy will be offered if indicated. For an oestrogen-dependent pathology the most appropriate treatment will be total abdominal hysterectomy and bilateral salpingo-oophorectomy and omentectomy, followed by adjuvant chemotherapy if necessary.

4. The use of outpatient hysteroscopy has negated the role of ultrasound in the management of women with postmenopausal bleeding. Do you agree with this statement? (20 marks)

Common mistakes

- The management of postmenopausal bleeding
- Day case versus inpatient hysteroscopy
- Avoid stating that hysteroscopy provides a histological diagnosis
- Both procedures are diagnostic, so do not state that one is and the other is not. Both procedures are also used for screening
- The question is not asking which is used first – hysteroscopy or ultrasound

A good answer will include some or all of these points

- There is no need to answer yes or no
- Both procedures are diagnostic
- Outpatient hysteroscopy:
  - Benefits – allows visualisation of the uterine cavity – directed biopsies may be taken at the same time – polyps may be removed, therefore may be therapeutic
  - Disadvantages – training – equipment – may not be feasible in all patients – stenosed cervix – may be associated with vasovagal attacks – risk of fluid overload – may not be acceptable to some patients – risks of perforation and infections
- Ultrasound: equipment; training; assess adnexal and endometrial cavity; not therapeutic; need to perform a separate biopsy to make a diagnosis; transvaginal scan may be more acceptable; evidence that it is effective in screening for postmenopausal bleeding; does not negate the need for hysteroscopy
- Conclusion – both procedures are complementary and not mutually exclusive. There is a role for both in the management of postmenopausal bleeding

Sample answer

These two procedures are important in the management of irregular vaginal bleeding, especially in postmenopausal women. In general, they complement each other.

Outpatient hysteroscopy allows visualisation of the endometrium; therefore directed biopsies may be taken from well-defined sites. Endometrial polyps cannot only be diagnosed but may also be removed during the hysteroscopy. The disadvantages of outpatient hysteroscopy include the need to train staff to perform the procedure and the cost of setting up units for this procedure. It may not be possible in some patients because of cervical stenosis. Vasovagal attacks may result from grasping the cervix in some cases and, where fluid is the distension medium, overload with resulting circulatory failure may occur, especially in those who are frail and who have cardiovascular compromise. Some patients may find it intrusive and there is always the risk of perforation of the uterus. Although uncommon, infection may occur as a complication of this procedure. In addition to these disadvantages, outpatient hysteroscopy does not allow the diagnosis of adnexal pathologies, which may be responsible for the post-menopausal bleeding, e.g. oestrogen-producing ovarian tumours.

Ultrasound, on the other hand, has the advantage of identifying adnexal pathologies and uterine pathologies, such as polyps. As endometrial thickness needs to be more than 4–5 mm for an endometrial biopsy to be performed, many women are spared the discomfort of unnecessary attempts at biopsy. Ultrasound scan, especially by the transabdominal route, may be more acceptable to some patients than hysteroscopy.

However, there are several disadvantages to the use of ultrasound in the management of patients with postmenopausal bleeding. Ultrasound, unlike hysteroscopy, does not offer an opportunity to treat some of the causes of postmenopausal bleeding. It must be accompanied by endometrial biopsy to be valuable in the diagnosis of endometrial carcinoma. The transabdominal approach requires a full bladder, which some patients may find unacceptable. The transvaginal approach, on the other hand, though better at defining endometrial and pelvic pathology, is considered by some as intrusive. Ultrasound machines are expensive and skilled manpower is necessary for the procedure to be reliable. Even in excellent hands, the reliability of this investigation depends on the individual undertaking the procedure and the route of scanning (transabdominal or transvaginal).

Outpatient hysteroscopy and endometrial biopsy, and ultrasound and endometrial biopsy, although very useful in the management of postmenopausal bleeding, are not interchangeable. Indeed, they complement each other and therefore the argument that one can negate the use of the other is unlikely to be tenable. It may be concluded that these procedures are complementary.

5. A 55-year-old woman is anxious about osteoporosis as she is not on HRT. (a) What are the risk factors for osteoporosis that you will want to exclude? (13 marks) (b) How will you screen her for this condition? (3 marks) (c) What advice will you give her with regards to reducing her risk of osteoporosis? (4 marks)

Common mistakes

- Discussing prevention of osteoporosis
- Pros and cons of HRT with regards to osteoporosis
- Diagnosis and treatment of osteoporosis
- Multidisciplinary team, including gynaecologists, physicians and GP
- Discussing the biochemical changes associated with osteoporosis

A good answer will contain some of all of these points

(a) What are the risk factors for osteoporosis that you will want to exclude? (13 marks)

- Genetic:
  - Positive family history, especially first-degree relative
  - Race – Caucasian versus Afro-Caribbean
- Constitutional:
  - Low body mass index (BMI)
- Endocrine disorders:
  - Hyperparathyroidism
  - Hyperthyroidism
  - Hypogonadism
  - Type I diabetes mellitus
  - Anorexia nervosa
  - Early menopause (<45 years)
- Drugs history:
  - Corticosteroids (>75 mg prednisolone or equivalent /day)
  - Gonadotropin-releasing hormone agonists
- Environmental:
  - Cigarette smoking
  - Alcohol abuse
  - Low calcium intake
  - Sedentary life style/immobilisation
  - Excessive exercise leading to amenorrhoea
- Diseases:
  - Chronic renal failure
  - Chronic liver disease
  - Neuromuscular disease

- Malabsorption syndromes
- Rheumatoid arthritis
- Post-transplantation bone loss

(b) How will you screen her for this condition? (2 marks)

- History
- Bone densitometry

(c) What advice will you give her with regards to reducing her risk of osteoporosis? (5 marks)

- Diet
- Exercise
- Bisphosphonates
- SERMs
- Calcium and vitamin D

Sample answer

(a) What are the risk factors for osteoporosis that you will want to exclude? (13 marks)

The risk factors for osteoporosis can be classified as genetic, constitutional, endocrine disorders, drug history, environmental and systemic diseases. Under genetic factors are a family history and race. It is more common in Caucasians compared to Afro-Caribbeans. Constitutional risk factors include BMI (greater risk in those with low BMI).

The endocrine risk factors include anorexia nervosa, early menopause and prolonged breastfeeding. Disorders such as hyperthyroidism, hypogonadism, hyperparathyroidism and type I diabetes mellitus increase the risk of osteoporosis.

Prolonged use of high doses of corticosteroids (e.g. equivalent of >75 mg prednisolone per day) significantly increases the risk. Lifestyle factors that are considered high risk include cigarette smoking, alcohol abuse, low calcium intake, sedentary lifestyle and excessive exercise leading to amenorrhoea.

Chronic systemic medical disorders that are considered high-risk factors for osteoporosis include chronic renal disease, chronic liver failure, neuromuscular disorders that limit mobility, malabsorption syndromes, rheumatoid arthritis and post-transplantation bone loss.

(b) How will you screen her for this condition? (3 marks)

Screening for osteoporosis is mainly by meticulous detailed personal and family history to exclude the risk factors highlighted in part (a). The presence of these factors will indicate a high risk and therefore further screening. The best tool available for screening for osteoporosis is bone densitometry. This is commonly of the hip, and wrist. The Z scores which quantify deviations from the norm for age identify those who are normal, and at risk. These dual-energy X-ray obsorptiometry results must be interpreted with references to the ethnicity and age of the patient.

(c) What advice will you give her with regards to reducing her risk of osteoporosis? (4 marks)

Prevention can be achieved through several approaches. Improvement of dietary calcium intake is an important factor associated with a reduction in the risk. Regular exercise and bisphosphonates should also be recommended if appropriate. Hormone replacement therapy is not recommended for the prevention or treatment of osteoporosis. However, SERMs such as raloxifene have been demonstrated to prevent osteoporosis and therefore this could be offered to this patient. Finally, calcium and vitamin D intake should be improved. Counselling must include modification of lifestyle factors that increase risk, such as smoking, alcohol and drugs.

12

Genital prolapse and urinary incontinence

1. A very obese, hypertensive, known asthmatic woman presents with urinary incontinence. Urogynaecological investigations have confirmed that she has significant urodynamic (genuine) stress incontinence (USI). (a) Critically appraise the non-surgical options for her management. (12 marks) (b) Evaluate the surgical options you may consider. (8 marks)

2. A 65-year-old woman has returned to the urogynaecology clinic with recurrent urinary incontinence 4 years after a successful colposuspension. (a) Comment critically on your initial evaluation of the patient. (10 marks) (b) How will you investigate her? (3 marks) Justify your subsequent management after this evaluation. (7 marks)

3. A 26-year-old woman with one child presents with genital prolapse. Critically appraise your management of this patient. (20 marks)

4. A 67-year-old woman who had an abdominal hysterectomy 10 years ago presents with vault prolapse. (a) Outline your approach to assessment prior to treatment. (8 marks) (b) Discuss the options for her treatment. (8 marks) (c) How would these differ if she had superimposed detrusor overactivity? (4 marks)

5. Mrs AB had a colposuspension operation 12 months ago. She comes to see you again complaining of USI, urgency and urge urinary incontinence. (a) Discuss your initial approach to her management. (6 marks) (b) Justify the investigations you will perform on the patient. (4 marks) (c) What are the likely causes of her symptoms? (4 marks) (d) Outline how you will treat her. (6 marks)

6. A 72-year-old woman presents with a dragging sensation in her vagina. There are no associated urinary symptoms. (a) How will you assess her symptom? (8 marks) (b) Briefly discuss the types of meshes and when you would use them in this patient. (4 marks) (c) What will influence the type of surgery you offer her? (4 marks) (d) What are the complications of using these suture materials in repairs? (4 marks)

1. A very obese, hypertensive, known asthmatic woman presents with urinary inconti-nence. Urogynaecological investigations have confirmed that she has significant USI. (a) Critically appraise the non-surgical options for her management. (12 marks) (b) Evaluate the surgical options you may consider. (8 marks)

Common mistakes

- Simply listing the diagnosis and management of USI – these must be related to the unique characteristics of the patient presented in this question
- Describing how the diagnosis of USI is made – this is unnecessary as the diagnosis has already been made
- Performing a urogynaecological investigation – same comment as above
- Concentrating on the treatment of her hypertension and asthma – these are already known problems, so you must assume that they are being treated. Even so, you should ask the appropriate specialists for advice
- Offering her surgery for genital prolapse without evidence of having diagnosed prolapse – making such an assumption without first confirming its presence is incorrect
- Assuming that she has mixed incontinence – she has USI and not mixed incontinence
- Treating for urinary tract infections (UTIs) only
- Failure to critically appraise

A good answer will include some or all of these points

(a) Critically appraise the non-surgical options for her management. (12 marks)

- Lifestyle modifications:
  - Weight loss
  - Exercise
  - Cessation of smoking
- Pelvic floor exercises (PFEs), with or without biofeedback or electrical stimulation:
  - Depends on motivation and how the exercises are undertaken:
    - 50 per cent of women do not know how to do PFEs, hence referral to physio-therapist is associated with better results
  - When lapsed or stopped, symptoms reoccur
- Devices to prevent urinary leakage:
  - Bladder neck support devices
  - Devices to block the external urethral meatus
  - Intraurethral devices
- Pessaries – if prolapse:
  - Ring pessary
  - Shelf pessary

- Drugs:
  - Selective serotonin reuptake inhibitor (SSRI) – duloxetine – 40 mg bd – effective but has side-effects (nausea, diarrhoea, constipation, dizziness, headaches) and anxiety about depression and suicide
  - Hormone replacement therapy – not proven to be very effective but improves the tissue of the genital tract in a menopausal women:
    - Unlikely to be beneficial to this obese woman if menopausal
    - Oestrogen cream – to improve integrity of pelvic structures – muscles and connective tissue – not very effective

(b) Evaluate the surgical options you may consider. (8 marks)

- Colposuspension – gold standard
- Tension-free transvaginal tape (TVT)
- Other sling procedures
- Anterior repair
- Periurethral bulking agents

Sample answer

(a) Critically appraise the non-surgical options for her management. (12 marks)

The first option is lifestyle interventions. These will include weight loss (especially as she is overweight), stopping smoking, early relief of constipation and exercise. Apart from weight loss in the morbidly obese, none of these other options has been shown to have a significant beneficial effect. Most of these will require motivation and for most patients, and especially this patient, this may not be possible.

The second option is PFEs. These can be offered either alone or combined with biofeedback or electrical stimulation. The success rate of PFEs will depend on the patient's motivation and how she does these exercises. Approximately 50 per cent of women cannot perform PFEs correctly and referral to a physiotherapist, especially an incontinence one, will be associated with a success rate in 40–60 per cent of cases. The combination with biofeedback or electrical stimulation has not been shown to offer any additional benefits.

The last non-surgical option to consider is the devices to prevent urinary leakage. Such devices are those that support the bladder neck, block the external meatus or are intraurethral. Bladder neck support will result in improvement, but has to be accepted by the patient who must have significant manual dexterity to insert them. Although the intraurethral devices are the most effective in this group, they are associated with significant morbidity including haematuria and UTIs.

Pessaries for the correction of prolapse may improve her symptoms especially as she is unfit.

If the patient is postmenopausal, oestrogen may be offered, locally or systemically. In this hypertensive patient, oestrogens may increase the risk of endometrial carcinoma unless she has had a hysterectomy.

The medical treatment option that has been shown to have promise is the SSRI duloxetine. At a dose of 40 mg twice a day, it has been shown to improve symptoms by approximately 50 per cent in 60–100 per cent of patients. In one study of women on the waiting list for surgery, treatment resulted in 20 per cent of the patients refusing surgery. However, the evidence for its long-term use is still scanty. The drug is associated with side-effects such a mild to moderate nausea, fatigue, dry mouth, constipation, insomnia, headaches, dizziness and diarrhoea. With appropriate counselling, these side-effects are well tolerated. The major drawback is the association with depression and suicide, leading to fatalities.

(b) *Discuss the surgical options you may consider. (8 marks)*

Although the surgical options are varied they include Burch colposuspension, Marshall–Marchetti–Kranz operation, abdominal paravaginal repair sling procedures (traditional pubovaginal, midurethral tapes and trans-obturator tapes), periurethral bulking agents and artificial urinary sphincters. Anterior repair and needle suspension procedures have virtually been superseded by these other procedures because of poor outcome.

Burch colposuspension is the gold standard but TVTs are associated with a similar success rate. The choice in this obese diabetic will be influenced by her suitability for surgery and the expertise available. Colposuspension is associated with increased morbidity and, for a patient with two medical complications, the morbidity may be more severe. In this situation, this will not be the treatment of choice. If her medical conditions are well controlled, this will be the surgical treatment of choice (if there is no available expertise) as it has the best 5-year success rate of approximately 85 per cent. Morbidity following an open colposuspension may be reduced by laparoscopic colposuspension but the success rate of this procedure is not as high as that following the open procedure. Where the expertise is available, the TVT will be considered the best option as it is easier to perform and has a quicker recovery.

Although the other sling procedures have been shown to have some advantages over TVTs, these have not been extensively investigated as the TVTs and should only be considered as alternatives. Periurethral bulking agents are best reserved for patients in whom other procedures have failed or in patients unfit for surgery. Therefore, this may be one option to consider in this patient. It has a low success rate, which varies with the material used and deteriorates to about 50 per cent after 2 years.

In the presence of genital prolapse, an anterior repair will be the treatment of choice if the prolapse is severe. This procedure is associated with a 60 per cent 5-year cure rate for USI. However, the morbidity following an anterior repair is less severe compared to that following a colposuspension. In the presence of a mild to moderate prolapse, unless the patient's medical conditions are severe, the treatment of choice will still be a colposuspension.

2. A 65-year-old woman has returned to the urogynaecology clinic with recurrent urinary incontinence 4 years after a successful colposuspension. (a) Comment critically on your initial evaluation of the patient. (10 marks) (b) How will you investigate her? (3 marks) (c) Justify your subsequent management after this evaluation. (7 marks)

Common mistakes

- Listing all the causes of urinary incontinence and detailing their treatment
- Assuming that she has recurrent USI
- Offering surgery for prolapse without confirming its presence
- Assuming she has already had a hysterectomy
- Failure to justify (i.e. giving reasons for any step taken in her management)

A good answer will include all or some of these points

(a) Comment critically on your initial evaluation of the patient. (10 marks)

- This patient has recurrent incontinence; therefore failure of previous treatment must be recognised in her management:
  - Obtain previous records for information on the degree of USI and any associated problems, e.g. prolapse, etc.
- There is need to obtain more information to help characterise the type of incontinence:
  - USI
  - Urgency and urge incontinence
  - Nocturia
  - Symptoms of prolapse – dragging sensation in the vagina, feeling of incompletely emptying the bladder or rectum
  - Constipation
- Physical examination:
  - To exclude prolapse
  - To assess mobility around the urethra as she may require surgery
  - Evidence of atrophic changes in the vagina

(b) How will you investigate her? (3 marks)

- Midstream specimen of urine (MSU)
- Blood glucose
- Frequency and volume chart
- Urodynamics

- Other investigations will depend on how fit she is and whether they are necessary as part of preoperative assessment (e.g. urea and electrolytes, chest X-ray and electro-cardiography)

(c) Justify your subsequent management after this evaluation. (7 marks)

- Treatment – depends on the cause of the incontinence:
  - Conservative – PFEs or physiotherapy
  - Drugs for detrusor overactivity – tolterodine (Detrusitol®), oxybutynin
  - Surgery – repeat colposuspension – need to be referred to urogynaecologist; TVT
  - Collagen implants

Sample answer

(a) Comment critically on your initial evaluation of the patient. (10 marks)

This patient has recurrent urinary incontinence and her management must start with obtaining more information to help identify the type of incontinence. Following the history, an appropriate physical examination and relevant investigations must be performed. Important questions to ask include associated symptoms, such as nocturia, urgency and urge incontinence. The presence of these symptoms will suggest either an associated detrusor overactivity or genital prolapse. If the patient has genital prolapse, she will, in addition, present with symptoms such as the feeling of a lump or a dragging sensation in the vagina. The type of incontinence is also important. If it is often precipitated by conditions that raise the intra-abdominal pressure, such as coughing, sneezing, etc., it is more likely to be USI. This will even be more so if there is no associated increased frequency of micturition and nocturia. The presence of dysuria will suggest an associated UTI. Other symptoms, which may not directly influence the diagnosis, but may affect the results of treatment, include coughing and constipation. In the presence of these symptoms, the urinary symptoms may become worse and response to surgical treatment may not be as successful.

Following the history, a general and pelvic examination must be undertaken. This aims, first, to ensure that the patient is fit for any surgical therapy if that is the correct option, and second, to rule out genital prolapse. The examination therefore must exclude chest signs and abdominal masses. A pelvic examination will exclude atrophy of the genital tract, associated urethrocele, cystocele, uterine prolapse if the patient has not had a hysterectomy, and an enterocele and a rectocele. Although only a cystocele may explain her symptoms, the presence of other types of genital prolapse may alter her treatment or may require additional procedures during surgery for the incontinence. A bimanual pelvic examination will identify any pelvic masses that could not be identified on abdominal examination. It will also enable the para-urethral vagina to be assessed for mobility, a factor that is extremely important if further surgery is necessary.

(b) How will you investigate her? (3 marks)

Relevant investigations to be performed include an MSU to exclude UTIs. This is common in women with prolapse and may make the symptoms of urinary incontinence worse. A random blood glucose will exclude diabetes mellitus, which is not uncommon in this age group and may present with symptoms mimicking urinary incontinence.

Urodynamic investigations will confirm the type of incontinence. However, before this, a frequency and volume chart will provide additional information on the possible causes of the patient's incontinence. It may, for example, suspect detrusor overactivity, a recurrent genuine USI or a combination. Rarely, the patient may have a low compliance bladder.

(c) Justify your subsequent management after this evaluation. (7 marks)

The treatment will depend on the findings on physical examination and the results of the urodynamic investigations. In the first instance, if the investigations only demonstrate a UTI and minimal prolapse, she could be offered antibiotics, physiotherapy and a local oestrogen cream to apply sparingly. For more severe forms of incontinence (USI), repeat surgery will be advisable. This must be performed by a urogynaecologist if possible. Alternatively, a sling operation may be performed. The complications should be discussed before surgery, with emphasis on the poorer success rate compared to that after a primary procedure. Surgical options include a repeat colposuspension or TVT. Whatever the treatment, the patient needs to be followed up for at least 5 years as the recurrence rate of incontinence following repeat surgery is of the order of 60 per cent after 5 years.

Where the cause of the incontinence is detrusor overactivity, the treatment of choice consists of anticholinergic drugs, e.g. tolterodine (Detrusitol®) or oxybutynin, or calcium-channel blockers. If the idiopathic detrusor overactivity (detrusor instability) coexists with genuine USI, surgery and medical treatment have to be offered. It may be advisable to initiate treatment for idiopathic detrusor overactivity (detrusor instability) prior to surgery, although surgery for USI may actually make idiopathic detrusor overactivity (detrusor instability) worse. If the diagnosis is a low compliance bladder, treatment will consist of collagen implants, bladder distension and clamp cystoplasty. The success rate of these procedures in the treatment of this type of incontinence is not good.

3. A 26-year-old woman with one child presents with genital prolapse. Critically appraise your management of this patient. (20 marks)

Common mistakes

- Take a history and perform a physical examination – this is too vague. You need to be more specific
- Offer vaginal hysterectomy and pelvic floor repair – this needs to be discussed critically
- Insert a pessary to treat her prolapse
- Offer investigations by electromyography
- Colposuspension and hysterectomy

A good answer will include some or all of these points

- This is an unusual presentation in a young woman
- More information is required about associated features of the prolapse, such as urinary symptoms
- Physical examination to determine the degree of prolapse
- Ascertain the patient's wishes for future pregnancies
- Further investigations of urinary symptoms, e.g. MSU
- Conservative management until family is complete
- Surgical management – options depend on the type of prolapse: Manchester repair; hysterectomy and repair; repair only
- Counselling about the future

Sample answer

In this young patient the difficulties arise if she has not completed her family. The fact that she has developed genital prolapse at such a young age indicates that the support of her pelvic organs is weak. However, trauma from childbirth must not be discounted. The first important step is therefore to obtain an adequate history about the onset of the prolapse and the precipitating factors. A recent traumatic delivery will be suggestive of a possible cause. However, it is unlikely to be the main reason for the prolapse. Further questioning may reveal a history of prolapse in other members of the family, suggesting a familial tendency. However, the absence of any precipitating factor or an affected family member does not exclude congenital weakness of the pelvic muscles. Other aggravating symptoms, such as chronic cough, constipation, abdominal swelling and an at-risk occupation, must be excluded.

A thorough general examination will exclude chest infection, hypertension and abdominal masses or ascites. During a pelvic examination, the perineum and its tone will be assessed as well as the type of prolapse (cystocele and rectocele or enterocele). These will determine to a large extent the management the patient will be offered. It is very likely that in this young woman the perineum will be demonstrated to be deficient.

Definitive management will depend on the examination findings. Management will be tailored to the patient's needs. Where her family is incomplete, surgery may have to be deferred until she has completed it. In that case, a pessary may be inserted after the pelvic examination as an interim measure. Retention of pessaries depends on a relatively intact perineum and pelvic muscle tone. If she has a defective perineum but the pelvic muscles are of a relatively good tone, a ring pessary may be retained. Once the patient has completed her family, definitive corrective surgery should be offered. In some cases, she may have to complete her family early to enable corrective surgery to be offered and in the long term this may result in regret if she later felt than her family was incomplete.

Another option is to offer the patient corrective surgery in the form of a Manchester operation. The operation consists of amputation of the cervix, shortening of the transverse cervical (Mackenrodt) ligament, anterior colporrhaphy and a colpoperineorrhaphy. Which of these components will be offered will depend on the type of prolapse. This procedure must only be undertaken after adequate counselling as its complications, such as cervical stenosis, infertility and cervical weakness (incompetence), may affect the patient's ability to have children.

The long-term management of this young woman is extremely important. It is most likely that she will become symptomatic in her later years even if corrective surgery is offered now or at a later date. An important part of her management should therefore include counselling about the prognosis and chances of success after corrective surgery and physiotherapy.

4. A 67-year-old woman who had an abdominal hysterectomy 10 years ago presents with vault prolapse. (a) Outline your approach to her assessment prior to treatment. (8 marks) (b) Discuss the options for her treatment. (8 marks) (c) How would these differ if she had superimposed detrusor overactivity? (4 marks)

Common mistakes

- Take a history and do a physical examination – this is too vague. You need to be more precise and relate this to the patient
- Offer a vaginal hysterectomy and pelvic floor repair!
- Offer a repair for enterocele
- Anterior and posterior repair
- Conservative surgery for urinary incontinence – you are making an assumption without explaining why

A good answer will include some or all of these points

(a) Outline your approach to assessment prior to treatment. (8 marks)

- History:
  - Associated symptoms:
    - Backache, constipation, urinary frequency, urinary incontinence, nocturia, USI, urgency or urge incontinence
    - Chest symptoms, e.g. chronic cough
    - Constipation and other bowel symptoms
    - Occupation
- Examine to rule out anterior and posterior wall prolapse:
  - Pelvic organ prolapse quantification (POPQ) assessment

(b) Discuss the options for her treatment. (8 marks)

- Surgery:
  - Sacrocolpoplexy
  - Sacrospinous fixation
  - Vault repair
  - Mesh repair
  - Colpocleisis
- Conservative:
  - PFEs
  - Pessaries

(c) How would these differ is she had superimposed detrusor overactivity? (4 marks)

- Treat medically before embarking on surgery:
  - Surgery, especially sacrocolpopexy, is associated with a 15 per cent increased risk of urinary incontinence
  - Urodynamics before offering treatment to exclude USI, whose presence will require a modified type of surgery
  - Retraining
  - PFEs – prior to surgery

Sample answer

(a) Outline your approach to assessment prior to treatment. (8 marks)

Vault prolapse is a complication that commonly occurs after a hysterectomy. The treatment will depend on the severity of the prolapse and associated symptoms. These have to be excluded from a history and the severity of the prolapse assessed by a vaginal examination.

Obtaining a history from this patient is one of the most important steps in her management. It is essential to establish the type of hysterectomy she had and whether it was associated with any repair procedures. If this information cannot be obtained from the patient, then her previous surgical notes must be reviewed, and if these are not available, contacts have to be made with the unit where her hysterectomy was performed for this additional information.

Associated factors of the vault prolapse should be determined. These include constipation and symptoms of a cystocele, such as frequency, nocturia and urinary incontinence. Urinary incontinence, for example, must be investigated before surgery. The history should exclude symptoms of cardiorespiratory and gastrointestinal disorders that may aggravate the prolapse. Following the history, a physical examination will be performed to define the degree of prolapse and the presence of an associated cystocele or rectocele. Mobility of the paraurethral vagina must also be assessed if the patient is to have any incontinence surgery as part of her treatment. The POPQ score should be used to assess any prolapse.

The investigations that will be performed will depend on the associated symptoms. In the presence of urinary symptoms, an MSU must be sent for microscopy, culture and sensitivity (M/C/S). This test should be performed even if there are no urinary symptoms but the patient has a cystocele. It is extremely valuable as treatment of any UTI will not only improve the symptoms of frequency, nocturia and urgency but will also reduce operative and postoperative morbidity. The treatment of UTIs with antibiotics to which the responsible organism is sensitive is inexpensive and does not require hospitalisation. In the presence of urinary incontinence, the most important investigation that will be performed on the patient will be a urodynamic assessment. This test is precise and available in most units. Uroflometry will identify the type of incontinence to which subsequent management will be tailored.

(b) Discuss the options for her treatment. (8 marks)

Once a complete assessment has been made, the patient will fall into one of several categories: (1) no associated vaginal wall prolapse, (2) associated vaginal wall prolapse with no urinary incontinence and (3) associated vaginal wall prolapse with urinary symptoms. Where there is no associated prolapse or symptoms of incontinence, treatment is either vaginal or abdominal. The vaginal treatment of choice is a simple repair or a sacrospinous fixation. The latter is not easy to perform. It may be associated with deviations of the vagina, haemorrhage from pudendal artery injury, pudendal nerve injury, USI and an enterocele. In experienced hands the success rate is good and, unlike the repair, it does not compromise the size of the vagina. A simple repair procedure involves isolation, excision and closure of the hernia sac at the vault and then closure of the vagina after excising the redundant part. Any associated cystocele and/or rectocele may then be corrected by either an anterior and/or posterior repair, respectively. The procedure has a poor success rate and, additionally, may result in a considerable shortening of the vagina.

The next operation of choice is a sacrocolpopexy. This is an abdominal operation in which the vault of the vagina is anchored to the anterior longitudinal ligament of the first sacral vertebra with a non-absorbable mesh. This has the advantage of correcting a cystocele and mild rectocele and the vault prolapse. However, it is associated with a high incidence of USI and backache. The incidence of urinary incontinence following this procedure is approximately 10–30 per cent. Appropriate counselling must therefore be offered before surgery.

(c) How would these differ is she had superimposed detrusor overactivity? (4 marks)

In the presence of idiopathic detrusor overactivity (detrusor instability), treatment will include anticholinergic drugs, but this must be offered as additional treatment as the patient's main symptom is prolapse. If she is surgically unfit, a pessary may be inserted, but the success of this conservative approach is poor. When intercourse is not intended, the vagina can be obliterated (colpocleisis) by purse-string sutures. Unfortunately, this procedure is also associated with a recurrence.

5. Mrs AB had a colposuspension operation 12 months ago. She comes to see you again complaining of USI, urgency and urge urinary incontinence. (a) Discuss your initial approach to her management. (6 marks) (b) Justify the investigations you will perform on the patient. (4 marks) (c) What are the likely causes of her symptoms? (4 marks) (d) Outline how you will treat her. (6 marks)

Common mistakes

- Candidates must resist discussing the following:
  - Why did the operation fail?
  - She had an incorrect operation or it was poorly performed
  - No need to describe the operation of colposuspension
  - Do not treat patient based on investigations performed 12 months ago
  - Do not state that if only detrusor overactivity, should not have had surgery

A good answer will include some or all of these points

(a) Discuss your initial approach to her management. (6 marks)

- Review notes, surgery and symptoms at the time of surgery
- Are her symptoms new?
- Any associated prolapse? Symptoms of prolapse – dragging sensation, frequency, nocturia
- Physical examination: mobility of the paraurethral vagina; prolapse – POPQ assessment

(b) Justify the investigations you will perform on the patient. (4 marks)

- MSU
- Frequency and volume chart
- Urodynamics
- Blood sugar

(c) What are the likely causes of her symptoms? (4 marks)

- USI
- UTI
- Detrusor overactivity
- Combination
- Low compliance bladder?

(d) Outline how you will treat her. (6 marks)

- UTIs – antibiotics (broad-spectrum until M/C/S results or clinical response to treatment)
- Idiopathic detrusor overactivity (detrusor instability):
  - Anticholinergic agents
  - Oestrogens
- USI:
  - Pelvic floor repair
  - TVT and other sling procedures e.g. trans-obturator tape (TOT)
  - Colposuspension – laparotomy or laparoscopic
- If both conditions, treat accordingly

Sample answer

(a) Discuss your initial approach to her management. (6 marks)

The initial management of this patient will involve enquiring after additional relevant information. It is important to determine whether these are new symptoms or persistence of the symptoms that she had before surgery. If the latter is the case, surgery may have been ineffective in the first instance. If they are new symptoms, she may have developed another type of urinary incontinence or the problems may have reoccurred in a different way, e.g. a mixed type of incontinence. It is also possible for the patient to have been cured of USI only to progressively develop symptoms of idiopathic detrusor overactivity (detrusor instability). The timing of the symptoms in relation to the previous surgery will suggest the relationship between surgery and her new symptoms. The symptoms need to be characterised, e.g. associated frequency, nocturia, urgency and urge urinary incontinence will be suggestive of idiopathic detrusor overactivity (detrusor instability). However, the type of urinary incontinence can only be diagnosed with certainty from uroflometry. It is also important to exclude symptoms of genital tract prolapse, such as a feeling of a lump in the vagina and or a dragging sensation in the lower abdomen.

A physical examination would identify any signs of obstructive airway disease and masses in the abdomen, both of which may contribute to genital prolapse. During a pelvic examination, genital prolapse has to be excluded using the POPQ score. Bimanual palpation for masses and ascertaining the mobility of the tissues around the urethra is essential. The latter may influence the type of surgical treatment the patient may be offered.

(b) Justify the investigations you will perform on the patient. (4 marks)

Investigations include an MSU to exclude UTIs, and a frequency and volume chart which she could keep for about 3–4 days before attending for urodynamic investigations. This will not only provide additional information about how much fluid the patient is taking, but also, more importantly, how severe her symptoms are. The most vital investigation is uroflometry.

This will not only diagnose the type of urinary incontinence but will provide some information about the likelihood of success if surgery is the treatment of choice. In some cases a random blood glucose should be performed. This may identify patients with diabetes mellitus.

(c) What are the likely causes of her symptoms? (4 marks)

The likely causes of this patient's symptoms include urinary stress incontinence, UTI, detrusor overactivity, a combination of these causes or a low compliance bladder. Most of these will present with USI. In USI, the typical presentation is that of USI without any additional symptoms. However, if there is superadded UTI, she may present with frequency, and urgency. These additional symptoms are typical of detrusor overactivity in addition to USI. A low compliance bladder will present with USI and frequency. If the patient has prolapse, she may well have a combination of these pathologies especially UTI, detrusor overactivity and USI.

(d) Outline how you will treat her. (6 marks)

Treatment will depend on the type of incontinence and other associated factors. If she has USI, she will be referred to a urogynaecologist. In the absence of this, a repeat colposuspension will be offered provided the paraurethral vagina is relatively mobile. The complications of this repeat operation must be explained to the patient. In addition, the lower success rate compared to that following primary surgery must be discussed. If the urinary incontinence is attributable to genital prolapse, this will be dealt with accordingly. Surgery for genital prolapse is often difficult if a colposuspension has been performed previously. Again, great care must be taken during surgery as it may be associated with severe complications. For a mixture of USI and idiopathic detrusor overactivity, anticholinergic agents such as oxybutynin hydrochloride should be initiated first and surgery performed later. Where there is a large cystocele, it may be possible to perform an anterior repair alone; however, the success rate of this operation in correcting USI is not as high as that following colposuspension and TVT. If she has recurrent USI, TVT or TOT is likely to be the best option. It is associated with a lower morbidity and a high success rate.

6. A 72-year-old woman presents with a dragging sensation in her vagina. There are no associated urinary symptoms. (a) How will you assess her symptom? (8 marks) (b) Briefly discuss the types of meshes and when you would use them in this patient. (4 marks) (c) What will influence the type of surgery you offer her? (4 marks) (d) What are the complications of using these suture materials in repairs? (4 marks)

Common mistakes

- Non-specific statement – take a history and do a physical examination
- Urinary symptoms – qualifying and quantifying them – she does not have urinary symptoms!
- Discussing the pathogenesis of prolapse and factors predisposing to prolapse
- Details about the management of urinary incontinence – discussing management of USI, etc.
- Details of what POPQ score is and how it is determined
- Hysterectomy and bilateral salpingo-oophorectomy for repair of prolapse – this is not correct as without pelvic floor repair, this will not resolve symptoms
- Discussing investigations and management of USI and detrusor overactivity

A good answer will include some or all of the following points

(a) How will you assess her symptom? (8 marks)

- History:
  - Previous surgery – hysterectomy or repair surgery?
  - Severity of symptoms and duration – reducibility (spontaneous or not)
  - Associated bowel symptoms
  - Quality of life evaluation using disease-specific quality of life questionnaire
- Physical examination:
  - Degree of prolapse – POPQ score
  - Assess for occult incontinence with a full bladder and having reduced the prolapse
  - Examine for defects in the pelvic floor especially if posthysterectomy – common
- Investigations:
  - Urine MSU – M/C/S
  - Any other investigations will depend on symptoms

(b) Briefly discuss the types of meshes and when you would use them in this patient. (4 marks)

- Two types of meshes – absorbable and non-absorbable
- Prolapse – recurrent prolapse – posthysterectomy (prehysterectomy – uncertainty about complications associated with mesh at the time of hysterectomy)

- Defects in the pelvic floor identified during assessment
- Specialised procedures:
  - Sacrospinous fixation
  - Prespinous colpopexy
  - Ileococcygeal fixation
  - Transabdominal sacrocolpopexy

(c) What will influence the type of surgery you offer her? (4 marks)

- The nature of the prolapse and associated symptoms
- Previous surgery
- Expertise available
- Facilities available
- Patient's desires

(d) What are the complications of using these suture materials in repair? (4 marks)

- Haemorrhage
- Infection
- Rejection
- Erosion
- USI

Sample answer

(a) How will you assess her symptom? (8 marks)

The severity of her symptom will be assessed from a thorough history, an appropriate physical examination and additional investigations. Useful information includes the duration of symptoms and how severe they are, e.g. does she feel a lump in her vagina? Is this lump reducible and does it get worse with time? A severe prolapse will be irreducible all the time or towards the end of the day. Where there is an associated bloody vaginal discharge, a decubitus ulcer is most likely; however, in view of her age, cancer of the endometrium should also be considered. Associated bowel symptoms such as constipation and inability to empty the bowel will indicate a coexisting rectocele or enterocele.

In this woman, it is important to also establish that this is her first presentation with symptoms of prolapse and that she has not had surgery before (either in the form of a hysterectomy, repair or incontinence surgery). This will have a significant influence on the type of treatment she may be offered. Finally, the severity of her symptoms should be gauged from the effect of the prolapse on her quality of life. This may be objectively assessed using quality of life disease-specific questionnaire or subjectively by asking the patient. The more severe the prolapse, the greater the effect it will have on her quality of life.

A thorough physical examination will then define the type and grade of the prolapse using the POPQ score standard quantifying tool. The degree of descent of the various anatomical parts of genital tract (singly or in combination) will help determine the type of treatment she will be offered. Where possible defects in the pelvic floor should be identified and defined.

Investigations that will help in her management include an MSU for M/C/S. The prolapse should be replaced and further assessments undertaken for occult urinary incontinence. There is no need for urodynamic investigations and even if occult stress incontinence is demonstrated, there is no agreement on surgically correcting it.

(b) Briefly discuss the types of meshes and when you would use them in this patient. (4 marks)

There are two types of meshes – the absorbable and non-absorbable type. The absorbable meshes such as polyglycolic acid (Vicryl®) are not recommended for repair unless they are being used for standard procedures such as anterior and posterior colporrhaphy. Where a hysterectomy is part of the surgical procedure, then these may be used.

The second type of mesh is the non-absorbable variety which incorporates or integrates into the patient's tissues. These are used for the specialised procedures for repair such as sacrospinous fixation, prespinous colpopexy, ileococcygeal fixation and transabdominal sacrocolpopexy. Where there are obvious pelvic floor defects, the meshes can be used to correct these defects. The main group of patients to benefit from these meshes are those with posthysterectomy vaginal wall prolapse.

(c) What will influence the type of surgery you offer her? (4 marks)

The type of surgery to be offered will be influence by several factors, including the nature of her prolapse and associated symptoms (especially bowel), the expertise available and the facilities in the unit. If, for example, she will benefit from the use of meshes and there is no local expertise, she will have to be referred to another unit. The wishes of the patient will ultimately determine the type of surgery she is offered. Since most of the surgical approaches will be under general anaesthesia, her suitability for anaesthesia will be an important influence. For example if she cannot withstand prolonged surgery, then the option of choice must be one that is short and effective.

(d) What are the complications of using these suture materials in her repair? (4 marks)

The complications include intraoperative haemorrhage, especially with sacrospinous fixation and sacrocolpopexy. The haemorrhage often results from damage to the pudendal arteries or presacral venous plexus or the medial sacral vessels. Mesh erosion occurs in approximately 8–12 per cent of cases. The factors that influence the erosion rate include the use of a large number of braided sutures, placement of the mesh at the vaginal apex (which is often devascularised), lack of fascia between the mesh and the thin vaginal wall and poor preoperative oestrogenisation. Attaching the mesh to the pubocervical fascia anteriorly and rectovaginal fascia posteriorly is recognised to reduce this complication. Using a single flap (thickness) mesh would reduce the amount of foreign material at the vaginal vault and hence the risk of erosion. The incidence of USI ranges from 1.3 to 12 per cent after mesh procedures. This may be because of the altered anatomy of the bladder neck. Finally, although rare, rejection is a recognised complication.

Further reading

Afffi R, Sayed AT (2005) Post-hysterectomy vaginal prolapse. *Obstetrician and Gynecologist* **7**: 89–97.
Karlovsky ME, Tharke AA, Rastinhead A, Kushner L, Badlani GH (2005) Biomaterials for pelvic floor reconstruction. *Urology* **66**: 469–75.
RCOG (2007) *Green-top Guidelines. The Management of Post Hysterectomy Vault Prolapse.* October 2007. London: Royal College of Obstetricians and Gynaecologists.
Thakur Y, Varma R (2005) Management of post-hysterectomy vaginal vault prolapse using posterior intravaginal slingoplasty. *Obstetrician and Gynecologist* **7**: 195–8.

13

Cervical malignancy

1. Cervical cancer remains an important cause of morbidity and mortality in gynaecology in the UK. (a) What factors are responsible for this? (8 marks) (b) Critically appraise how the incidence may be reduced. (12 marks)

2. All women with abnormal cervical smears should be referred for colposcopy. Debate this statement. (20 marks)

3. A 25-year-old nulliparous woman has been referred for colposcopy on account of a severe dyskaryotic smear. (a) Under what circumstances will you consider the colposcopy unsatisfactory? (6 marks) (b) Discuss the management options for this patient. (10 marks) (c) What complications may she have following a knife cone biopsy? (4 marks)

4. A 25-year-old nulligravid woman is diagnosed with invasive carcinoma of the cervix. (a) Justify the investigations you will undertake on this patient. (8 marks) (b) What factors will influence the treatment she receives? (12 marks)

5. A 26-year-old woman with carcinoma of the cervix has been offered radiotherapy. (a) Outline the complications of this treatment modality. (6 marks) (b) What steps will you take to minimise these complications? (14 marks)

1. Cervical cancer remains an important cause of morbidity and mortality in gynaecology in the UK. (a) What factors are responsible for this? (8 marks) (b) Critically appraise how the incidence may be reduced. (12 marks)

Common mistakes

- Discussing the aetiology of cervical cancer
- Detailing the screening programme and how to take a cervical smear
- Emphasising the success of the screening programme in the reduction of mortality from cervical cancer

A good answer will include some or all of these points

(a) What factors are responsible for this? (8 marks)

- Sexual promiscuity – most cases are due to infection with human papillomavirus HPV-16 and -18 (sexually transmitted)
- Screening problems:
    - Take-up – some people do not take up screening
    - False negatives and poor follow-up
    - Inaccurate screening methods – obtaining smears and reading them
    - Unpredictable course of some of the abnormal patterns identified from screening
    - Failure to communicate results to patients and general practitioners (GPs)
    - Immigration and communication failure (language and refugees)

(b) Critically appraise how the incidence may be reduced. (12 marks)

- Improvement in screening:
    - Technique of obtaining smears – liquid-based cytology should improve the quality of smears
    - Reporting – automated systems should reduce human errors
    - Computer systems of reading
    - Population – screening (attempts to screen every susceptible woman)
    - Mechanisms to identify those who fail to take up screening and encourage them to do so
- Management of abnormal smears:
    - Communication of all results with patients
    - Pathways for managing all abnormal smears
    - Direct access to colposcopy clinics and oncologists
    - Training of colposcopists
    - Education of GPs and nurse practitioners on how to obtain smears

- Vaccination:
  - Adolescent vaccination – Gardasil® (HPV-16 and -18)
- Education:
  - Prevention of sexually transmitted infections (STIs)
  - Contraception – barrier methods
  - Promiscuity

Sample answer

(a) What factors are responsible for this? (8 marks)

Cervical cancer is now considered by some as an STI. The most important factor for its continuing to be an important cause of morbidity and mortality is an increase in sexual promiscuity and genital tract infections with HPV. Most of these infections (especially HPV-16 and -18) are asymptomatic. The decreasing age at first sexual intercourse, multiple sexual partners and lifestyle factors (e.g. smoking) have contributed to the persistence of this malignancy.

A second and equally important factor is related to screening. There remains a group of women who will not take up screening or fail to attend for follow-up screening. Additionally, problems with the screening itself remain. These include inappropriate sampling from the cervix, incorrect interpretation and failure to communicate results with women and their GPs. The problems with sample collection and the reporting of smears result in false-negative and false-positive results, which offer false reassurance or unnecessary treatment. The traditional wooden spatula is well known to be associated with poor sample collection.

The last factor is the impact of immigration. A larger number of immigrants fail to take up screening, partly because of language barriers and also because of cultural differences to accepting screening – especially one that may be seen as intrusive.

(b) Critically appraise how the incidence may be reduced. (12 marks)

The first approach is education on the causes of cervical cancer. This could be provided in schools, by GPs, in family planning clinics and in the media. An understanding of this may results in modification of sexual behaviour, improved used of barrier methods of contraception and modification of lifestyle factors that increase the incidence of cervical cancer.

Improvements in screening methods, including the technique of collection, reading and reporting, and communication with women and GPs will reduce the number of false results and failure to act on results. The introduction of liquid-based cytology will improve sample collection, while automation of reading of smears will eliminate human error and therefore the risk of abnormal tests. Current computer approaches to reading smears go a long way to addressing this problem. Currently, screening is voluntary and all eligible women should be encouraged to attend for routine screening. Information on screening should be provided in different languages and attempts made to understand reasons why some women do not take up screening, and solutions should be found to these obstacles.

Timely and appropriate management of abnormal smears will reduce the incidence of cervical cancer. This can be achieved if there is effective communication between the cytology laboratory and GPs and women. There should be clear pathways for managing abnormal smears in every community. There should be ready access to trained colposcopists who should not only perform colposcopies but should also be able to treat local premalignant lesions. All those involved in screening must be trained on how to obtain smears, and regular quality control systems instituted with regular quality audits.

The advent of vaccination against cervical cancer (e.g. Gardasil®) will hopefully reduce the incidence. The vaccines, which are for teenagers (12–16 years), will reduce infections from HPV-16 and -18 which are responsible for approximately 70–80 per cent of all cervical cancers. This reduction is anticipated to be higher since the vaccine also protects to an extent against some of the cancers caused by other HPV subtypes. The introduction of this vaccine will therefore radically reduce the prevalence of this condition.

2. All women with abnormal cervical smears should be referred for colposcopy. Debate this statement. (20 marks)

Common mistakes

- Only extorting the virtues of cervical screening
- Discussing the cervical screening programme
- Details of colposcopy
- Discussing the local treatment of abnormal cervical smears

A good answer should include some or all of these points

- Cervical screening programme aimed at reducing the incidence of carcinoma of the cervix
- Screening itself does not identify cancer, but a precancerous state
- Cytology is different from histological diagnosis
- Need for further assessment of the women with abnormal smears
- Current thinking – opinion divided: colposcopy recommended mainly to women with repeated mild dyskaryosis and moderate to severe dyskaryosis; based on the premise that progression to carcinoma from mild dyskaryosis takes a long time; most mild smears will revert to normal on observation only; the burden on resources if all had colposcopy
- Progression of cervical dysplasia (cervical intraepithelial neoplasia) CIN I to CIN III within 2 years in up to 26 per cent of cases. Some may have been within 6 months
- Cervical cytology an imprecise science – 50 per cent of women with CIN II–III have mild dyskaryosis on cytology
- Conclusion – ideal for every woman with an abnormal smear to be offered colposcopy. This may frighten women with mild abnormality and put enormous strain on manpower and other resources. Ultimately, will significantly reduce the progression of mild dyskaryosis to CIN II and CIN III

Sample answer

The cervical screening programme introduced into the UK in the 1980s is aimed at reducing the incidence and mortality from cervical cancer. For this programme to be successful it must exist alongside a colposcopy service. This is primarily because, although cytology may identify abnormality, it does not define the histological grade of the abnormality, the extent of the lesion and the need for further treatment. In fact, there is evidence to suggest that cervical cytology could be unreliable in up to approximately 50 per cent of cases. In one study, it was shown that approximately 50 per cent of patients with CIN II or CIN III had mild dyskaryosis on cervical cytology. The logical argument, therefore, is that all women with abnormal cervical smears should be offered colposcopy and directed biopsies to ensure that all those with inaccurate reports are identified and treated.

How realistic is this approach? Opinion is divided among the experts. Currently, the most common approach is for those with moderate to severe dyskaryosis to be offered colposcopy, directed biopsy and treatment, whereas those with mild dyskaryosis have a repeat smear 6 months later and only after a repeat abnormal smear are they referred for colposcopy. Such an approach has been questioned, especially in view of the imprecise nature of the cytological reports. Counter arguments put forward are that only 26 per cent of women with CIN III progress to cancer after 20 years' follow-up. The precancerous stage of the disease is therefore very prolonged. This may not necessarily be the case as there are patients who develop cancer soon after normal smears. In such cases, either the cytology is unreliable or the disease manifests an unusually quick progression through to cancer from a precancerous state. Those who advocate colposcopy for all women with abnormal smears argue that since cytological examination of smears is not very precise the best results can only be achieved if all women with abnormal smears are further screened by colposcopy. Such an approach would place a significant burden on already stretched resources and manpower.

Another argument for not offering colposcopy to all women with abnormal smears has been that a large proportion of women with abnormal smears undergoing colposcopy do not have any significant pathology that warrants treatment. Such an approach may therefore frighten the women and could become counterproductive – a point that the authors of an ideal screening programme ought to consider before it is set up. It could be counter-argued that if the screening were only to be for the abnormal cases, it would no longer be a screening programme, but a selective investigation. Currently, there are some data to support colposcopy for every woman with an abnormal cervical smear. There are also data to support limiting colposcopy to those with moderate to severe dyskaryosis. In an ideal world, all these women ought to have colposcopy to reassure them and also to provide an opportunity to identify those cases where cytology is incorrect and to offer more specific treatment. Although such an approach may reduce the incidence of progression to cancer, it is impracticable as rationing which governs contemporary practice is an integral part of the National Health Service.

3. A 25-year-old nulliparous woman has been referred for colposcopy on account of a severe dyskaryotic smear. (a) Under what circumstances will you consider the colposcopy unsatisfactory? (6 marks) (b) Discuss the management options for this patient. (10 marks) (c) What complications may she have following a knife cone biopsy? (4 marks)

Common mistakes

- No need to discuss the equipment for colposcopy
- Discussing the training and accreditation of colposcopists
- Details of colposcopy – how to perform a colposcopy
- Complications of colposcopy
- Relating management to pregnancy and desire for more babies
- Cone biopsy and laser as outpatient procedures

A good answer will include some or all of these points

(a) Under what circumstances will you consider the colposcopy unsatisfactory? (6 marks)

- Conditions for a satisfactory colposcopy
  - False squamocolumnar junction (SCJ) caused by abrasion
  - SCJ in the canal (within the endocervical canal)
  - Inspected from too acute an angle (assessment of both the length of the endocervical canal involved with CIN and the severity of the lesions becomes unreliable)
  - Previously treated cervix resulting in an alteration to the topography of the transformation zone (area of metaplasia, CIN, invasive disease in the canal or covered by new squamous epithelium – cervical glands may have escaped destruction)
  - Failure to define the upper limit of abnormal glandular lesions: the rules of colposcopy do not always apply
  - Adenocarcinoma in-situ (AIS) and small adenocarcinomas cannot be identified colposcopically, so cone biopsy an essential investigation

(b) Discuss the management options for this patient. (10 marks)

- Degree of abnormality defined and treatment offered:
  - If satisfactory colposcopy – large loop excision of the transformation zone (LLETZ)
  - Inconclusive or other features – cone biopsy under general anaesthesia (GA)
- Malignancy found – treat accordingly:
  - Stage disease and manage according to stage
  - Early stage disease and family not complete – cone biopsy, trachelectomy
  - Early invasive stage – Wertheim's hysterectomy

- Advanced disease – unlikely as this will be obvious at pelvic examination
- Need for follow-up after management of abnormal cervical smears

(c) What complications may she have following a knife cone biopsy? (4 marks)

- Haemorrhage – primary and secondary
- Cervical stenosis – dysmenorrhoea
- Cervical weakness – miscarriages, preterm labour
- Infertility – complete excision of the internal cervical canal

Sample answer

(a) Under what circumstances will you consider the colposcopy unsatisfactory? (6 marks)

A satisfactory colposcopy is one in which the SCJ is clearly seen and is not in the canal, any lesion present does not extend into the canal and there are no glandular lesions. Wherever these criteria are not fulfilled, then the colposcopist must consider a cone biopsy. The indications for such a biopsy therefore include cases where the SCJ is not seen in its entirety, e.g. when it is in the canal. Occasionally, the upper part of the SCJ is inspected from too acute an angle, making an assessment of both the length of the endocervical canal involved and the severity of the lesion difficult.

In the presence of abrasions within the cervix, a false SCJ may be created resulting in misinterpretation of the colposcopy findings. Both CIN and metaplastic epithelium can be detached easily from the underlying stroma. During the colposcopy, the SCJ should be identified by observing the lower limit of normal columnar epithelium rather than the upper limit of squamous epithelium.

A cervix that has been previously treated for any reason has an altered topography of the TZ. Areas of metaplasia, CIN or invasive disease in the canal or in the cervical gland may have escaped destruction and may persist as isolated iatrogenic skip lesions surrounded by columnar epithelium or covered by new squamous epithelium. These patients are therefore best treated by excision.

The last group of patients in whom a knife cone biopsy should be considered are those in whom there is suspicion of glandular lesions. This is because adenocarcinoma or AIS cannot be identified colposcopically.

(b) Discuss the management options for this patient. (10 marks)

This young woman will no doubt be exceptionally anxious and worried about cancer when confronted with an abnormal smear. Therefore, in the first instance, she must be given an explanation of the findings. She must be reassured that cancer has not been diagnosed and that the findings suggest the need for further investigation to be able to define the abnormality accurately and offer adequate treatment. She needs to be told that abnormal smears are common and their presence is the *raison d'être* for the cervical cytology programme.

The patient must next be referred for colposcopy. This should be performed at the next available time. The importance of minimising delay is purely on the basis of the psychological consequences of a long delay on the patient. At colposcopy, 5 per cent acetic acid will be applied to the cervix to identify the abnormal cells. In addition, the vascular pattern of the cervix will be studied as other tell-tale features of severe abnormality or frank malignancy.

At the colposcopic examination, a biopsy would be performed. For most patients, this can be performed under paracervical block by use of a local anaesthetic. Where the colposcopy is complete, i.e. the colposcopist is satisfied, treatment may be offered in the form of a LLETZ. This will usually be sufficient for the treatment of the abnormal areas on the cervix. Complications of this procedure include haemorrhage and infections. The advantages of this inexpensive procedure are that it is performed on an outpatient basis, and that there is material for histology. The histology will also determine whether the margins of the excision were well clear of the abnormal areas on the cervix. If any of the following are present, LLETZ may not be the most appropriate method of treatment: (1) suspicion of invasion, which can usually be obvious from the vascular pattern before the application of acetic acid, (2) any suspicion of glandular abnormality, (3) failure to visualise the SCJ and (4) in some cases, a history of previous cervical surgery or AIS. For any of these, the treatment of choice will be cold knife cone biopsy, which is preferably performed under GA and on an inpatient basis because of the complications of intraoperative and postoperative haemorrhage.

Lastly, it must not be forgotten that, in some cases, colposcopy may identify frank malignancy, which needs to be confirmed on histology. Following this, staging will determine the treatment option. For early disease (1a1) and if the woman's family is not complete, the options to consider include cone biopsy and trachelectomy. For early invasive disease (stage 1a2–11a), a Wertheim's hysterectomy followed by adjuvant radiotherapy if indicated, is the treatment of choice, although it is unlikely that more advanced disease would not have been picked up by clinical examination.

(c) What complications may she have following a knife cone biopsy? (4 marks)

The complications of a cone biopsy include haemorrhage which may be primary, reactionary or secondary. The risk of reactionary and secondary haemorrhage is the reason why women are often admitted for at least 24 hours after a knife cone biopsy. Cervical stenosis is another complication which may present with severe dysmenorrhoea, rarely amenorrhoea with haematocolpos and cervical dystocia in labour. Overexcision of the cervix may result in difficulties conceiving, mid-trimester miscarriages and preterm labour. Infections are a recognised complication and this may result in secondary haemorrhage and occasionally pelvic inflammatory disease (PID), especially if the pathogens present in the vagina at the time of the biopsy were those that could ascend and cause PID.

4. A 25-year-old nulligravid woman is diagnosed with invasive carcinoma of the cervix. (a) Justify the investigations you will undertake on this patient. (8 marks) (b) What factors will influence the treatment she receives? (12 marks)

Common mistakes

- Assuming that the patient has a defined stage of disease, e.g. stage I, and discussing only the management of this stage
- Failure to discuss treatment according to stage of disease
- Other treatment options, e.g. cisplatin. Chemoreduction is the treatment of choice now
- Advocating colposcopy – no place once carcinoma has been diagnosed
- Considering fertility as a factor in determining treatment of choice – this is at a very early stage and should be mentioned only for early stage disease
- Listing cone biopsy as treatment determined by complete or incomplete family
- Radical surgery – what does it stand for?
- Listing investigations and not explaining why (failure to justify)

A good answer will include some or all of these points

(a) Justify the investigations you will undertake on this patient. (8 marks)

- Full blood count (FBC) – determine haemoglobin (Hb)
- Group and save
- Urea and electrolytes
- Clinical staging to an extent determines management:
  - Examination under anaesthesia (EUA) (parametrial, vaginal and rectal), cystoscopy
- Radiological investigations to exclude distant metastases:
  - Chest X-ray (CXR)
  - Magnetic resonance imaging (MRI)
  - Ultrasound scans of the abdomen and urinary tract

(b) What factors will influence the treatment she receives? (12 marks)

- Only 25 years old – therefore surgery is preferred if possible. Preserves ovaries and avoids acquired gynatresia
- Stage of the disease is one of the most important factors:
  - Trachelectomy if wants to preserve fertility and early stage disease, laparoscopic surgery and node dissection and recognise the limitations of these new techniques
  - For stage I and IIa – offer Wertheim's hysterectomy and adjuvant therapy for positive nodes
  - For advanced disease (stages IIb–IIIa), radiotherapy – external and intracavitary. Node involvement, complete excision of tumour possible?

- More advanced disease – palliative care, e.g. exenteration
- Expertise available – multidisciplinary approach – gynaecological oncologist, radiotherapist, oncologist
- Facilities available, e.g. radiotherapy

Sample answer

(a) Justify the investigations you will undertake on this patient. (8 marks)

Investigations to be performed before the initiation of treatment include a FBC and a renal function test. These will determine the patient's Hb, as she could be anaemic if the presenting symptom is bleeding. In the presence of anaemia surgery will be more risky and, if radiotherapy is the primary therapy, response to radiation will be poor. In addition, blood must be grouped and saved as the patient may require blood transfusion either to correct anaemia or following haemorrhage, which is a very common complication of surgery in such patients. An abnormal renal function test may indicate more advanced disease. An ultrasound scan or MRI of the renal tract can confirm this. A CXR is essential, not only to ensure that she is fit for surgery if this is the treatment of choice but also to exclude secondaries in the chest.

An important step in the management of this patient is to stage the cancer, as this will determine the type of primary treatment to be offered. In addition, it will facilitate counselling the patient about the 5-year survival rate. The staging process will include a radiological examination of the chest and the liver for secondaries and the urinary tract for obstruction to the ureters. If there are secondaries in the chest or the liver, or the ureters are obstructed, the disease is advanced and surgery will not be the best option. If these have been excluded, clinical staging must be performed. Ideally, this should be by means of an EUA, cystoscopy and rectal examination. During this procedure, the parametrium must be assessed to exclude involvement.

(b) What factors will influence the treatment she receives? (12 marks)

Treatment will depend on the stage of the disease. For stages I–IIa, the treatment of choice in this young woman will be a Wertheim's hysterectomy. This involves an abdominal hysterectomy, removal of the parametrium and pelvic nodes and also a cuff of the vagina (usually the upper third of the vagina). Subsequent management will depend on the presence of positive nodes. If the nodes are negative, there is no need for adjuvant therapy but if they are involved, radiotherapy, usually in the form of external beam radiation, is the preferred adjunctive treatment. The advantage of surgery in this woman is that is allows the ovaries to be preserved and therefore avoids the complications of premature menopause. In addition, gynatresia, which is a complication of radiation, is absent.

For advanced stage disease (stages II–III) the treatment is radiotherapy. This is usually by a combination of external and intracavitary radiotherapy. The most commonly used source of radiotherapy is caesium 137. This is the chosen method because complete excision of the disease is impossible. In the more advanced disease, curative treatment is not an option. The therapy in this case is palliative. This may consist of anterior exenteration, posterior exenteration or complete exenteration. This therapy is often accompanied by supportive and psychological terminal care, which may best be offered in a hospice. The complications of radiotherapy and surgery must always be borne in mind when discussing these treatment options.

Recent developments in the treatment of carcinoma of the cervix are worth considering, especially in this nulliparous young woman. If she has early stage disease and wishes to have children, radical trachelectomy and dissection of pelvic lymph nodes may be an acceptable treatment option. It is important to stress that although preliminary results in some centres are encouraging, long-term follow-up in a large series is not yet available. Therefore, before considering this option the patient must be properly counselled. The place of chemotherapy as adjuvant treatment for carcinoma of the cervix is increasingly being recognised and this may be the adjuvant treatment of choice in this young woman if she has positive nodes. The advantage of this is that it bypasses the complications of radiotherapy.

Irrespective of the stage, the choice of treatment will depend on the facilities available and the expertise in the unit. In the UK, this will be in the regional oncology units where the multidisciplinary oncology teams are based; however, some of the smaller units have gynaecological oncologists and these units are also able to offer appropriate treatment to these women.

5. A 26-year-old woman with carcinoma of the cervix has been offered radiotherapy. (a) Outline the complications of this treatment modality. (6 marks) (b) What steps will you take to minimise these complications? (14 marks)

Common mistakes

- Not asked about the success of radiotherapy
- What are the reproductive wishes of the patient – stating that these will influence therapy
- Discussing the indications for radiotherapy
- Detailing how radiotherapy is administered
- Not asked for the various methods of treating carcinoma of the cervix
- Do not discuss staging of carcinoma of the cervix

A good answer should include some or all of these points

(a) Outline the complications of this treatment modality. (6 marks)

- Systemic and psychological:
  - Nausea
  - Vomiting
  - Depression
- Rectal
- Bladder and urinary tract infections (UTIs)
- Bowel
- Skin
- Vaginal
- Consequences of oestrogen deficiency

(b) What steps will you take to minimise these complications? (14 marks)

- Treating systemic side-effects: analgesics; antidiarrhoeal agents; evacuate bowel before radiotherapy; FBC – correct anaemia before radiotherapy – improves responsiveness to radiotherapy and general wellbeing of the patient
- Systemic – antiemetic agents
- Rectal and bladder – packing/shielding these from applicators – ovoids in the vaginal fornices
- Bowel – adequate dose/shielding
- Perineal skin – shielding
- Vaginal – stenosis – dilators and regular intercourse when feasible
- Psychological – support and education

Sample answer

(a) Outline the complications of this treatment modality. (6 marks)

The complications of radiotherapy are systemic, local and psychological. Therefore, before and during therapy, all attempts must be made to minimise these side-effects to alleviate the pain and distress that such therapy may cause. Systemic side-effects include radiation cystitis and colitis, skin radiation burns, nausea and vomiting. Often, radiation to the bowels will result in diarrhoea, whereas that to the bladder will result in frequency and dysuria. The psychological effects of radiotherapy are difficult to specify, but most patients will be anxious and may even be depressed, irritable and have sleepless nights and palpitations. Radiotherapy will induce premature menopause in this woman and the oestrogen deficiency state may cause all the symptoms of menopause, including night sweats, irritability, hot flushes, reduced libido and the long-term consequences on the cardiovascular and skeletal system.

(b) What steps will you take to minimise these complications? (14 marks)

The first step to minimise these effects is to ensure that the patient is not anaemic before radiotherapy. This will ensure a general improvement in her health and a feeling of wellbeing will lead to a better psychological tolerance of radiotherapy. Urinary tract infections should be treated to minimise the risk of cystitis. A midstream specimen of urine should be performed and appropriate antibiotics given before radiotherapy. Since diarrhoea is a recognised effect of radiotherapy, it is often advisable to evacuate the bowels before the treatment. In addition, nausea may be minimised by the administration of antiemetic agents, usually systemically.

During the radiotherapy itself, side-effects may be minimised by ensuring that exposure of the bladder and bowels to radiation is kept to a minimum. To achieve this, the bladder and bowel are packed away from the radiation source. The ovoids, which support the applicator for the caesium, are kept well away from the bladder by gauze packs. Shielding the perineum from the radiation will also reduce the complication of radiation burns to the skin. The bladder should be catheterised during radiation to ensure that it is constantly empty.

Psychologically, the patient needs to be supported and before therapy she should be seen by a nurse oncologist who will educate her on the entire process and the possible complications. Adequate preparation will minimise the psychological complications. After radiotherapy there is an increased risk of vaginal stenosis. To minimise this, the vagina may be dilated or, once it is possible, regular sexual intercourse resumed. It must be remembered that once a patient is diagnosed as having cancer, psychotherapy becomes an important therapeutic modality. This is even more important in a patient receiving radiotherapy, especially when the cancer is advanced.

Oestrogen-deficiency symptoms can be minimised by hormone replacement therapy. Since carcinoma of the cervix is not oestrogen dependent, this will not be contraindicated in this patient. Appropriate counselling about this will reduce the morbidity associated with the symptoms.

14

Uterine malignancy

1. A hysterectomy was performed on a 45-year-old woman with irregular vaginal bleeding 5 days ago. The histology has been reported as endometrial carcinoma. (a) What factors will affect the prognosis of the carcinoma? (14 marks) (b) How may her survival be improved? (6 marks)

2. (a) Evaluate the options for the treatment of a woman with atypical endometrial hyperplasia presenting with abnormal uterine bleeding at 56 years of age. (14 marks) (b) How would your treatment differ if she were 36 years old and wanted to have children? (6 marks)

3. Critically appraise your management of a 65-year-old woman with a diagnosis of endometrial carcinoma. (20 marks)

4. During surgery for endometrial carcinoma, you discover that the tumour has extended to the cervix. (a) What steps will you take at the time of surgery? (10 marks) (b) Justify your subsequent management of the patient. (10 marks)

1. A hysterectomy was performed on a 45-year-old woman with irregular vaginal bleeding 5 days ago. The histology has been reported as endometrial carcinoma. (a) What factors will affect the prognosis of the carcinoma? (14 marks) (b) How may her survival be improved? (6 marks)

Common mistakes

- Take a history and do a physical examination of the patient
- Discussing the management of endometrial cancer
- Listing the risk factors for endometrial cancer
- Diagnosis of endometrial cancer – this will not improve survival
- There are two parts to the question so answer both – do not ignore the other

A good answer will include some or all of these points

(a) What factors will affect the prognosis of the carcinoma? (14 marks)

- Prognostic factors:
  - Stage of the disease – myometrial invasion? Cervical extension?
  - Grade of disease – well or poorly differentiated
  - Histological type – adenocarcinoma, adenoacanthoma, adenosquamous? – serous, clear (papillary – poor prognosis)
  - Ploidy status
- Type of surgery: total abdominal hysterectomy + bilateral salpingo-oophorectomy + ? Nodes (A Study in the Treatment of Endometrial Cancer (ASTEC) Trial)
- Surgeon (oncologist)?
- Radiotherapy – preoperatively or postoperatively
- Chemotherapy – progestogens
- Follow-up to detect early recurrences and persistence of disease
- Endometrial cancer prognostic index. For stage I – depth of invasion, DNA ploidy and morphometric parameters, such as mean short axis

(b) How may her survival be improved? (6 marks)

- Timing of surgery
- Oncologist is associated with a better prognosis
- Histology to define the stage
- Adjuvant therapy – radiotherapy
- Comorbidity – treating it (e.g. diabetes mellitus)
- Follow-up in a multidisciplinary team

Sample answer

(a) What factors will affect the prognosis of the carcinoma? (14 marks)

Early stage disease is associated with a better prognosis. This is one of the most important prognostic factors in this patient. If the carcinoma has invaded less than 50 per cent of the myometrium, then it is early stage and the prognosis is considered to be good. Extension to the cervix, invasion of blood vessels and spread to other pelvic structures, the liver or chest are poor prognostic factors. Stage I disease has the best prognosis, whereas stage IV disease has the worse. The 5-year survival for stage I disease is 86 per cent and this falls to 16 per cent for stage IV.

Another important prognostic factor is the grade of the disease. Well-differentiated carcinomas tend to have a better prognosis than poorly differentiated ones. Histological type is also significant. Adenocarcinomas have the best prognosis followed by adenoacanthoma, whereas adenosquamous carcinomas have the worse prognosis. Other prognostic factors include the age of the patient, the ploidy and the endometrial prognostic score. The older patient has a poorer prognosis. In this case her age may, therefore, be a good prognostic factor. The ploidy status of the cancer can only be determined cytogenetically. It is also important to determine whether the patient's carcinoma is serous, clear or papillary. The last variety has the worse prognosis compared to the serous type, which has the best prognosis. For stage I disease, the endometrial prognostic index can be used to gauge prognosis. This index includes the depth of myometrial invasion, DNA ploidy and morphometric parameters, such as mean short axis.

The prognosis of the carcinoma may be improved in a variety of ways ranging from the most appropriate treatment to adjuvant therapy. The best prognosis is obtained if the patient's surgery is performed by a gynaecological oncologist. The surgery of choice is a hysterectomy and bilateral salpingo-oophorectomy. The role of adenectomy in surgery for carcinoma of the endometrium has been assessed by the ASTEC trial, which has concluded that this does not improve prognosis and may, in fact, make it poorer.

For early stage diseases, surgery is enough for a good outcome. However, for advanced disease, adjuvant radiotherapy improves the prognosis. What is uncertain is whether preoperative or postoperative radiotherapy has a better effect on the prognosis. For most people, postoperative radiotherapy seems to be the best option as it is only offered to those in whom histology reveals significant myometrial invasion and/or invasion of blood vessels. Chemotherapy with progestogens has not been shown to improve prognosis, although it may be of limited value in those with recurrent disease.

After surgery, meticulous follow-up to identify early recurrences and institute timely and appropriate therapy is associated with a better prognosis. Such follow-up is in the form of regular clinical examinations and identification of signs of secondaries or metastasis.

(b) How may her survival be improved? (6 marks)

The survival rate of this patient may be improved by early surgical treatment, preferably by a gynaecological oncologist. The sooner the surgery is performed after diagnosis, the less likely the risk of invasion as most would have been in an earlier stage. A surgery performed by an oncologist is said to have a better prognosis than one done by a general gynaecologist. This is also the recommendation of the Royal College of Obstetricians and Gynaecologists. Appropriate histology, not only to define the type of cancer but also to determine the degree of invasion, will help in staging the disease and therefore determine the need for adjuvant therapy. Where the disease has invaded blood vessels, lymph nodes and/or is beyond the inner 50% of the myometrium, adjuvant therapy with radiotherapy is associated with an improved prognosis. Finally, treatment by a multidisciplinary team consisting of a gynaecological oncologist, a medical oncologist with an interest in gynaecology, specialised nurses and the general practitioner (GP) is associated with better outcome. Treating comorbidities such as diabetes mellitus improves the patient's ability to withstand not only the disease but also the therapy.

2. (a) Evaluate the options for the treatment of a woman with atypical endometrial hyperplasia presenting with abnormal uterine bleeding at 56 years of age. (14 marks)
    (b) How would your treatment differ if she were 36 years old and wanted to have children? (6 marks)

Common mistakes

- Discussing the aetiological factors of endometrial carcinoma
- Discussing the management of endometrial carcinoma
- Treating endometrial hyperplasia rather than atypical hyperplasia
- Offer hysteroscopy and ultrasound to make a diagnosis
- Treatment depends on the age of the patient and her desire for more children
- Chemotherapy is the treatment of choice
- Failure to evaluate the options

A good answer will include some or all of these points

(a) Evaluate the options for the treatment of a woman with atypical endometrial hyperplasia presenting with abnormal uterine bleeding at 56 years of age. (14 marks)

- Endometrial atypical hyperplasia is a premalignant condition – risk of progression to malignancy up to 22–88 per cent in some cases
- Coexistent carcinoma in 25–50 per cent of cases
- Expectant management, therefore, is not an option
- History to exclude exogenous oestrogens, tamoxifen and physical examination to exclude ovarian masses. Investigations to exclude possible causes of the hyperplasia
- Treatment options need to be discussed and depend on the general health of the patient, i.e. how fit she is for surgery
- Total abdominal hysterectomy + bilateral salpingo-oophorectomy
- Progestogens – high doses (duration of treatment not uniformly agreed)
- Levonorgestrel intrauterine contraceptive system (Lng-IUCS)
- Long-term follow-up after treatment
- Radiotherapy – disadvantage
- If not treated by surgery, need for close follow-up

(b) How would your treatment differ if she were 36 years old and wanted to have children? (6 marks)

- Progestogens:
  - Local in the form of the Lng-IUCS (Mirena®)
  - Systemic – tablets or Depo-Provera® – high doses
  - Follow-up after 6 months

- Complete family, offer hysterectomy
- Hysteroscopic resection of the area of abnormality? How is this identified?

Sample answer

(a) Evaluate the options for the treatment of a woman with atypical endometrial hyperplasia presenting with abnormal uterine bleeding at 56 years of age. (14 marks)

Atypical hyperplasia of the endometrium is a premalignant condition with the risk of progression to frank malignancy reported to vary from 22 to 88 per cent (Soutter, 2003). In the management of this patient it is essential to exclude a coexistent carcinoma of the endometrium, which may be present in between 25 and 50 per cent of patients with atypical hyperplasia of the endometrium. Important causes of this diagnosis may be excluded from a history. These include unopposed exogenous oestrogen therapy as hormone replacement therapy or tamoxifen for breast cancer. Following this, a hysteroscopy and a thorough pelvic examination should be performed. This is only necessary if the patient has not already had such investigations. An ultrasound scan will identify an ovarian tumour, which may be the source of oestrogens responsible for the atypical hyperplasia. A CA125 will be performed if there is a suspected ovarian tumour or if this has been confirmed on ultrasound scan. An abnormally high CA125 will raise suspicion of ovarian malignancy.

In view of the increased risk of progression to malignancy or the high coexistence risk of carcinoma, there is no place for expectant management of this patient. The options available to this 56-year-old woman are surgery, systemic progestogens or locally administered progestogens. The best option will be a hysterectomy and bilateral salpingo-oophorectomy. This ensures that the endometrial pathology is removed as well as a possible source of oestrogens (the ovaries). This option provides cure and removes any occult carcinoma, which may not have been identified from an endometrial biopsy. After surgery, there will be no need to follow up the patient, and even if she had a malignancy, which does not usually involve more than a superficial invasion of the myometrium, this treatment will be effective.

The second option is treatment with progestogens. These can be administered systemically or locally. Systemic progestogens should be given in high doses for about 3–6 months. There is no generally agreed duration of therapy with systemic steroids. However, after the treatment, the patient needs to be followed up for a long time as the recurrence of atypical hyperplasia and malignancy has been reported after a long interval following such therapy. This is not the preferred option unless the patient is unsuitable for surgery or does not wish to have surgery. If she does not wish to have systemic steroids, the LnG-IUCS may also be used. This delivers levonorgestrel locally and avoids some of the systemic effects of progestogens. Since progestogen therapy (systemic and local) may be associated with irregular vaginal bleeding, the occurrence of this complication may be confused with persistence/recurrence of the atypical hyperplasia.

Another option worth considering, if none of the above, is applicable is intrauterine radiotherapy. It induces endometrial atrophy and is therefore effective, but it is associated with radiation complications and may induce vaginal stenosis. The recurrence of the disease may therefore not be easily recognised.

(b) How would your treatment differ if she were 36 years old and wanted to have children? (6 marks)

The options would include the progestogens, locally delivered to the uterine cavity or systemic. The local option is the LnG-IUCS, while the systemic options include oral (medroxyprogesterone acetate or norethisterone acetate) or depot injections (depot medroxyprogesterone acetate). These have to be given in high doses and for at least 6 months. This conservative treatment option requires regular monitoring of the endometrial thickness by ultrasound scan and biopsies after a period of treatment. If the area with the pathology was localised on hysteroscopy, directed biopsy could be applied. Once the woman has completed her family, a hysterectomy and bilateral salpingo-oophorectomy should be considered.

Reference

Soutter WP (2003) Premalignant disease of the lower genital tract. In: Shaw RW, Soutter WP, Stanton SL (eds) *Gynaecology*, 3rd edn. Edinburgh: Churchill Livingstone, pp. 561–82.

3. Critically appraise your management of a 65-year-old woman with a diagnosis of endometrial carcinoma. (20 marks)

Common mistakes

- Take a history and perform a physical examination
- Hysteroscopy/ultrasound to make diagnosis
- Listing the treatment options for endometrial carcinoma
- Wertheim's hysterectomy
- Vaginal hysterectomy and pelvic floor repair
- Chemotherapy/radiotherapy
- Progestogens only

A good answer will include some or all of these points

- Diagnosis already made but investigations need to be performed to define extent of disease
- Clinical assessment to determine whether she is suitable for surgery
- Planned surgery with oncologist or involve gynaecological oncologist
- Total abdominal hysterectomy + bilateral salpingo-oophorectomy with or without lymphadenectomy
- Postoperative radiotherapy
- Preoperative radiotherapy
- Chemotherapy with progestogens
- Follow-up clinically with GP or hospital?
- Conclusion

Sample answer

The mainstay of treatment is surgery and this is more so with early stage disease. In late stage disease, surgery has to be supported by adjuvant chemotherapy or radiotherapy. Therefore, the first step in the management of this 65-year-old woman is to try to define the extent of the disease.

A clinical assessment is paramount to determine the extent of the disease but also to exclude systemic diseases (e.g. chest infections) which may affect her fitness for surgery. An abdominal and pelvic examination may demonstrate masses arising from the pelvis (uterine or ovarian) and ascites, which may indicate the presence of peritoneal secondaries. Although examining the abdomen is important, it is often negative and, indeed, does not define the true extent of the disease. This is better done at surgery and, most importantly, will have to be confirmed following histological examination. Clinical examination is also unlikely to identify metastases to nodes, the liver and other distant sites unless they are symptomatic.

Ancillary investigations such as a chest X-ray (CXR) and an ultrasound scan will be more useful in identifying secondaries in the liver and the chest. These may not, however, identify lymph node secondaries but magnetic resonance imaging (MRI) may. Urea and electrolytes (U&Es) and serum creatinine are essential to assess renal function. Since endometrial carcinoma is more common in women with diabetes mellitus, urinalysis for glucose is important. A full blood count and group and save serum will establish the patient's haemoglobin level and will also ensure that, if she requires transfusion during surgery or due to anaemia caused by vaginal bleeding (a possible primary symptom of the patient), blood is easily cross-matched.

The treatment of choice is a total hysterectomy and bilateral salpingo-oophorectomy. Although the hysterectomy is commonly performed abdominally, there is no evidence to suggest that mortality and morbidity are greater after a vaginal hysterectomy. However, an abdominal approach is preferred if lymphadenectomy is to be performed. If her disease is considered to be early stage, a laparoscopically assisted vaginal hysterectomy and bilateral salpingo-oophorectomy will be effective treatment, offering benefits of reduced morbidity, shorter hospital stay and recovery. However, if there is any suspicion of extension beyond the uterus, this approach will be unsuitable.

At surgery, peritoneal washings have to be performed and lymph nodes either removed or biopsied. Management after surgery will depend on the histological diagnosis, myometrial invasion and the presence of positive nodes. Positive nodes or myometrial invasion of more than 50 per cent, or a poorly differentiated tumour, will be an indication for radiotherapy. This is preferred to preoperative radiotherapy as it is restricted to women with nodes and other poor prognostic factors. About 5 per cent develop complications of radiotherapy and therefore restricting postoperative radiotherapy limits the number of women exposed to these complications.

Apart from radiotherapy, chemotherapy with progestogens may be considered for advanced disease. This is often given for recurrent cases. There are no randomised controlled trials to evaluate the efficacy of progestogens in the adjuvant therapy of endometrial carcinoma, but it is the treatment of choice for recurrent disease, since over 80 per cent of progestogen-receptor-positive and 70 per cent of oestrogen-receptor-positive tumours respond to progestogen therapy. After surgery, this patient will need to be followed up for at least 5 years. During this time any recurrence will be treated with progestogens or radiotherapy for vault disease. Her follow-up would be provided by her GP and the gynaecologist.

4. During surgery for endometrial carcinoma, you discover that the tumour has extended to the cervix. (a) What steps will you take at the time of surgery? (10 marks) (b) Justify your subsequent management of the patient. (10 marks)

Common mistakes

- Counsel the patient and obtain consent about more extensive surgery!
- Total abdominal hysterectomy and bilateral salpingo-oophorectomy and offer radio-therapy
- Abandon surgery and treat with radiotherapy
- Take a history and perform an examination
- Review the notes and the results of all the investigations
- Inform relatives and obtain consent before proceeding with surgery

A good answer will include some or all of these points

(a) What steps will you take at the time of surgery? (10 marks)

- Once carcinoma has extended to the cervix, it must be treated as cancer of the cervix
- Involve gynaecological oncologist
- Define the extent of disease
- May need to do a cystoscopy
- Wertheim's hysterectomy if possible and considered appropriate; otherwise, hysterectomy followed by radiotherapy

(b) Justify your subsequent management of the patient. (10 marks)

- Postoperative counselling – inform of the findings and treatment
- Await histology including that of nodes if Wertheim's
- If only hysterectomy, radiotherapy afterwards
- Follow-up with multidisciplinary team
- Further investigations:
  - CXR
  - Abdominal ultrasound or MRI
  - U&Es

Sample answer

(a) What steps will you take at the time of surgery? (10 marks)

This will depend on the precise time when recognition of cervical involvement if made. If it is made at the time of pelvic examination following catheterisation of the bladder, then the two options are (1) abandoning the procedure (surgery for endometrial carcinoma is different from that of carcinoma of the cervix and once endometrial carcinoma has involved the cervix, treatment is that for carcinoma of the cervix) and (2) referring the patient to a gynaecology oncology team or calling the team to come and stage the disease while the patient is still under anaesthesia. The advantage of the second approach is that the patient will not have to be exposed to a second anaesthetic with its associated risks. For the first option, staging will have to be done at a latter date. Staging, whether done at the time of surgery or later, will include a cystoscopy and rectal examination.

Since the current recommendation is that only ovarian and cervical cancers should be treated by gynaecological oncologists, this patient may well be having surgery performed by a general gynaecologist. Once the disease has spread to the cervix, the treatment must then become that for carcinoma of the cervix. This is because involvement of the cervix would imply possible spread to the parametrial tissues and vessels, which may have implications for the prognosis of the disease. If the recognition is at the time just before of after removal of the uterus and cervix, then the oncologist should be asked to come and review the patient and her surgery.

The subsequent management will depend on the extent of the disease. Surgical treatment for early carcinoma of the cervix is Wertheim's hysterectomy. If this were to be performed on this patient, her ovaries would have to be removed as the primary cancer is oestrogen dependent. This may not be possible but if this option were possible, then removal of the parametrium, dissection of the lymph nodes and removal of the upper cuff of the vagina will be the minimum. This will be on the assumption that the cancer of the cervix is restricted to stages I and IIa. If it is more advanced, the surgery will be inadequate. If a Wertheim's hysterectomy was not possible, then the hysterectomy and bilateral salpingo-oophorectomy should be completed and adjuvant radiotherapy offered.

(b) Justify your subsequent management of the patient. (10 marks)

After surgery, subsequent management will be tailored according to the histological extent of the disease (i.e. positive nodes). It is essential to investigate the patient and exclude secondaries. The essential investigations will include U&Es, a CXR and an abdominal MRI or computerised tomography scan to exclude chest secondaries, liver and abdominal (liver and nodes) secondaries. Ultrasound scan of the renal tract will exclude hydronephrosis, the presence of which will indicate at least stage III disease. If the pelvic nodes are involved, radiotherapy in the form of external beam will be the adjuvant treatment of choice. This must be offered by a team consisting of a clinical oncologist and a gynaecological oncologist. Endometrial cancer is not as sensitive to radiotherapy as squamous carcinoma of the cervix. The prognosis for this patient after adjuvant radiotherapy will therefore not be as good as that following squamous carcinoma of the cervix.

If distant metastases are suspected, chemotherapy with progestogens may be considered. This will be effective in 80 per cent of progestogen-receptor-positive and 70 per cent of oestrogen-receptor-positive tumours. The duration of chemotherapy is uncertain but careful follow-up is necessary to identify recurrent disease. Any recurrence in the vagina should be treated by radiotherapy.

15

Ovarian malignancy

1. A schoolteacher presented with vague abdominal symptoms and following investigations had surgery for an ovarian mass. This was suspected to be malignant at the time of surgery. (a) Describe her management at the time of surgery. (4 marks) (b) What factors will govern her prognosis? (12 marks) (c) How will she be followed up if the histology is borderline? (4 marks)

2. Screening for ovarian cancer is not as effective as that for cervical cancer. Justify this statement. (20 marks)

3. A 44-year-old woman presents with an abdominal mass that is thought to be ovarian in origin. (a) How will you clinically determine that this mass is malignant? (12 marks) (b) What additional information will you require to counsel the woman and her family about risks? (8 marks)

4. An 18-year-old girl presented with intermittent right-sided abdominal pain and a mass of rapid onset. Ultrasound scan demonstrated a unilocular large ovarian cyst measuring $10 \times 12 \times 14$ cm with no associated ascites. The serum alpha-fetoprotein (AFP) was described as raised. Outline your management of this patient. (20 marks)

1. A schoolteacher presented with vague abdominal symptoms and following investigations had surgery for an ovarian mass. This was suspected to be malignant at the time of surgery. (a) Describe her management at the time of surgery. (4 marks) (b) What factors will govern her prognosis? (12 marks) (c) How will she be followed up if the histology is borderline? (4 marks)

Common mistakes

- Monitoring serum markers for ovarian cancer
- Diagnosis of ovarian cancer
- History and physical examination
- Discussing the management of ovarian cancer
- Listing the risk factors for ovarian cancer

A good answer will include some or all of these points

(a) Describe her management at the time of surgery. (4 marks)

- Call a gynaecological oncologist to complete the surgery
- Peritoneal washings (pelvis and paracolic gutters for cytology)
- Thorough surgical staging – unilateral?; capsule intact?; presence of ascites?
- Frozen section if facilities are available
- Total abdominal hysterectomy (TAH) and bilateral salpingo-oophorectomy (BSO), omentectomy

(b) What factors will govern her prognosis? (12 marks)

- Stage of the disease
- Histological type
- Treatment
- Adjuvant therapy
- General state of health of the patient
- Residual disease after surgery
- Multidisciplinary team (MDT) involvement in her care
- Facilities for treatment and follow-up

(c) How will she be followed up if the histology is borderline? (4 marks)

- Clinical – regular examination (6-monthly)
- CA125

- Ultrasound
- Doppler scans have no role

Sample answer

(a) Describe her management at the time of surgery. (4 marks)

Once a malignancy is suspected, the gynaecological oncologist should be involved in the subsequent management of this patient. The first stage of her management will be a thorough surgical staging. This involves collecting peritoneal fluid from the pouch of Douglas and the paracolic gutters and if there is none, peritoneal washings should be collected for cytology. The tumour itself should be inspected to determine whether the capsule has been breached and whether it is bilateral or unilateral. The consistency of the tumour should also be noted. A partly solid and cystic tumour is more likely to be malignant. If the facilities are available, a frozen section should be considered. The limitations of this must be recognised as the section may not necessarily represent the whole pathology of the tumour. If the tumour is unilateral, a section of the contralateral ovary should also be taken. The next stage is definitive surgery, which in this case will be a TAH, BSO and omentectomy.

(b) What factors will govern her prognosis? (12 marks)

Ovarian cancer is the most common cause of mortality from gynaecological cancer in the UK. The overall 5-year survival rate is approximately 23 per cent. This is because most present late, usually in stage III. The prognosis of ovarian cancer is guided by several factors. These vary from the histological type to the treatment that the patient is offered.

The 5-year survival for ovarian cancer varies with the stage of the disease. For stage I disease, the 5-year survival is 60–70 per cent, whereas for stages III–IV it is 10 per cent. The fact that the overall 5-year survival is only between 15 and 23 per cent suggest that most patients present with advanced disease. A chest X-ray (CXR) and an abdominal ultrasound will help in the staging, as it will exclude secondaries in the chest and liver respectively.

The histological type and grade of the disease influence prognosis significantly. For example, in stage I disease, 5-year survival in those with grades I or II disease is 90 per cent, compared with lower rates for poorly differentiated diseases. This is an important factor in early stage disease. For advanced tumours, stage is a more important prognostic factor than grade, even for well-differentiated tumours. In addition to the histological type, ploidy is an important prognostic factor in early and advanced stage disease. Diploid tumours tend to have a better prognosis than aneuploid tumours in both early and advanced stage disease.

The younger and therefore healthier patient has a better prognosis than the older woman. However, age tends to be associated with other factors. In addition, another important prognostic factor is the surgeon. It is now well recognised that the prognosis is better if surgery is performed by a gynaecological oncologist. More important is the size of residual disease following surgery. Where residual disease is minimal, medium-term survival tends to be longer. Adjuvant therapy is a prognostic factor for ovarian cancer. If it is offered by a team consisting of a clinical oncologist, a gynaecological oncologist and an oncology nurse, the prognosis tends to be better. In addition, a combination including cisplatin has a better prognosis than one without. Very recently, the value of oncogenes in the prognosis of ovarian cancer has been assessed. Oncogenes that have been studied include epidermal growth factor receptor, insulin-like growth factor-1 receptor, *cerb-2*, *c-ras* and *c-myc*. Overexpression of one of these oncogenes, especially epidermal growth factor receptor, was considered a poor prognostic factor. In patients with borderline tumours, the most important prognostic factor is tumour ploidy.

(c) How will she be followed up if the histology is borderline? (4 marks)

The follow-up will be by a combination of regular (6-monthly) clinical, radiological and bio-chemical parameters. The clinical parameters include abdominal masses, ascites and secondaries in the chest and liver. Ultrasound examination of the abdomen and pelvis will screen for masses and ascites and secondaries in the liver while a rising CA125 will be suspicious of recurrence or progression. There is no role for Doppler scans in the follow-up of this patient.

2. Screening for ovarian cancer is not as effective as that for cervical cancer. Justify this statement. (20 marks)

Common mistakes

- Not asked to describe the diagnosis of ovarian cancer or cervical cancer screening
- Not asked to discuss the risk factors for the two cancers
- Avoid treating the two screening programmes in isolation
- Focusing mainly on why cancer of the ovary cannot be screened and why cancer of the cervix has been successfully screened
- Describing the treatment of ovarian cancer and carcinoma of the cervix
- Failing to justify (i.e. give reasons for what you do)

A good answer will include some or all of these points

- Ovarian cancer – most common gynaecological killer
- Screening for cancer of the cervix – has reduced mortality from it. Failure to improve 5-year survival for ovarian cancer is secondary to inadequate screening
- Ideal screening – sensitive, predictive of condition, inexpensive and cost effective, applicable to the general population
- Cervix accessible, premalignant stage defined, natural history of premalignant stage
- Ovary – inaccessible, natural history (premalignant stage poorly defined)
- Screening methods – targeted – inapplicable to the general population: pelvic examination
- Ultrasound examination – cysts? What are the characteristics?
- CA25 and other tumour markers, e.g. melanocyte-stimulating factor, ovarian cancer antigen, AFP, beta-human chorionic gonadotropin (βhCG) – not specific
- Doppler ultrasound – how useful?
- Breast cancer antigens BRCA1 and BRCA2
- Conclusion

Sample answer

Ovarian cancer is the most common cause of mortality from gynaecological malignancy. There are about 5800–6000 new cases every year in the UK. Although carcinoma of the cervix used to be the most common gynaecological malignancy, the introduction of the cervical screening programme has significantly reduced mortality from cervical cancer, although the overall incidence of cancer of the cervix has not decreased significantly. If mortality from cervical cancer has fallen significantly due to screening, then screening from ovarian cancer should aim to reduce mortality from this dreadful disease. Unfortunately, screening for ovarian cancer has not been as successful as cervical cancer screening. Several factors are responsible for this big difference. They vary from the screening methods and accessibility of the ovaries to early diagnosis and treatment of cancer.

The ovaries, by virtue of their location, are inaccessible to early diagnosis of pathology. In addition, there is no well-recognised premalignant stage of ovarian cancer. Even where a premalignant stage is known, as in borderline disease, the natural progression of this to malignancy is unknown. This is in contrast to the cervix, which is accessible to inspection and therefore screening, has a well-defined premalignant state and a well-understood natural progression from the premalignant state to frank cancer. This difference has been responsible for the development of a screening test and programme for carcinoma of the cervix. Failure to develop a screening programme and test for carcinoma of the ovary, therefore, has been a major contributor to the failure of any screening methods at reducing the mortality from this condition.

The screening methods for ovarian cancer themselves are insensitive, poorly predictive and, in most cases, inapplicable to the general population. In addition, they are not cost effective and most are not cheap. These screening methods primarily fail to meet the World Health Organization criteria for a screening test. For example, pelvic examination in postmenopausal women is inexpensive, but is very non-specific and depends on the clinician's ability to identify an adnexal mass. Even if the ovary is palpable in a postmenopausal woman, it will not suggest the presence of a premalignant state of ovarian cancer. Another important factor is how frequently this examination has to be undertaken. This difficulty is common to all screening tests for ovarian cancer.

Radiological screening has been advocated and is being offered to some women. Ultrasound of the ovaries and/or Doppler scanning of the ovarian vessels have been shown to be of poor sensitivity and unpredictable, even in the high-risk population. Again, for these to be effective, various characteristics of abnormality have to be defined and be universally acceptable. Unfortunately, there are difficulties defining these criteria. However, in a high-risk population this may be useful as it will identify increased vascularity of ovaries and cysts.

The use of biochemical screening has been tried and is still being offered to women at risk of ovarian cancer. The problem with this test is that most are non-specific and cannot be offered to the whole population. For example, CA125 is raised in all epithelial tumours, infections and endometriosis. However, other markers may be more specific but these (e.g. βHCG and AFP) cannot be used as screening tools for ovarian cancer.

Recently, genetic markers have been used to identify those at risk of ovarian cancer and subsequently to screen them. The most specific markers are the breast cancer antigens BRCA1 and BRCA2. However, to use these, two relatives must be known to have died of ovarian cancer or the patient must have one dead relative and one alive with ovarian cancer. Again, these are non-specific in the general population. In affected families, the presence of these genes will indicate a high risk and may therefore increase the chances of identifying early cancer.

Although there is no acceptable screening test for ovarian cancer, the history of ovarian cancer provides a reliable means of identifying the at-risk population. The lifetime risk of ovarian cancer is 1.4 per cent in the UK. If one close family relative has ovarian cancer, this risk is increased to 2.5 per cent and for two close family relatives, it rises to 30–40 per cent. Therefore, this is probably the most useful method of identifying the at-risk group. However, it does not allow the diagnosis of the premalignant stage of the disease and only prophylactic oophorectomy offered to these high-risk women may reduce the incidence of ovarian cancer.

3. A 44-year-old woman presents with an abdominal mass that is thought to be ovarian in origin. (a) How will you clinically determine that this mass is malignant? (12 marks) (b) What additional information will you require to counsel the woman and her family about risks? (8 marks)

Common mistakes

- Not asked about how to manage ovarian cancer
- You have not been asked to discuss the various histological types of ovarian cancer
- No need to discuss frozen sections
- The role of CA125 is limited and so, too, is the role of Doppler ultrasound
- Discussing chemotherapy and hormone replacement therapy
- You have not been asked how to reduce the risk of ovarian cancer in her family; therefore no need to discuss prevention of ovarian cancer

A good answer will include some or all of these points

(a) How will you clinically determine that this mass is malignant? (12 marks)

- Clinical:
  - Rapid onset
  - Associated feature of malignancy – weight loss, anorexia
  - Examination – fixed, bilateral, irregular masses, ascites
- Radiology – magnetic resonance imaging (MRI), computerised tomography (CT) – nodes and nature of masses
- Doppler – increased vascularity
- Surgery:
  - Fixed, ruptured capsule, bilateral
  - Secondaries on the liver, omentum and para-aortic nodes
  - Cytology
  - Histology: haematoxylin and eosin stains of sections

(b) What additional information will you require to counsel the woman and her family about risks? (8 marks)

- Family history of the following cancers and the degree and age of relative involved. Any tissues available:
  - Breast
  - Ovary
  - Colon
  - Stomach

- Type of cancer – epithelial or not – 5 per cent of epithelial cancers have a genetic component
- BRAC1 and BRCA2; Lynch syndrome screening – has any been done?
- BRCA1 increases risk by 40–50 per cent and BRCA2 by 25 per cent

Sample answer

(a) How will you clinically determine that this mass is malignant? (12 marks)

A malignant ovarian tumour is most likely to be rapidly growing and associated with features of malignancy, such as anorexia, dyspepsia and weight loss. If there is a longstanding history of a swelling in the abdomen and there are no tell-tale features of malignancy, this is unlikely to be malignant. Clinical features suspicious of malignancy include weight loss, secondaries in the chest, ascites, bilaterality of the tumour and fixity in the pelvis. Radiologically, there may be features of malignancy, such as secondaries in the chest and liver on X-ray or ultrasound scan, and adenopathy on MRI of the abdomen. Irregularly enlarged ovarian masses with mixed echogenicity demonstrated in growths on the wall of the tumours on ultrasound scan and associated ascites will be suggestive of malignancy. A Doppler examination of the ovarian pedicle and ovary showing increased vascularity is suggestive of malignancy.

At the time of surgery, specific features that may suggest malignancy include blood-stained ascites, ruptured capsule, secondaries on the liver surface and bowel, and bilateral tumours that are partly solid, partly cystic, irregular in nature and fixed to the pelvis. Malignant cells in ascitic fluid sent for cytology will be suggestive of malignancy. The ultimate distinction between a benign and a malignant ovarian tumour will be from a histological examination. Such examinations are performed on haematoxylin and eosin stains. Since histological examinations are only of specific sections prepared for the examination, there is the possibility (though slim) that early disease may be missed. Therefore, this distinction does not completely guarantee the accuracy of diagnosis.

(b) What additional information will you require to counsel the woman and her family about risks? (8 marks)

Counselling will focus mainly on the risk of relatives developing cancer and the woman's risk of developing other cancers, such as colon and breast. Such counselling will require crucial information about her family history of these cancers. If any of her relatives have had cancer, it is important to ascertain whether any tissues from the cancer are available and whether there has been any screening for syndromes that are cancer related, e.g. Lynch syndrome. Inheritance plays a role in 5 per cent of epithelial ovarian cancers and these tumours are usually serous. The lifetime risk for a woman with an affected relative depends on her own age and the relationship with the affected relative. For her sisters, their risk of developing ovarian cancer is 4 per cent. If another relative had ovarian cancer, then her risk will be 14 per cent. If the family are screened for the *BRCA1* and *BRAC2* gene mutations, *BRAC1* mutation will increase the risk of ovarian cancer by 40–80 per cent and that of breast cancer by 60–80 per cent while *BRAC2* will increase the risk of ovarian cancer by 25 per cent.

4. An 18-year-old girl presented with intermittent right-sided abdominal pain and a mass of rapid onset. Ultrasound scan demonstrated a unilocular large ovarian cyst measuring $10 \times 12 \times 14$ cm with no associated ascites. The serum AFP was described as raised. Outline your management of this patient. (20 marks)

Common mistakes

- History and physical examination
- Screen for ovarian cancer
- Measure various markers for malignancy
- Treatment will depend on age and desire for more children
- Diagnostic laparoscopy to determine extent of disease
- Obtain consent for oophorectomy and, if necessary, speak to parents at laparotomy on type of surgery

A good answer will include some or all of these points

- The most likely diagnosis is a germ cell tumour
- Management must take her age into consideration
- Further investigations:
    - CXR – any secondaries in the lungs?
    - Abdominal ultrasound – secondaries in the liver?
    - Urea and electrolytes (U&Es) – chemotherapy may be nephrotoxic
    - Full blood count (FBC) and group and save – may require transfusion at the time of surgery
- MDT meeting to discuss before counselling and surgery
- Adequate counselling is an important initial step:
    - Type of surgery that may be offered – depends on the findings
    - May lose both ovaries and/or uterus
- A laparotomy is the treatment of choice – to be done by gynaecological oncologist
- Define the extent of the lesion
- Surgical removal of the ovarian tumour and consider the other side – frozen section?
- Follow-up – chemotherapy, subsequent management

Sample answer

The most likely diagnosis in this young girl is a germ cell tumour. In view of the rapidly developing nature of her symptoms and the raised AFP levels, the most likely type of germ cell tumour she may have is an endodermal sinus tumour. This is the second most common germ cell tumour. The presence of pain suggests a complication, such as haemorrhage into the cyst or necrosis within the cyst. If she has not already had a CXR and CT scan of the abdomen, this must be performed. These are necessary to determine any spread to the chest, liver and para-aortic lymph nodes. A FBC and a group and save will ensure that blood is available for surgery if required and that anaemia prior to surgery is corrected. A U&E and liver function test will form the baseline for monitoring toxicity to chemotherapeutic agents.

Once this is suspected, the definitive management is a laparotomy performed by a gynaeco-logical oncologist. In this young girl, appropriate counselling before surgery is extremely important. An MDT meeting to discuss the patient will provide a solid basis for counselling. The counselling must include the diagnosis and the implications. An endodermal sinus tumour is typically unilateral, well encapsulated and solid. However, in some cases, there may be spread to the contralateral ovary or other sites. In view of her age, it is essential to aim to preserve the other ovary and her uterus unless the disease is outside the affected ovary. She must be counselled about the possible surgical options and the possibility of adjuvant chemotherapy. This is preferred to radiotherapy as is does not affect future fertility. In this patient a vertical abdominal incision would be preferred as it offers better exposure and allows a more thorough exploration of the abdomen and also the possibility of extension if required.

If the tumour is confined to one ovary and the capsule is intact, an oophorectomy and biopsy of the omentum and para-aortic nodes, and the contralateral ovary should be per-formed. If the disease has extended to the contralateral ovary, a bilateral oophorectomy, ome-mentectomy and lymphadenectomy will be the treatment of choice. In some cases, although the disease may be confined to one ovary, the capsule may appear breached by the tumour or there may be ascites. In such cases, a frozen section of the contralateral ovary must be per-formed and sent along with ascitic fluid for urgent histology and cytology, respectively.

Subsequent management of the patient will depend on the presence of malignant cells in the contralateral ovary or the ascitic fluid. In most cases, the logistics of a frozen section are diffi-cult. However, subsequent management needs to be influenced by the histological findings. Although in the past, patients with these tumours were treated by hysterectomy and BSO if the tumour involved both ovaries or the patient did not want to have children, there is now a place to consider BSO and preserving the uterus. This allows the patient an opportunity to have children at a later date by use of donated ova. It is important to discuss all these options before surgery. If the patient is certain about not wanting a family, a TAH and BSO may be the treat-ment of choice. However, at the age of 18 years, this may be a difficult decision to make and therefore consideration ought to be given to future regrets.

Follow-up management by an oncology team would depend on the histology of the biopsy from the contralateral ovary and the para-aortic nodes. Whatever the histology of the samples obtained at surgery, the patient would benefit from postoperative chemotherapy. In the past this consisted of vincristine, actinomycin D and cyclophosphamide. More contemporaneous treatment consists of cisplatin compounds given in combination with bleomycin and etopo-side. In some case, radiotherapy may be offered but this tumour is not very radiosensitive. The disadvantage of radiotherapy is its effect on the remaining ovary and therefore the patient's future fertility. It was suggested in the past that once the patient had completed her family, she should subsequently be offered a hysterectomy and removal of the other ovary. However, this approach is being questioned by some oncologists who feel that adequate follow-up with ser-ial AFP and clinical symptoms is all that is required.

16

Gestational trophoblastic disease

1. A 27-year-old patient has been diagnosed with choriocarcinoma. (a) Comment on the prognostic factors in this patient. (12 marks) (b) What advice will you give her about pregnancy? (8 marks)

2. A 27-year-old woman is being followed-up after a miscarriage of a complete hydatidiform mole. (a) Justify the contraceptive advice you will offer her. (10 marks) (b) When will you initiate chemotherapy in this patient? (10 marks)

3. A 28-year-old woman presented with an incomplete miscarriage, for which an evacuation was performed. Histology of the products of conception concluded that she had a hydatidiform mole. (a) What will be your immediate management? (8 marks) (b) Justify your long-term management of this patient. (8 marks) (c) How will you manage her in her next pregnancy? (4 marks)

1. A 27-year-old patient has been diagnosed with choriocarcinoma. (a) Comment on the prognostic factors in this patient. (12 marks) (b) What advice will you give her about pregnancy? (8 marks)

Common mistakes

- Discussing the genetics of molar pregnancy
- Discussing chemotherapy
- Increased risk of prophylactic chemotherapy
- Details of chemotherapy
- Take a history and physical examination
- Details of the complications of choriocarcinoma and chemotherapy

A good answer will include some or all of these points

(a) Comment on the prognostic factors in this patient. (12 marks)

- Prognostic factors are important in categorising patients into low-, medium- or high-risk groups for the purpose of chemotherapy
- The various risk factors include:
  - Age
  - Antecedent pregnancy
  - Interval between antecedent pregnancy and start of chemotherapy
  - Beta-human chorionic gonadotropin (βhCG) level at the time of initiation of chemotherapy
  - Blood group
  - Largest tumour
  - Uterine tumour; site of metastases
  - Number of metastases identified
  - Prior chemotherapy

(b) What advice will you give her about pregnancy? (8 marks)

- Best avoided for at least 12 months after completion of chemotherapy
- Treatment does not affect fertility
- Contraception:
  - Avoid the combined oral contraceptive pill while receiving treatment and βhCG high – may delay return of βhCG to normal
  - Barrier methods – ideal

- Avoid progestogen-only pill (POP) and intrauterine contraceptive devices (IUDs) – irregular bleeding from the contraceptives will be confused with that from the disease
- Once pregnant, arrange an early ultrasound scan
- At the end of pregnancy, should have a follow-up test (βhCG) at the regional centre 6 weeks later.

Sample answer

(a) Comment on the prognostic factors in this patient. (12 marks)

These factors are used to classify the patients into low, medium and high risk. Chemotherapy and prognosis is then based on this classification.

The patient's age is an important prognostic factor. Women over the age of 39 years are of a higher risk than younger women. The antecedent pregnancy is one of the most important prognostic risk factors. The prognosis of choriocarcinoma after a normal pregnancy is worse than that following a miscarriage and this, in turn, is worse than that after a hydatidiform mole. Since intensive monitoring is often initiated only after a molar pregnancy, progression to choriocarcinoma is most likely to be identified early. However, after a normal delivery, there is usually no follow-up and the diagnosis of choriocarcinoma is therefore unlikely to be made until after a prolonged interval when secondaries might have developed.

It follows that the shorter the interval between the antecedent pregnancy and the initiation of chemotherapy, the better the prognosis. The longer the interval, the more likely it is that secondaries will have developed, especially in the chest, brain and the liver. Traditionally, this interval has been classified as: <4 months carrying the best prognosis; 4–12 months an intermediate prognosis and >12 months the worst prognosis. The blood group of the patient as well as that of the father of the antecedent pregnancy are considered important prognostic factors. The exact reasons for this are uncertain. Patients with blood group B (female) and AB (male) have the worst prognosis, whereas those with blood group O (female) and O (male) have a better prognosis.

Closely related to interval are the βhCG levels prior to the commencement of chemotherapy; the higher the levels, the poorer the prognosis. Levels below 1000 IU/L are associated with the best prognosis and those above 100 000 IU/L with the worse prognosis. The largest tumour, including the uterine tumour, and the number and sites of metastases are prognostic factors. These are invariably linked to the βhCG levels prior to the initiation of chemotherapy. Tumours measuring between 3 and 5 cm have the best prognosis, whereas those >5 cm have a poor prognosis. Secondaries in the brain have the worst prognosis, whereas those in the gastrointestinal tract and liver have a moderate effect on prognosis. Where the number of metastases is fewer than four, a prognostic score of one out of four is awarded to the patient; if the number of secondaries is between four and eight, the score is two and for more than eight secondaries, the score is four. Prior chemotherapy is an important prognostic risk factor, with single-agent chemotherapy having a better prognostic influence than two or more chemotherapeutic agents.

(b) What advice will you give her about pregnancy? (8 marks)

She is best advised to avoid pregnancy for at least 12 months after the completion of chemotherapy. This is not only because chemotherapy is teratogenic but also because the βhCG produced by the pregnancy will interfere with monitoring of treatment. Treatment does not affect fertility *per se*. An effective contraceptive is advisable to avoid pregnancy. The combined oral contraceptive pill is not recommended while βhCG levels have not returned to normal as they may delay the return. The POP is also not recommended as this is associated with irregular and unpredictable bleeding, which could be confused with persistent disease. The IUD is not recommended because of the risk of perforation during insertion and the irregular bleeding it may cause. The best contraceptive is therefore the barrier method.

Once pregnant, an early ultrasound scan is advisable as this will confirm the presence of a viable intrauterine pregnancy (if there is recurrence of a molar pregnancy, this may be identified early). Finally, at the end of each pregnancy, serum βhCG or urinary βhCG should be checked approximately 6 months later to ensure that there is no persistent disease.

Further reading

Bagshawe KD (1963) Risk and prognostic factors in trophoblastic neoplasia. *Cancer* **38**: 1373–85.

2. A 27-year-old woman is being followed-up after a miscarriage of a complete hydatidiform mole. (a) Justify the contraceptive advice you will offer her. (10 marks) (b) When will you initiate chemotherapy in this patient? (10 marks)

Common mistakes

- Discussing chemotherapy in patients with choriocarcinoma
- Details of the different types of hydatidiform mole
- Monitoring procedure – referral to tertiary centres and routine ultrasound scan of the ovaries as follow-up
- Details of the World Health Organization categorisation of patients requiring chemotherapy into various risk groups and details of the different chemotherapeutic combinations to use
- Monitoring of various therapeutic protocols
- Failure to justify methods of contraception

A good answer will include some or all of these points

(a) Justify the contraceptive advice you will offer her. (10 marks)

- Avoid combined oral contraceptive until βhCG returns to normal
- Avoid IUD and progestogens as these may cause irregular bleeding, which will be confused with persistent disease
- IUD – increased risk of perforation
- Barrier methods – most appropriate
- Avoid pregnancy for at least 6 months
- Once period missed, early ultrasound scan

(b) When will you initiate chemotherapy in this patient? (10 marks)

- High level of βhCG 4 weeks after evacuation of mole (serum βhCG >20 000 IU/L; urine levels >30 000 IU/L)
- Progressively increasing βhCG values at any time after evacuation
- Histological identification of choriocarcinoma at any site, or evidence of central nervous system (CNS), renal, hepatic or gastrointestinal metastases, or pulmonary metastases >2 cm in diameter or more than three in number
- Persistent uterine haemorrhage with an elevated βhCG levels stationary for 2–3 or more conservative weeks? Others levels elevated after 8–10 weeks?

Sample answer

(a) Justify the contraceptive advice you will offer her. (8 marks)

The contraceptive advice to be offered is to ensure that she is not pregnant for at least 6 months after βhCG levels have returned to normal. The combined oral contraceptive pill is not recommended while βhCG levels are still high, as this may delay their return to normal and therefore increase the risk of initiating chemotherapy. The IUD is also not recommended because the risk of perforation during insertion is higher than that in women with non-molar pregnancies. Additionally, the irregular bleeding which may accompany the IUD, especially during the first few months, may be confused with persistent disease. The progestogen-only contraceptive pill is also not advisable for similar reasons of unpredictable irregular vaginal bleeding. An ideal contraceptive is therefore the barrier method with spermicides. Once the βhCG levels have returned to normal, the combined oral contraceptive can be used.

(b) When will you initiate chemotherapy in this patient? (12 marks)

Initiation of chemotherapy is indicated if serum βhCG levels are more than 20 000 IU/L or urine levels are more than 30 000 IU/L 4 weeks after the evacuation. Occasionally, the levels may not be this high but may continue to rise after the evacuation, even though the uterus is empty. This indicates persistent trophoblastic disease and is therefore an indication for chemotherapy.

If there is histological evidence of choriocarcinoma from the tissue obtained from an evacuation (a primary evacuation or a repeat evacuation), chemotherapy will be initiated irrespective of the βhCG levels. The histological distinction is made from the absence of chorionic villi in choriocarcinoma.

Although these biochemical and radiological factors are the common indications for the initiation of chemotherapy, clinical evidence of secondaries in the CNS, liver or kidneys or the presence of more than three secondaries in the lungs measuring >2 cm are also considered an indication for chemotherapy. Other indications for chemotherapy include persistent uterine bleeding with elevated βhCG or stationary βhCG levels on at least two occasions. When to commence chemotherapy in such patients with persistently high or static βhCG levels remains controversial. Some centres, for example, recommend chemotherapy when the levels are elevated 8–10 weeks after evacuation, whereas others initiate chemotherapy when levels are static for 2, 3 or more consecutive weeks after evacuation.

Irrespective of the indications for chemotherapy, this must not be treated in isolation. It is important that, for this patient, the whole clinical picture is kept in perspective. A combination of factors will certainly affect the indication for chemotherapy more than each of them singly.

3. A 28-year-old woman presented with an incomplete miscarriage, for which an evacuation was performed. Histology of the products of conception concluded that she had a hydatidiform mole. (a) What will be your immediate management? (8 marks) (b) Justify your long-term management of this patient. (8 marks) (c) How will you manage her in her next pregnancy? (4 marks)

Common mistakes

- The chromosomes of the parents must be determined
- Management should be by the local oncology centre
- Follow-up must be for a defined period of 2 years
- Offer evacuation as hydatidiform moles always need evacuation!
- Bleeding may require surgery
- Quoting incorrect incidences, e.g. recurrence risk, and risk of progression to cancer if untreated
- Cross-match blood – why?

A good answer will include some or all of these points

(a) What will be your immediate management? (8 marks)

- Review the report for the type of mole – prognosis and length of follow-up will be determined by this – complete or partial mole?:
  - Need for chemotherapy – 15 per cent following a complete mole and 0.5 per cent following a partial mole
- Explain the diagnosis to the patient and her partner
- Discuss need for follow-up – persistent disease, invasive disease, choriocarcinoma – all treatable
- Risk of progression to invasive mole is 16 times more after a complete mole than after a partial mole

(b) Justify your long-term management of this patient. (8 marks)

- Register patient with one of three centres: Sheffield, Dundee or London
- Follow-up process
- Postal samples – frequency, if uncertain please do not quote
- Need to avoid pregnancy – why?
- Complete mole and partial mole 6 months after βhCG levels have returned to normal
- Contraception – avoid hormonal until βhCG levels return to normal. Avoid IUD – risk of bleeding. Best method – barrier methods (not too reliable though). Depo-Provera® – avoid – risk of irregular vaginal bleeding. May be confused with recurrence of disease

(c) How will you manage her in her next pregnancy? (4 marks)

- Subsequent pregnancies: early ultrasound scan – why? – to rule out recurrence. What is the recurrence risk? (1:55) and >98 per cent of those who become pregnant will not have a molar pregnancy. If recurrence, 68–80 per cent will have the same histological type
- Postdelivery – follow-up sample

Sample answer

(a) What will be your immediate management? (8 marks)

Hydatidiform mole has a risk of progression to choriocarcinoma in approximately 3 per cent of cases in the absence of follow-up and chemotherapy for persistent trophoblastic disease. The risk of developing choriocarcinoma depends on the type of molar pregnancy, hence the need for chemotherapy is different following each type of hydatidiform mole. It is higher after a complete (15 per cent) than a partial (0.5 per cent) hydatidiform mole. Therefore, the first step in the management of this patient is to determine the type of hydatidiform mole.

The diagnosis, and the need for prolonged follow-up, should be explained to the patient. This is mainly to prevent the development of choriocarcinoma by the early identification of persistent disease, which may be treated effectively with chemotherapy. Where choriocarcinoma has developed (especially if identified early), chemotherapy is effective without affecting fertility.

(b) Justify your long-term management of this patient. (8 marks)

Her long-term management will include immediate registration at one of three centres in the UK: Sheffield, Dundee or Charing Cross in London. These centres will initiate follow-up monitoring of urinary βhCG by sending sample bottles to her through the post. The frequency with which these bottles are sent for urine collection will be determined by the centre. Briefly, this is every 2 weeks until βhCG levels from the samples reach the limit of detection and thereafter every month until it is back to normal, and for another 3 months after it has returned to normal.

The minimum follow-up period has traditionally been 6 months for a partial hydatidiform mole and 1 year for a complete mole. However, since progression of a partial mole to choriocarcinoma is uncommon, this may no longer be the best advice. The reasons why patients are advised to avoid pregnancy during the follow-up period is to ensure that rising levels are not confused with pregnancy and therefore delay treatment. During the follow-up period, a barrier method of contraception is offered until 3 months after βhCG levels have returned to normal. This is because the combined oral contraceptive pill slows the return of the βhCG levels to normal values. An IUD is inadvisable as it may perforate the uterus and may also cause irregular vaginal bleeding, which may be confused with features of persistent disease.

(c) How will you manage her in her next pregnancy? (4 marks)

Subsequent pregnancies must be confirmed early by ultrasound scan to exclude a recurrence of a molar pregnancy. The patient has a 20-fold increased risk of recurrent hydatidiform mole following one molar pregnancy. Even after the pregnancy has been completed she will need to be followed up, as the risk of a placental site trophoblastic tumour is higher in this patient.

17

Operative gynaecology

1. Critically comment on the types of abdominal incisions that gynaecologists use. (20 marks)

2. A 47-year-old woman, who is protein S deficient, is scheduled for a hysterectomy and bilateral salpingo-oophorectomy. (a) Justify your pre- and intraoperative management. (10 marks) (b) What postoperative measures will you take to reduce the risk of venous thromboembolism (VTE)? (10 marks)

3. During a vaginal hysterectomy and repair on a 67-year-old obese woman, you discover (after the hysterectomy) a large, partly solid, partly cystic (10×8 cm) ovarian mass. (a) Justify your subsequent surgical management of the patient. (10 marks) (b) How will you manage her after surgery? (10 marks)

4. During an abdominal hysterectomy, you suspect that the ureter has been damaged on the right side. Outline the steps you will take (a) in theatre (14 marks) and (b) after surgery. (6 marks)

5. How might bladder injuries be prevented during gynaecological surgery? (20 marks)

6. Twenty-four hours after a vaginal hysterectomy, a 43-year-old woman is noted to have a blood pressure (BP) of 85/50 mmHg, a pulse of 123 bpm and poor urinary output. (a) What are the most likely causes of her shock? (10 marks) (b) Outline how you will manage her. (10 marks)

1. Critically comment on the types of abdominal incisions that gynaecologists use. (20 marks)

Common mistakes

- Discussing different types of major and minor gynaecological procedures
- Details of how to make the various surgical incisions
- Complications of the incisions

A good answer will include some or all of these points

- The types of incisions
- Advantages and disadvantages of these incisions

Sample answer

Abdominal incisions for gynaecological surgery are, to a large extent, determined by the type of operation. The fundamental principles governing the type of incisions used are adequate surgical exposure and cosmetic acceptability. Whether surgery is laparoscopic or laparotomy also influences the type of abdominal incisions; therefore they may vary from small to large.

The most common incision for major gynaecological surgery is the Pfannenstiel incision. This is a transverse incision above the pubic symphysis. Exposure of the pelvis with this incision is considered adequate for most benign gynaecological operations. However, there are some limitations of this type of incision. It does not provide adequate exposure to large pelvic masses. In addition, it is not easily extendable and therefore when indicated to facilitate surgery, this is either not possible or the extension is inadequate. The advantage of this incision is the associated lower risk of incisional hernia. It heals properly and is more cosmetically acceptable to patients. This type of incision is considered inadequate for ovarian cancer surgery.

The vertical incision is the second most common approach for major gynaecological surgery. It offers a better exposure for the surgeon and is also easy to extend. Vertical incisions are commonly used for gynaecological cancer surgery and surgery for large pelvic masses, such as large fibroids and ovarian cysts. Where there is the risk of bladder damage during entry into the abdominal cavity (as in cases of severe adhesions), this incision allows superior entry and therefore minimises this risk. Disadvantages include the high risk of burst abdomen, especially in obese patients in whom postoperative infections are more likely. It is also associated with an increased risk of incisional hernia.

Other incisions that may be used are those for laparoscopic surgery. These tend to be infraumbilical or oblique incisions in the iliac fossae. Occasionally, a small suprapubic incision may be employed. These incisions have the advantage of being very cosmetic. However, they are very small and are unsuitable for any other type of surgery. If not closed properly, these incisions may be complicated by Richter's hernia.

Although these are the most common types of abdominal incisions in gynaecological surgery, occasionally other types may be used. These include an oblique abdominal incision in the iliac fossa. This does not permit good access and also is not cosmetically acceptable to patients.

2. A 47-year-old woman, who is protein S deficient, is scheduled for a hysterectomy and bilateral salpingo-oophorectomy. (a) Justify your pre- and intraoperative management. (10 marks) (b) What postoperative measures will you take to reduce the risk of VTE? (10 marks)

Common mistakes

- Discussing deep vein thrombosis (DVT) or pulmonary embolism (PE) – investigations, diagnosis and treatment
- Discussing alternatives to surgery in this patient
- Discussing the indications for surgery
- History and physical examination
- Past medical history of DVT and PE

A good answer will include some or all of these points

(a) Justify your pre- and intraoperative management. (10 marks)

- Patient is at an increased risk by virtue her thrombophilia
- Reduction of DVT risk:
  - Involve haematologist
  - Assess and modify other risk factors, e.g. obesity, smoking, concurrent infections
  - Prophylactic heparin/Fragmin®/tinzaparin preoperatively and postoperatively; pneumatic stockings and thromboembolic deterrent stockings
  - Good hydration at the time of surgery
  - Prophylactic antibiotics to minimise the risk of postoperative infection

(b) What postoperative measures will you take to reduce the risk of VTE? (10 marks)

- Continue with thromboprophylaxis:
  - Pneumatic stockings, low-molecular-weight heparin (LMWH), early mobilisation, antibiotics
  - Early identification and treatment of complications such as infections (chest, wound, urinary tract, etc.)
- Hormone replacement therapy (HRT) – if ovaries removed – need for HRT; benefits versus side-effects and risk of DVT; on balance will need HRT
- Need to monitor for warning signs of DVT/PE
- Preoperatively, counsel patient about these risks and educate on warning signs
- If taking warfarin, change to heparin before surgery is undertaken

Sample answer

(a) Justify your pre- and intraoperative management. (10 marks)

This patient, by virtue of her thrombophilia, is at an increased risk of VTE. The focus on her management must be to reduce her risk of VTE perioperatively and postoperatively. From the outset, a haematologist should be involved in her perioperative care. Although this is unlikely to significantly alter her planned surgery, advice on the most effective thromboprophylaxis will be provided. This will take the form of heparin or LMWH before surgery. Preoperatively, risk factors for DVT need to be identified and attempts made to modify them. Such risks include obesity, smoking and concurrent infections. At the time of surgery, pneumatic stockings should be used. The duration of surgery must be kept to a minimum, whilst blood loss must be carefully controlled. Adequate hydration must also be maintained at the time of surgery and prophylactic antibiotics prescribed to reduce the risk of postoperative infection.

(b) What postoperative measures will you take to reduce the risk of VTE? (10 marks)

Postoperatively, adequate hydration and early mobilisation are essential. The patient should have compression stockings during her time in hospital and the anticoagulants initiated perioperatively should be continued for at least 5 days after surgery. Early identification and treatment of complications such as chest, urinary tract and wound infections, will reduce morbidity and reduce immobility, hence a reduction in the risk of VTE.

An important aspect of the management of this patient will involve HRT. This will take the form of oestrogens since she will have had a hysterectomy and oophorectomy. The need for HRT, with emphasis on its risks versus its benefits, should to be discussed before initiating it. On balance, it may be more beneficial for the patient to start HRT as she is only 47 years old. The early warning signs for DVT and PE need to be discussed in a careful and non-frightening manner and advice given on the need to report early if they occur.

In some cases, the patient might have already been taking warfarin before surgery. If this is the case, the oral thromboprophylaxis should be converted to a parenteral form before surgery. This switch is preferably done a day before surgery.

3. During a vaginal hysterectomy and repair on a 67-year-old obese woman, you discover (after the hysterectomy) a large, partly solid, partly cystic (10 × 8 cm) ovarian mass. (a) Justify your subsequent surgical management of the patient. (b) How will you manage her after surgery?

Common errors

- Take a history
- Investigate – BRCA1, CA125, ultrasound, etc.
- Obtain consent for more extensive history
- Perform a laparoscopy
- Wrongly managed and therefore a serious mistake
- Management will depend on her age and desire for further pregnancies
- Staging laparotomy and then planned definitive surgery
- No further action for now, as patient cannot consent
- Not asked to outline management of patient with ovarian cyst
- Preoperative information given: not legal to remove ovary without patient's consent
- Heavy periods – indication for a vaginal hysterectomy and repair?

A good answer will include most or all of these points

(a) Justify your subsequent surgical management of the patient. (10 marks)

- Appearances of the ovarian pathology are highly suspicious of malignancy (i.e. malignancy needs to be ruled out). This can only be achieved by an adequate exploration, which cannot be offered vaginally
- Proceed to a laparotomy (and involve gynaecological oncologist if uncertain, or if a malignancy is the working diagnosis): midline incision; explore and take peritoneal fluid for cytology; bilateral salpingo-oophorectomy and omentectomy if suspicion of malignancy; palpate para-aortic and pelvic nodes and biopsy if necessary
- Frozen section if available

(b) How will you manage her after surgery? (10 marks)

- Postoperatively, explain findings and procedure to patient
- Counsel appropriately and wait for histology
- Histology:
  - Benign – no need for follow-up unless for the prolapse
  - Malignant – refer to gynaecological oncologist
- Malignancy – investigate to exclude secondaries – chest X-ray, abdominal ultrasound or magnetic resonance imaging

- Commence on chemotherapy after discussion at the multidisciplinary team meeting
- Planned follow-up with oncologists
- Conclusion

Sample answer

(a) Justify your subsequent surgical management of the patient. (10 marks)

The appearances of this ovarian mass require a malignancy to be excluded. Indeed, this tumour must be considered malignant until proved otherwise. Subsequent management must be geared towards this tentative diagnosis and must aim to provide the best results for the patient. The only way this can be achieved is by a laparotomy and subsequent surgery, preferably by a gynaecological oncologist.

The next stage is to perform a laparotomy by use of a midline incision. This incision will allow a better assessment of the tumour, its bilaterality, associated secondaries in the liver, omentum and lymphadenopathy. It will also allow completion of the surgical treatment for ovarian cancer. This consists of bilateral salpingo-oophorectomy, omentectomy and other necessary surgery. If there are any secondaries the ultimate aim must be to ensure that the residual disease is minimal (<1.5 cm if possible). Peritoneal fluid and washings must be collected and sent for cytology. If there are facilities for frozen sections, this may be offered but it is unlikely to significantly change the type of surgery she will be offered. If her primary surgery was for prolapse, it would be advisable for a repair to be performed after the abdominal procedure to avoid her returning with the symptoms of prolapse.

(b) How will you manage her after surgery? (10 marks)

Postoperatively, the patient must be offered adequate counselling about the findings and the nature of the surgery she has undergone. Whatever the case, the ultimate counselling will have to await histology on the ovarian tumour and other tissues removed at surgery. Further management will depend on the type of cancer, if she does have cancer, and the need for adjuvant chemotherapy. If the histology is benign, there is no need for chemotherapy. However, if it is a malignancy then adjuvant chemotherapy should be offered by a team consisting of a gynaecological oncologist and a medical oncologist. The patient should be followed up for at least 5 years to identify early recurrence.

4. During an abdominal hysterectomy, you suspect that the ureter has been damaged on the right side. Outline the steps you will take (a) in theatre (14 marks) and (b) after surgery. (6 marks)

Common mistakes

- Discussing bladder/kidney injury
- Postoperative suspicion of ureteric injury
- Description of the procedure of a hysterectomy
- Prevention of ureteric injury – do not discuss: preoperative intravenous urogram (IVU) or ultrasound to outline course of ureters; postoperative catheterisation of the bladder; complications of vesicovaginal fistula; what steps will you take to minimise bowel injury during gynaecological surgery

A good answer will include some or all of these points

(a) Outline the steps you will take in theatre. (14 marks)

- Ureteric injuries are difficult to recognise, but common in difficult gynaecological cases. Index of suspicion must therefore be high
- Suspicion is during surgery – therefore: call for help – senior gynaecologist or urologist; ensure left kidney is present and left ureter is normal
- Has any injury or damage actually occurred?: trace ureter; identify site of possible injury or damage; may need the help of cystoscopic retrograde catheterisation of the ureter – IVU may be useful where cystoscopic retrograde catheterisation is not possible
- Management of injury if confirmed: end-to-end anastomosis; reimplantation; raising a Boari flap; splint with ureteric catheter

(b) Outline the steps you will take after surgery. (6 marks)

- Postoperative management: complications – urinary peritonitis?; IVU later
- Counsel patient appropriately
- Incident reporting
- Antibiotics
- Follow-up to review and ensure that there are not complications

Sample answer

(a) Outline the steps you will take in theatre. (14 marks)

Ureteric injuries are rare and very difficult to identify, both at the time of surgery and afterwards. A high index of suspicion is therefore important in patients at risk of ureteric injury during surgery. This injury is likely to occur in patients with adhesions, large uterine fibroids and ovarian tumours, especially malignancies, and in those undergoing Wertheim's hysterectomy.

Once a ureteric injury is suspected, a key step in the management is to call for help if the surgeon does not have the expertise to recognise this injury. The contralateral ureter must be identified to ensure that this is present. Sometimes this may be absent, in which case very great care must be exercised during the repair of the damaged side.

The next stage is to confirm that an injury has indeed occurred. This can be confirmed by observing urine welling in the operative field. However, this may not be easy. Ancillary measures may be taken to confirm the diagnosis. These include retrograde catheterisation of the ureter, retrograde cystoureteroscopy and dye injection. The advantage of a dye injection is it allows the site of the lesion to be localised. Intraoperative IVU has a role in defining the site and nature of the injury but this is time consuming.

Once the damage has been confirmed, various procedures may be undertaken to repair the injury. These will depend on the type of injury. Immediate anastomosis will be ideal if this is possible. In addition to end-to-end anastomosis, a ureteric stent is essential to splint the site of anastomosis. In some cases, this may not be easy. Another option is to raise a Boari flap. This ensures that the ureter remains functional and reduces the chances of kidney damage. In some cases, reimplantation of the ureter into the bladders may be the treatment of choice. However, in others, an ileal conduit may be the best approach. Most of these procedures need to be performed by a urologist. Where the injury is a crushing type or the ureter was transfixed, simply removing the stitch and stenting it may be considered adequate. However, if the crushed segment is judged to be necrotic, it has to be excised and end-to-end anastomosis undertaken as described above.

(b) Outline the steps you will take after surgery. (6 marks)

Postoperatively, the patient should be placed on prophylactic antibiotics and monitored for the early warning signs of urinary peritonitis. She should be counselled about the injury and the course of management after. An incident form should be completed for risk-management purposes. Once the healing is thought to be complete, the ureteric stent should be removed. It may then be advisable to offer the patient an IVU to confirm the patency of the ureter and a functioning kidney.

5. How might bladder injuries be prevented during gynaecological surgery? (20 marks)

Common mistakes

- Describing the operative procedures in detail
- Discussing renal tract abnormalities
- Radiological investigations
- Discussing the details of each type of injury

A good answer will include some or all of these points

- Injuries most likely to occur at laparoscopy, laparotomy, during dissection with distorted pelvic anatomy and at the time of vaginal surgery
- Preoperative precautions – empty bladder or intraoperative needle emptying
- Identification of at-risk patients – previous difficult pelvic surgery, history of pelvic inflammatory disease, review notes for these
- Surgical technique – laparoscopy/dissection/vaginal/abdominal – meticulous approach
- Expert help if bladder adherent
- Good knowledge of anatomy
- Entry to abdomen – modify incisions depending on anticipated difficulties
- Recognition: at the time of surgery – urine welling up; suspect but uncertain – methylene blue into the bladder; postoperatively – incontinence – haematuria

Sample answer

Bladder injuries are not uncommon during gynaecological surgery. These are most likely to occur either during introduction of the laparoscopic port or dissection of the bladder away from the uterus, from adhesions, and during a colposuspension abdominally or vaginally during a hysterectomy or anterior repair. Prevention of these injuries must start with recognising those patients who are at risk of such injuries, followed by meticulous surgery and early recognition and management when they occur.

The patients at risk of bladder injuries during gynaecological surgery include those with large abdominopelvic masses undergoing surgery, pelvic adhesions from infections and endometriosis, or from previous pelvic surgery, such as Caesarean section. Patients undergoing laparoscopic surgery and those undergoing a vaginal procedure are also at risk. In these patients, various important steps need to be taken to prevent bladder injuries. For all abdominal procedures, the most important single step to take is to empty the bladder. This must be done before laparoscopy. For other operations, this may be done once the abdomen has been opened. The only disadvantage with this approach is that if the patient's bladder is already very full, it may actually be damaged during entry into the peritoneal cavity. Those advocating this approach argue that suprapubic drainage with a needle reduces the risk of urinary tract infections.

The surgical technique itself must be systematic and meticulous. During laparoscopy, it is important to direct the Verre's needle and the trocar towards the pelvis but away from the bladder. Similarly, if adhesions are suspected, a more superior approach to entering the abdomen will bypass an adherent bladder. Blunt dissection will be safer than sharp dissection. If there is any bleeding around the bladder base, this must be clearly identified before haemostasis is secured. Blind diathermy or suturing may result in bladder injuries. The best weapon available for avoiding bladder injuries (apart from surgical skill) is in-depth knowledge of the anatomy of the pelvis. An understanding of the relationship of the bladder to the uterus and the anterior abdominal wall is essential to minimise the risk of injury. If the surgeon encounters adhesions and lacks the expertise to deal with them, prudence demands that senior help is summoned.

Prevention of injuries must not only be limited to inflicting the injury itself, but also early recognition and correction when it occurs. Once an injury is suspected, it must be confirmed. This could be done by filling the bladder with a dye, such as methylene blue. Alternatively, the operation site welling with clear fluid must raise the suspicion of a bladder or ureteric injury. During colposuspension, filling the bladder with methylene blue before dissecting the para-urethra tissues away from the proximal urethra and neck of the bladder will allow for early identification of any injuries and repair. The closure of the peritoneum during a vaginal hysterectomy and buttressing of the bladder base must be done with extreme caution as injuries are more likely to occur at this time. Postoperatively, the injuries may be recognised from haematuria or incontinence. These must be investigated and early treatment offered to prevent further deterioration.

6. Twenty-four hours after a vaginal hysterectomy, a 43-year-old woman is noted to have a BP of 85/50 mmHg, a pulse of 123 bpm and poor urinary output. (a) What are the most likely causes of her shock? (10 marks) (b) Outline how you will manage her. (10 marks)

Common mistakes

- Take a history
- Discussing the management of cardiac shock
- Failure to manage the patient
- Concentrating on the management of haemorrhage and ignoring other possible causes

A good answer will include some or all of these points

(a) What are the most likely causes of her shock? (10 marks)

- Haemorrhage
- Drug reaction
- Infection – Gram-negative septicaemic shock
- Ureteric injury
- Hypovolaemia from poor replacement

(b) Outline how you will manage her. (10 marks)

- Examination
- Intravenous line – large cannulae
- Intravenous fluids – start with volume expanders
- Group and cross-match at least 4 units of blood
- Call senior on-call
- Inform theatre
- Exploratory laparotomy
- Rectify problem – depend on the cause
- If other organs involved involve appropriate specialty

Sample answer

(a) What are the most likely causes of her shock? (10 marks)

This patient is in shock and the possible causes include drugs, haemorrhage, infections, injury to viscera and hypovolaemia due to inadequate fluid replacement. Haemorrhage can be concealed or revealed. In the latter, the degree of shock will be reflected by the amount of blood lost. In this case, no obvious bleeding was observed, hence if this was the cause it is most likely to be concealed/or internal. An examination will reveal fluid in the peritoneal cavity or a bulge vaginally where the blood has accumulated above the vault.

Drug reactions as a cause of the hypovolaemic shock will be typified by the onset of the symptoms. It may be possible to relate them to the initiation of treatment. The most common reaction will be to opiates, which are commonly used as postoperative analgesia. Other drugs may cause shock, hence the medication she is on would have to be reviewed thoroughly. Infections, especially Gram-negative bacteria, may cause septicaemia. In addition, there may be hypothermia and rashes, which characterise Gram-negative septicaemia.

Poor fluid replacement may also be a cause. This will be diagnosed by examining the deficit between fluid input and output in an input and output chart. Although a rare cause of shock, injury to the bowel may present for the first time after surgery with features of shock.

(b) Outline how you will manage her. (10 marks)

The first step in her management is to set up an intravenous line with a large-bore cannula if none is already in place. If there is one already sited, a second one should be inserted. If there are difficulties, the anaesthetist should be involved. A thorough physical examination should then be undertaken looking for the features of the various differentials discussed above. The most important of these will be an abdominal and pelvic examination where features of fluid collection may be recognised. An urgent full blood count is essential and blood should be grouped and at least 4 units cross-matched.

It is important that a senior colleague is involved, especially as the likely treatment for this patient will be surgery. An exploratory laparotomy will be required for suspected haemorrhage or bowel injury. Appropriate steps will be taken for each of these procedures (i.e. involvement of other specialties such as bowel surgeons, urologists, etc.) for the specific type of injury. Adequate fluid replacement before or after surgical correction of any injury will reduce the risk of renal failure.

18

Ethics, medico-legal, clinical governance

1. It has been suggested that *in vitro* fertilisation (IVF) may be used to provide organ or marrow donors to siblings suffering from diseases that require transplantation. Can you debate this statement? (20 marks)

2. What steps will you take to reduce the rising litigation in gynaecology in the UK? (20 marks)

3. Selective feticide is unjustified in the twenty-first century. Debate this statement. (20 marks)

4. Treatment for infertility should not be offered on the National Health Service (NHS). Do you agree with this statement? (20 marks)

5. How will you set up a risk-management team in your unit? (20 marks)

1. It has been suggested that IVF may be used to provide organ or marrow donors to siblings suffering from diseases that require transplantation. Can you debate this statement? (20 marks)

Common mistakes

- Extolling the virtues of IVF, or the history of IVF, or the indications for IVF
- Discussing human rights and how the fetus and newborn have rights
- Discussing killing babies so others can survive
- Cloning of humans
- Research on embryos
- Avoid being emotional and depersonalise your answer

A good answer will include some or all of these points

- This debate crosses ethical, moral, religious and legal boundaries
- Advantages: long waiting lists for donors – overcome; risk of incompatibility – reduced; family is the source of donor and therefore feels involved in the cure of patient
- Disadvantages: expensive; complications of IVF to the mother; failure of IVF and attendant disappointment; even if successful, no guarantee of compatibility; legal and other obstacles; may be abused
- Conclusion: well-defined role to avoid abuse

Sample answer

This is a problem that crosses ethical, religious, moral and legal jurisdictions. The radical developments in assisted reproductive techniques will no doubt continue to cause an increasing number of demands on the techniques. The use of IVF to produce tissues or organs for siblings must be examined from the different perspectives above.

There are consistent problems with donor organs. These include long waiting times for suitable donors, the problem of compatibility and often the psychological feeling by the recipient that he or she has an organ of no genetic or biological relationship. The provision of organ donors from family members, even if these were from IVF programmes, would overcome some of these obstacles, e.g. they would significantly reduce the problems of rejection or compatibility. In addition, the donor would be a member of the recipient's family. This latter advantage overcomes the psychological problems of recipients never knowing any details of their organ donor. The family is the source of the donation and so feels involved in the treatment that requires the donation.

However, there are several disadvantages of such an approach. The IVF procedure is expensive and fraught with complications, especially to the mother. There is the risk of multiple pregnancy and consequently the problems of prematurity and its possible sequelae of neurodevelopmental disability. Embarking on a pregnancy mainly to provide a donor for a sibling may be perceived as morally unjustified. In addition, such actions may have significant effects on both the donor and recipient siblings.

There is no guarantee that if IVF is successful, there would be compatibility between the donor and the recipient. The family may raise their hopes just to have them dashed. Although such an approach may be extremely beneficial to some families, there is the risk of it being abused for other non-medical reasons. There are various legal, ethical and religious obstacles that must be overcome before this technique is made available. An important aspect of this treatment is counselling. This needs to be undertaken before treatment.

Although there is a place for offering such treatment to families with no other options, it must not be seen as the primary approach to obtaining donor organs. In most cases, the procedure has to be highly regulated to ensure that it is not abused. In addition, the process of counselling must be extensive and tailored to the needs of the family before and after the donor process.

2. What steps will you take to reduce the rising litigation in gynaecology in the UK? (20 marks)

Common mistakes

- Discussing the legal aspects of obstetrics/gynaecology
- Details of audit
- Concentrating on structures to counteract litigation claims

A good answer will include some or all of these points

- Litigation costs rising. Obstetrics – 60 per cent of the total cost in the NHS
- Causes of litigation
- How to minimise risks: training; audit; openness; documentation; risk-management teams; incident reporting; more senior input in care of patients

Sample answer

Litigation is increasingly becoming an important problem in gynaecology. Although there is more litigation in obstetrics than gynaecology, there is no doubt the problems exist. The principles involved in reducing litigation in any discipline are essentially the same. Increasing litigation is an important drain on resources and causes untold stress to staff. Significantly, in most cases this is preventable. The process of reducing litigation must include training, adequate communication between patients, and documentation. Most of these principles are well expounded in the clinical governance document.

Adequate training is an important first step in reducing the rising incidence of litigation. Training programmes must be set up to identify the needs, or rather deficiencies, of all gynaecologists and to ensure that these deficiencies are rectified. Training must be patient-focused and should address the concerns of patient care, the aim being to improve dialogue/communication between patients, staff and between careers.

Most problems resulting in litigation are easily identified. Poor communication between patients and hospital staff is a major constituent. In this regard, adequate training sessions for junior doctors and nurses, and other members of the team, must be undertaken. Communication must be transparent and directed to the right person and at the right level. Communication between general practitioners (GPs) and hospitals should be detailed enough to ensure that GPs are able to relate to the patient information emanating from the hospital.

There must also be appropriate documentation in patients' notes. All discussions with patients, colleagues and others involved in patient care should be well documented. Efforts to write contemporaneous notes will eliminate the potential difficulties of recall and obvious bias in documentation.

Patients who often complain are those most likely to seek legal redress. Early recognition of these patients and prompt action to minimise the consequences of any accidents or lack of communication will significantly reduce the numbers doing so. Although a few patients set out to seek monetary compensation, a large proportion wants to ensure that mistakes are not repeated and that there is someone to take responsibility and apologise for errors. Transparency in dealing with at-risk patients is therefore very important. In this regard, there is a need for a risk-management team, which will deal with potential complainants and offer adequate explanations and apologies when necessary. In addition, incident reporting protocols will ensure that incidents are recognised early and dealt with, in some cases proactively.

If the unit does not have a transparent patients' complaints procedure, this must be established. This will ensure that patients see the transparency and speed with which their complaints are dealt. It is important to make sure that these processes are not seen as witch hunting, as this may drive a wedge between good and responsible practice, and defensive medicine.

3. Selective feticide is unjustified in the twenty-first century. Debate this statement. (20 marks)

Common mistakes

- Discussing the procedure of feticide
- Criticising the process itself on moral or religious grounds
- Failure to debate but simply stating the indications for feticide

A good answer will include some or all of these points

- Advantages: reduces the risk of prematurity; complications of pregnancy; beneficial when one fetus is abnormal; more acceptable to parents – financial constraints on bringing up more than one child
- Disadvantages: complications; how do you select the fetus to kill? Complications of the retained intrauterine death on the surviving fetus; ethics of this; abuse – selection of ideal sex and genetic make-up?
- Conclusion: well-balanced cases, with adequate counselling may be a procedure to be offered

Sample answer

Selective feticide has increasingly become an important procedure in obstetrics, especially in the early stages of pregnancy. This procedure involves the killing of one or more fetuses to offer a greater chance of survival to the other(s). Although the Human Fertilisation and Embryology Authority 1991 guarantees that not more than three embryos are replaced in any assisted reproduction technique to reduce the problems of multifetal gestations, these still occur. Selective reduction may also be offered in natural pregnancies or in those pregnancies following ovulation induction for various reasons.

The primary indication for selective feticide is to reduce the number of fetuses in multifetal gestations and therefore significantly reduce the incidence of prematurity and its complications. It has been shown that by reducing the number of fetuses, the pregnancy can be prolonged significantly and increase the survival of the fetus(es). Selective feticide may be performed as early as 7–8 weeks. However, it is advantageous to do this in the late first trimester as most of the fetuses that will not survive for other reasons would naturally have been miscarried or died *in utero*.

Another indication for feticide is if one fetus is abnormal. However, there is increasing social demand for feticide where the parents are unable to cope with a twin or triplet pregnancy. There have been some cases where it has been performed for sex selection. The justification of this procedure may not be morally or religiously acceptable to some patients. Therefore, the introduction of this topic must be made with extreme caution and sensitivity.

The procedure itself has several disadvantages. It results in the retention of a dead fetus during pregnancy, which may cause problems, especially of coagulopathy and neuropathy in the surviving fetus(es). During the procedure, if there is anastomosis between the fetuses, the drug administered to affect the feticide may be transferred to the other fetus and may cause its demise as well.

An important difficulty is which fetus(es) to select in the absence of an obvious abnormality. Moralist will argue that we have no right to select one fetus on the basis of chance. This argument is buttressed by the recent cases of a wealthy family choosing feticide of a twin pregnancy as the parents did not want two babies to cause a significant inconvenience to their lifestyle. Such an attitude may be perceived as an abuse of the system and there is, therefore, a need for tougher regulation of selective feticide. Abuse may extend to the choice of the sex of the baby or babies not conforming to various physical characteristic desired by the parents. With the unmapping of the human gene, it is conceivable that parents may start studying the characteristics of their future offspring and use selective feticide to choose the right babies.

On balance, therefore, selective feticide has an important role to play in modern-day obstetrics and gynaecology. However, it must be offered in a well-regulated environment where ethical, religious, moral and legal considerations are always taken into account. Without tight regulation and moderation, this may be subject to significant abuse.

4. Treatment for infertility should not be offered on the NHS. Do you agree with this statement? (20 marks)

Common mistakes

-   Details of infertility treatment
-   Complications of infertility treatment
-   Rationale for treating infertile couples
-   Centres for treatment
-   The law on infertility treatment

A good answer will include some or all of these points

-   Infertility is a disease
-   Treatment is both necessary and important
-   World Health Organization's (WHO) definition of disease (not only the absence of infirmity)
-   Cost implications deter ready availability of this treatment on the NHS
-   Other mundane conditions being treated – stripping varicose veins, plastic surgery, sex-change operations, etc.
-   Rationing in other disciplines
-   Problem of making it available to all on the NHS
-   Abuse
-   Diverting scarce resources from other important areas to infertility
-   Ideal – combining funding?
-   Conclusion – may be a place for investigating and treating, but not for all cases, and not every unit should offer advanced assisted reproduction techniques – to ensure compliance with the law and improved success

Sample answer

Infertility affects about 15 per cent of couples in the UK. There are many causes of this condition, most of which can be corrected at the primary and secondary levels. However, in some cases, more extensive and advanced investigations and treatment are required. The controversy about treating couples with infertility is often focused on these advanced therapeutic modalities. Infertility is a disease and deserves to be treated like any other disease. The WHO defines a disease as not merely the absence of an infirmity but complete psychological, physical and mental wellbeing. Couples with infertility, although they may not have a physical disability, have a psychologically disabling condition which deserves the same treatment offered to others with depression, anxiety and physical disorders.

The arguments for or against treating patients with infertility concentrate on the absence of physical disability and, therefore, failure to conform with the definition of disease. More importantly, because of the rapidly advancing technology in this field, cost implications for various health authorities are quite enormous. Another point often advanced against offering treatment is the low success rates, especially that following the advanced infertility treatments. Are these really justified?

Not all cases of infertility require advanced treatment methods. For those cases where the cause can easily be identified and adequate treatment offered, the results are very good. In fact, the treatment is often considered by most as being cost effective. However, for the advanced therapies, the success of the regimens varies, but is usually in the region of approximately 15–25 per cent 'baby take-home' rate. The suggestion that all infertility treatment should not be offered on the NHS is therefore not valid for the cases that can be managed at the primary and secondary levels. For the cases requiring advanced treatment, the cost argument needs to be supported.

Within the NHS, rationing is an important process and allows prioritisation of treatment because of inadequate resources. However, there are many minor medical conditions that are treated, despite the need for rationing, e.g. stripping varicose veins, cosmetic plastic surgery and sex-change operations. It could be argued that most of these treatments are not essential and are unnecessary. However, the reasoning behind treating these conditions is the severe psychological consequences that failure to treat may have on patients. Infertility is known to consume the whole life of couples, affecting their work, relationships with colleagues and families, and has been known to cause marital disharmony and psychiatric illness. Therefore, treating couples with infertility indirectly treats these associated problems.

The NHS aims to treat all, irrespective of the problem. Infertility is a disease and therefore deserves to be treated within the NHS. But is it life-threatening compared to other conditions, such as cancer and cardiac diseases? This argument is unsubstantiated as many other illnesses being treated in the NHS are not life-threatening. If the arguments against offering tertiary treatment for infertility are that limited resources for important health conditions will be diverted to the treatment of this condition, a similar argument could be advanced for the treatment of other non-debilitating conditions.

Therefore, the argument about treatment must be similar to that for other conditions. In an ideal world where resources are limitless, this would not arise. It is important to acknowledge that rationing is an integral part of the NHS and will remain so for a long time to come. Where resources are limited, there may be a place to limit the treatment of couples with infertility to that offered at primary and secondary levels. However, tertiary treatment must be made available but in a few designated centres where expertise and wide experience exists in order to improve the success rates. Regulating practice is important to prevent abuse. The principles of rationing require that all cases are assessed on merit and treatment offered when it is considered to be necessary. Couples with infertility being refused treatment on the NHS are being treated unfairly and that undermines the fundamental principles of the NHS.

5. How will you set up a risk-management team in your unit? (20 marks)

Common mistakes

- Details of what a risk-management team consists of
- Role of risk-management team
- Audit cycle and risk management
- The process of risk management

A good answer will include some or all of these points

- What is a risk-management team?
- Who should be in the team?
- What should be the remit of the team?
- How should it work?
- Description of the role of the team?
- Effect of the team on care
- Integration with other aspects of perinatal care
- Assessment/evaluation of the effectiveness of the team

Sample answer

Risk management is increasingly being recognised as an important component of clinical governance. This is more so in the light of the rising cost of litigation in medicine. In obstetrics and gynaecology, this is even more important in view of the fact that although the discipline contributes only a small proportion of cases, its litigation bill comprises about 60 per cent of the NHS litigation bill. It is, therefore, not surprising that the Clinical Negligence Scheme for Trusts requires all units to have risk-management teams. Setting up these teams is imperative. How these units are set up will define their effectiveness.

In setting up a risk-management team, the first consideration must be the composition of the team. Within each unit, there should be a risk manager working within the team with the remit of minimising risk. Team membership should reflect the multidisciplinary nature of patient care within the unit. It should include a midwife/nurse, physicians (junior and senior) and an anaesthetist. This will ensure that all members of staff feel represented. The members of the team should have an interest in risk management and must be educated on the importance of risk management as a means of improving care rather than as a punitive process.

The remit of the team must be clearly defined. The team should aim to identify risk-management issues within the unit, set up guidelines on how to deal with these and, importantly, how to minimise risk-management issues within the unit. There may be a place for the introduction of incident reporting so that various risk-management issues could be identified and a process set in place on how to deal with any deficiencies. The role of the team within the unit must be clear. In addition, there must be channels of communication between the team, members of staff and management. This communication must be two way and efforts made to ensure that the staff in the unit do not perceive the team as a fault-finding and blame team but one whose role is constructive, aiming for a risk-free service within the unit.

Once the team has been established, there has to be a mechanism by which information is disseminated to the unit. This may be through meetings and other fora where information on risk-management issues is presented. The ultimate objectives of the risk-management team are to ensure that complaints are dealt with quickly and early, that potential problems are identified early, dealt with and that members of staff are educated where weaknesses are identified in their practices. Members of risk-management teams must be seen to work in collaboration with all aspects of the services provided within the team.

Section Three
Multiple-choice questions (MCQs)

1

Sample MCQs

Answer true or false

Concerning autosomal recessive inheritance

1. If the carrier has an affected partner, there is a 50 per cent chance of the children being affected.
2. There is an association with consanguinity.

Concerning X-linked inheritance

3. More females than males show the recessive phenotype.
4. The disease is transmitted by a carrier female, who is usually asymptomatic.
5. A carrier mother will have a 50 per cent chance of her sons being affected and a 50 per cent chance of her daughters being carriers.
6. Affected males may have unaffected parents but will often have an affected maternal uncle.

The following disorder(s) is/are correctly associated with the mode of inheritance

7. Tay–Sachs disease   Autosomal recessive.
8. Marfan's syndrome   Autosomal recessive.
9. von Willebrand's disease   Autosomal dominant.
10. von Recklingausen's disease (neurofibromatosis)   Autosomal dominant.

In adolescent pregnancies

11. The incidence of sudden infant death syndrome is higher than in older women.
12. The interval between pregnancies is influenced by whether or not the first pregnancy is planned.
13. Preterm labour is less common than in older women.

Concerning pregnancies in ethnic minorities

14. Sickle cell disease rarely occurs in women of non-African origin.
15. When there is non-engagement of the head in a black British woman at 38 weeks' gestation, cephalopelvic disproportion needs to be excluded.
16. Glucose-6-phosphate dehydrogenase deficiency is more common in women from the Mediterranean and African region than in those from south-east Asia.

With regards to miscarriages

17. Disseminated intravascular coagulation (DIC) is not a recognised complication.
18. Gas gangrene is a complication of septic miscarriages.
19. The treatment of an incomplete miscarriage should include a broad-spectrum antibiotic.
20. *Clostridium welchii* is a recognised cause of the recurrent variety.
21. Misoprostol, when used to medically evacuate the uterus, is successful in 90 per cent of cases with incomplete miscarriages.

A 36-year-old woman was admitted at 36 weeks' gestation with vaginal bleeding and abdominal pain. An ultrasound scan performed at 20 weeks' gestation had located the placenta to be posterior and fundal. Which of the following statements about her management is/are correct?

22. The diagnosis of placental abruption is confirmed by the presence of abdominal pain.
23. An ultrasound scan is unnecessary as placenta praevia has been excluded.
24. If DIC is suspected, delivered by Caesarean section is recommended.

Concerning ultrasound in pregnancy

25. The finding of an isolated echogenic bowel suggests a high risk of Down's syndrome.
26. The presence of two or more soft markers increases the risk of aneuploidy.
27. When undertaken at 20 weeks' gestation, more than 70 per cent of cardiac anomalies are detected.
28. About 20 per cent of fetuses with an nuchal translucency (NT) of 5 mm will be aneuploid.

Which of the following statement(s) about human immunodeficiency virus (HIV) infection in pregnancy is/are correct?

29. The median time between exposure to the virus and the development of detectable antibody is about 2 months.
30. Transplacental transfer to the fetus is reduced by Caesarean section.
31. The rate of vertical transmission to the fetus is increased by the presence of co-infection with other sexually transmitted infections.
32. Approximately 20 per cent of infected children born to untreated Europeans will develop the symptoms of autoimmune deficiency syndrome within the first year of life.

With regards to neural tube defects

33. Recurrence tends to be concordant.
34. They may be associated with Meckel–Gruber syndrome.
35. A previously affected child increases the risk of recurrence to about 1–3 per cent.
36. The presence of acetyl cholinesterase in amniotic fluid is diagnostic of an open defect.

Which of the following is/are recognised to be associated with an abnormally large NT?

37. Diaphragmatic hernia.
38. Gastroschisis.
39. Cardiac abnormality.

Soft markers for chromosomal abnormalities include

40. Cerebellar hypoplasia.
41. Pyelectasis.
42. Cerebral ventriculomegaly.
43. Choroid plexus.

Complications of chorionic villus sampling include

44. Transverse limb reduction deformities.
45. Preterm labour.
46. Placental abruption.

Routine amniocentesis is

47. Associated with an increased risk of orthopaedic deformities.
48. Complicated by chorioamnionitis in 5 per cent of cases.

The following is/are true about stillbirths

49. Most occur in labour.
50. At least 50 per cent are preventable.
51. Fetal growth restriction (FGR) is an associated factor in approximately 50 per cent of unexplained cases.

Maternal smoking in pregnancy is associated with

52. Reduced blood flow to the fetal brain.
53. Diminished fetal breathing movements.
54. Neonatal hypoglycaemia.
55. An increased incidence of amniorrhexis.

Neonatal complications of FGR include

56. Respiratory distress syndrome.
57. Hypothermia.

With regards to polyhydramnios, which of the following is/are correct?

58. The cause is identifiable in more than 60 per cent of cases.
59. Acute cases are more likely in twin-to-twin transfusion syndrome.
60. The incidence of unexplained stillbirth is higher when the aetiology is unexplained.

Oligohydramnios

61. Is associated with renal agenesis in most cases.
62. Is associated with congenital malformations in about 15 per cent of cases.
63. When its onset is before 25 weeks' gestation, neonatal mortality is of the order of approximately 90 per cent.

Complications in the surviving twin of a monozygotic pregnancy with one intrauterine fetal death include

64. Bilateral renal cortical necrosis.
65. Multicystic encephalomalacia.
66. Hydrocephalus.

With regards to fetal hydrops

67. The diagnosis is based on the presence of fluid within at least one fetal cavity.
68. Non-immune hydrops is five times more common than the immune type.
69. The prognosis depends on the cause and the time of diagnosis.
70. Perinatal mortality is of the order of 30 per cent.

Maternal autoimmune thrombocytopenia is

71. Associated with an increased risk of fetal thrombocytopenia if it is symptomatic.
72. Associated with an increased risk of neonatal thrombocytopenia to about 40 per cent if splenectomy has been performed.
73. Associated with haemorrhagic complications if the maternal platelet count is 30×10^9/L.
74. A contraindication to instrumental vaginal deliveries.

Fetal bradycardia if

75. Uncomplicated is most likely to be secondary to hypoxia.
76. Unprovoked should be managed by immediate delivery.

With regards to congenital heart diseases

77. They complicate about 1 per cent of all pregnancies.
78. The best time for antenatal diagnosis is at the 20 weeks' anomaly ultrasound scan.
79. More than three-quarters are diagnosed from the four-chamber view of the heart.

With respect to parvovirus B19 infection

80. It is the most commonly treatable cause of non-immune hydrops.
81. Viraemia develops 1 week after exposure.
82. The virus has a predilection for haematopoietic sites.

Congenital infection with cytomegalovirus is

83. Associated with cerebral calcifications.
84. A recognised cause of microcephaly.
85. Associated with polyhydramnios.
86. Associated with FGR.
87. Associated with thrombocytopenia.

Concerning tuberculosis in pregnancy

88. It is a notifiable disease.
89. Breastfeeding is contraindicated.
90. Infected patients must be screened for HIV.

With regards to malaria infection in pregnancy

91. It is most commonly due to *Plasmodium falciparum.*
92. Convulsions are a recognised clinical presentation.
93. Placental infestation occurs in as many as 40–50 per cent of cases.

Neonates of drug-addicted mothers

94. Classically develop withdrawal symptoms after 4–5 days.
95. Suffer from more severe withdrawal symptoms when breastfed.

The following drugs are considered teratogenic

96. Lithium.
97. Zidovudine (AZT).
98. Thiazide diuretics.

In a woman with severe pre-eclampsia

99. Creatinine clearance is raised.
100. Fibrinogen degradation products are normal.

Recognised effects of the administration of the calcium-channel blocker atosiban in the third trimester include

101. Increased maternal pulse pressure.
102. Reduced urine output.

Concerning shoulder dystocia

103. It occurs more frequently in macrosomic fetuses of diabetic mothers.
104. Erb's palsy is a recognised complication.
105. Brachial plexus injury involves cranial nerve roots 5 and 6 more frequently than 7 and 8.

Pregnancy exacerbates the clinical features associated with

106. Sickle cell haemoglobinopathy.
107. von Recklingausen's disease.
108. Peptic ulceration.
109. Bronchial asthma.
110. Eisenmenger's syndrome.

Regarding peripartum cardiomyopathy

111. The maternal mortality rate within the first year is more than 80 per cent.
112. Cardiac transplantation is not an appropriate treatment.
113. Epidural analgesia is contraindicated in labour.

Endometrial ablation

114. Is effective in the treatment of menorrhagia secondary to adenomyosis.
115. Has a better patient satisfaction rate compared to that after hysterectomy.
116. Should only be performed in women who have completed their families.

After an abdominal hysterectomy, there are difficulties in waking up the patient from general anaesthesia. Which of the following may be responsible?

117. Use of hypotensive agents.
118. Pulmonary oedema.

Concerning damage to viscera during gynaecological surgery

119. A crushing damage of the ureter should be corrected by resecting the damaged portion and re-anastomosis.
120. Damage to the bladder should be repaired with a non-absorbable suture material and a catheter left *in situ* for 7–10 days.
121. A defunctioning colostomy is required after repair of damaged small bowel.
122. Following suspected perforation of the uterus, a laparotomy is essential.

Following massive haemorrhage

123. Hyperkalaemia is a recognised complication of blood transfusion.
124. Fresh frozen plasma which contains the protein constituents of plasma, including the clotting factors, should be given.
125. Hypothermia is a recognised complication of treatment.
126. Cryoprecipitate should be given if the fibrinogen level is <1.0 g/dL.

In a fetus with 5-alpha-reductase deficiency

127. There is failure of conversion of testosterone to dihydrotestosterone in target tissues.
128. Masculinisation at puberty is secondary to high circulating levels of androgens.
129. Partial androgen insensitivity may be associated with partial masculinisation and breast growth.
130. There is no need to remove the gonads.

During the menstrual cycle

131. The luteinising hormone (LH) surge begins at the same time as the follicle-stimulating hormone (FSH) surge.
132. The mean duration of the LH surge is 36 hours.
133. Ovulation occurs 24 hours after the LH surge.

The following is/are recognised cause(s) of precocious puberty

134. Hypothyroidism.
135. Craniopharyngioma.
136. McCune–Albright syndrome (polyostotic fibrous dysplasia).
137. Neurofibromatosis.

A child presents with labial adhesions

138. Reassure the mother and leave the child alone.
139. Prescribe topical oestrogen preparations after separating the labia.
140. Exclude congenital malformations of the upper genital tract.

A 21-year-old presented with primary amenorrhoea. She is one of three sisters – the others attained menarche at 11 and 13 years, respectively. On examination, the secondary sexual characteristics are normal. Some investigations were undertaken and the results are as follows: FSH = 7 IU/L, LH = 5 IU/L, 17-beta-oestradiol = 350 pmol/L, testosterone = 0.7 nmol/L, prolactin = 350 IU/L, chromosomes = 46XX. Which of the following is/are correct?

141. An obstruction to the lower genital tract is the most likely cause of her amenorrhoea.
142. If she suffers from cyclical pain, the diagnosis is an imperforate hymen.
143. Ultrasound scan of the pelvis is more reliable than a magnetic resonance imaging in diagnosing the cause.
144. The progesterone challenge test is an option in the evaluation of the cause of the amenorrhoea.

Concerning precocious puberty

145. Treatment with gonadotropin-releasing hormone agonists results in atrophy of the breast.
146. It is a recognised cause of short stature.
147. Cyproterone acetate is an acceptable treatment option.

The following is/are recognised causes of galactorrhoea in a 36-year-old woman

148. Phenothiazines.
149. Metoclopramide.
150. Cimetidine.

Bromocriptine treatment

151. Causes postural hypotension.
152. Improves libido.

Premature ovarian failure

153. Is associated with a negative progesterone challenge test.
154. Occurs in 10–15 per cent of women presenting with secondary amenorrhoea.

In unexplained infertility

155. Spontaneous conception rates close to 80 per cent are achievable if the duration is less than 3 years.
156. Treatment with clomifene citrate will improve conception rates.

A 26-year-old woman undergoing superovulation for infertility presents with severe ovarian hyperstimulation syndrome (OHSS)

157. She is at an increased risk of venous thromboembolism (VTE).
158. Renal function is normal in most of such patients.
159. The presence of a pleural effusion is an indication to abandon the infertility treatment.
160. If she becomes pregnant, she should be given human chorionic gonadotropin to support the pregnancy.

Antisperm antibodies can be detected by

161. Mixed agglutination reaction test.
162. Immunobead test.
163. Postcoital test.
164. Immunoabsorbent assay of the antibodies in semen.

Which of the following statements regarding male reproduction is/are correct?

165. Testosterone administration improves semen quality when there is oligozoospermia.
166. *Ureaplasma urealyticum* infection does not impair fertility.
167. Cystic fibrosis is a recognised cause of infertility.

With regards to OHSS

168. The risk is related to the total number of mature and immature follicles.
169. The incidence does not correlate with conception cycles.
170. Avoidance of sexual intercourse when there is a significant risk is an acceptable advice.
171. Spontaneous resolution is unlikely to occur without treatment if there is a successful pregnancy.

Features associated with a failed pregnancy (missed abortion) include

172. Breast tenderness.
173. A brown vaginal discharge.

A 4-year-old presented with a persistent vaginal discharge that causes significant vulval irritation and staining of the underwear. The following statement(s) about her management is/are correct

174. Sexual abuse should be considered as a cause.
175. Most cases are characterised by recurrence until puberty.
176. A broad-spectrum antibiotic should be prescribed.
177. Examination under anaesthesia is indicated if the discharge is bloodstained.

Patients with polycystic ovary syndrome are more likely to

178. Achieve regular cycles if they lose approximately 1–2 per cent of their weight.
179. Be hyperinsulinaemic.

Medroxyprogesterone acetate

180. Is effective in the treatment of endometriosis.
181. Is associated with breakthrough bleeding.
182. Induces regression of endometrial hyperplasia.

A pelvic abscess is associated with

183. Diarrhoea.
184. Bacteraemia.
185. Swinging pyrexia.

Carcinoma of the cervix

186. Is characteristically preceded by human papillomavirus infection.
187. Characteristically originates from the transformation zone.
188. Is adenocarcinoma in <10 per cent of cases.
189. Involves obstruction of the ureter in most cases of stage II disease.

The diagnosis of premenstrual syndrome can confidently be made from

190. A symptom diary chart.
191. A gonadotropin analogue therapeutic trial test.
192. A general health questionnaire.
193. Blood hormone assays performed throughout the ovarian cycle.

With regard to the menopause

194. It is premature when cessation of menstruation occurs before the age of 40 years.
195. Hypothalamic–pituitary activity changes are not obvious until 2–3 years before menopause.
196. During the phase of ovarian failure, the ovarian stroma ceases production of hormones.
197. The symptoms are related mainly to the levels of FSH and LH.

Risk factors for osteoporosis include

198. Cortisol therapy.
199. Chronic renal failure.
200. Prolonged lactation.
201. Hyperparathyroidism.

Hormone replacement therapy after the age of natural menopause

202. Increases the risk of VTE by 2–4-fold.
203. Decreases the risk of cardiovascular disease.
204. Is contraindicated in patients with previous VTE.
205. Increases the relative risk of breast cancer after 5 years.

If a woman on the combined oral contraceptive pill experiences breakthrough bleeding

206. Reassure her if the bleeding occurs within the first 6 months on the pill.
207. Exclude a coexisting gynaecological disorder if it persists.
208. Change from a 50 mg containing pill to a 30 mg containing pill.
209. Stop the pill immediately and observe for persistence of the bleeding as a means of excluding a coexisting cause.

Concerning female sterilisation

210. The failure rate with Filshie clips is higher than with diathermy.
211. Up to 10 per cent of women regret their decision to undergo the procedure.
212. The failure rate is 3 per 1000.
213. There is an increased gynaecological consultation for menstrual problems following sterilisation.

There is an increased incidence of postoperative burst abdomen with

214. Steroid therapy.
215. Smoking.
216. Non-closure of the peritoneum.

The following procedures have been shown to significantly reduce the risk of adhesion formation after myomectomy:

217. Plication of the round ligament.
218. Instillation of concentrated solutions of dextran after surgery.
219. Use of oxidised regenerated cellulose in the peritoneal cavity after surgery.

With regards to cervical intraepithelial neoplasia (CIN)

220. It rarely affects the gland crypts.
221. Cellular atypia is the most important abnormality when assessing CIN.
222. The squamocolumnar epithelium must be present for an adequate diagnosis to be made.
223. The proportion of the thickness of the epithelium showing differentiation is important in assessing the degree of severity.

Concerning surgery for urodynamic stress incontinence

224. Anterior colporrhaphy is associated with a 5-year cure rate of 70 per cent.
225. Colposuspension is commonly complicated by detrusor overactivity.

2

Answers to the MCQs

1. T   2. T

Autosomal recessive (AR) genes or traits are only expressed in homozygotes for the gene. Horizontal inheritance occurs and affected individuals usually have normal parents. Mating between heterozygotes will produce individuals with a 25 per cent risk of being affected. Both sexes are equally affected, although AR genes may show a sex influence, e.g. haemochromatosis is AR but has a higher incidence in males due to a lower dietary iron intake and menstruation in females. There is an association with consanguinity.

3. F   4. T   5. T   6. T

Sex-linked defects are located on either the X or Y chromosomes. Y-linked inheritance is very rare. For X-linked inheritance, more males than females show the recessive phenotype; the disease is transmitted by a carrier female, who is usually asymptomatic. Sons of a carrier mother will have a 50 per cent chance of being affected, while her daughters will have a 50 per cent chance of being carriers. Affected males usually have no affected offspring but all the daughters will be carriers and, in turn, 50 per cent of their sons will be affected.

7. T   8. F   9. T   10. T

Autosomal recessive conditions include cystic fibrosis, phenylketonuria, Tay–Sachs disease, sickle cell disease, Gaucher's disease, thalassaemia and congenital adrenal hyperplasia. Autosomal dominant conditions include achondroplasia, retinoblastoma, tuberous sclerosis, Marfan's syndrome, von Willebrand's disease and familial hypercholesterolaemia.

11. T   12. F   13. T

In adolescent pregnancies, the incidence of sudden infant death syndrome is higher and the Caesarean section rates are not significantly higher but preterm labour is more common. Whether or not the pregnancy is planned does not influence the interval between pregnancies. Anaemia is more common. The incidence of abnormal presentations is no different from that in older women.

14. T   15. F   16. T

Sickle cell disease is more common in black individuals but may occur in other races. The fetal head commonly enters the pelvis during labour in black women, hence failure of the head to engage after 36 weeks' gestation is not an indication to exclude disproportion. Glucose-6-phosphate dehydrogenase deficiency is more common in the Mediterranean region and Africa than south-east Asia.

17. T   18. T   19. F   20. F   21. F

Clostridium welchii is not a recognised cause of recurrent miscarriages. However, gas gangrene is a recognised complication of incomplete miscarriages, especially those that become septic. Other complications of septic miscarriages include disseminated intravascular coagulation and septicaemia. There is no need to administer antibiotics to women undergoing evacuation for incomplete miscarriages unless there is a suspicion of genital infections or the miscarriage is complicated by infection (i.e. it is septic). Medical management of failed pregnancies is successful in about 80–85 per cent of cases.

22. F   23. F   24. F

Placental abruption presents with abdominal pain. The diagnosis cannot be excluded by ultrasound scan and it is associated with an increased risk of congenital malformations. Disseminated intravascular coagulation is a recognised complication and is not an indication for Caesarean section. In its presence, regional anaesthesia is contraindicated.

25. F   26. T   27. F   28. F

Most babies with echogenic bowels on ultrasound scan are normal. Other associated soft markers need to be excluded. This may be associated with cystic fibrosis, bowel obstruction, cytomegalovirus (CMV) infection and aneuploidy. In isolation, it is not an indication for karyotyping. The presence of two or more soft markers is an indication for karyotyping as this increases the risk of aneuploidy. Routine anomaly scans are able to identify between 40 and 60 per cent of cardiac malformations. Most fetuses with an abnormal nuchal translucency (NT) will be normal.

29. F   30. F   31. T   32. F

The median time between exposure to the human immunodeficiency virus (HIV) and development of antibodies is approximately 6 months. Vertical transfer of the HIV virus to the fetus is facilitated by other genital tract infections, especially the sexually transmitted infections. However, transplacental transfer can be minimised by antiviral treatment. Delivery by Caesarean section and the avoidance of breastfeeding will also reduce the risk of vertical transmission. Without treatment, approximately 15–25 per cent of babies will acquire the virus. The interval to development of autoimmune deficiency syndrome tends to be much longer than 12 months.

33. T   34. T   35. T   36. T

The recurrence of neural tube defects (1–3 per cent) tends to be concordant. They may be part of the abnormalities in Meckel–Gruber syndrome. Others include a posterior fossa cyst and renal malformations. Amniocentesis is not indicated to diagnose neural tube defects, but the presence of acetyl cholinesterase in amniotic fluid is diagnostic of an open neural tube defect.

37. T   38. F   39. T

An abnormal NT may be associated with thoracic malformations, cardiac malformations, aneuploidy and various poorly defined syndromes. However, most fetuses with a value of more than 3 mm are normal.

40. F   41. T   42. T   43. F

Soft markers of aneuploidy include pyelectasis, cerebral ventriculomegaly, choroid plexus cyst, echogenic focus in the chest, short femur and Sandal gap. A choroid plexus is present in every fetus and is not a soft marker for aneuploidy.

44. T   45. F   46. F

Chorionic villus sampling (CVS) may theoretically be complicated by transverse limb defects, especially when performed before 10 weeks' gestation, miscarriages and Rhesus isoimmunisation. Mosaicism is reported in approximately 1 per cent of cases. Preterm labour is a recognised complication of amniocentesis rather than CVS.

47. F   48. F

Routine amniocentesis is not associated with orthopaedic deformities; however, amniocentesis performed before 14 weeks (which is not routine) is associated with a 10-fold increase in the risk of talipes equinovarus). Chorioamnionitis is the most common cause of miscarriages, which complicate 0.5–1 per cent of cases. Isoimmunisation may complicate amniocentesis.

49. F   50. F   51. T

Most stillbirths occur antenatally and fetal growth restriction (FGR) is a common association. Most are unexplained and in this population, approximately 50 per cent of the fetuses are growth restricted from customised charts.

52. F   53. T   54. F   55. F

Maternal smoking is associated with a reduction in the incidence of pre-eclampsia (PET) and reduced fetal breathing movements but not blood flow to the brain. It is not associated with fetal hypoglycaemia or amniorrhexis. It is a risk factor for stillbirth and venous thromboembolism (VTE) but not for amniorrhexis.

56. T   57. T

Neonatal complications of FGR include hypoglycaemia, polycythaemia, thrombosis, hypothermia and necrotising enterocolitis. Respiratory distress syndrome is a complication in those delivered preterm.

58. F   59. T   60. T   61. F   62. F   63. T

Acute polyhydramnios is more likely in monozygotic twin pregnancies. Most cases of polyhydramnios are idiopathic, are associated with unexplained stillbirths and may be diagnosed clinically by the present of a fluid thrill and a uterine fundus larger than dates. Oligohydramnios, on the other hand, may be due to renal failure or congenital infections. When it occurs early, mortality is over 90 per cent, because of pulmonary hypoplasia. Renal agenesis tends to be associated with an hydramnios.

64. T   65. T   66. T

Following the death of one twin, the surviving twin has an increased risk of renal cortical necrosis, multicystic encephalomalacia and hydrocephalus. The risk of neurodevelopmental abnormality is considerably higher.

67. F   68. F   69. T   70. T

Fetal hydrops is diagnosed when fluid is present in at least two fetal cavities. The non-immune type is more common and the prognosis depends to an extent on the timing of the diagnosis – the earlier the diagnosis, the poorer the outcome. Alloimmunisation may be assessed by the Coombs test.

71. T   72. T   73. T   74. F

Maternal autoimmune thrombocytopenia complicates about 8 per cent of all pregnancies. It may be associated with haemorrhagic complications in the fetus. Instrumental deliveries are contraindicated only if the count is less than 30×10^9/L.

75. F   76. F

Uncomplicated fetal bradycardia is more likely to be related to maternal hypotension rather than fetal hypoxia. Hypoxia will induce complicated bradycardia. Where the bradycardia is unprovoked, other measures, such as turning the patient from the dorsal to the lateral position, should be attempted first. However, attempts must be made to limit the delay in rectifying this and therefore delivery should be considered if the bradycardia is persistent.

77. T   78. F   79. F

Congenital cardiac disease complicates approximately 1 per cent of all pregnancies. The best time of diagnosis is 22–24 weeks. The five-chamber view will diagnose close to 60 per cent of all cases. Tachycardia may cause hydrops from heart failure.

80. T   81. F   82. T

Fetal hydrops may be caused by parvovirus B19. The virus has a preference for the haematopoietic system and causes anaemia, which is correctable by intrauterine transfusion.

83. T   84. T   85. T   86. T   87. T

Cytomegalovirus infections *in utero* may cause echogenic bowel, cerebral calcifications, microcephaly, hydrocephalus and FGR. The CMV may be detected in the urine of the infant. Most viral infections may cause polyhydramnios, FGR and thrombocytopenia in the fetus.

88. T   89. F   90. F

Tuberculosis is a notifiable disease, caused by *Mycobacterium tuberculosis*. Infected mothers may breastfeed. Although its presence should increase the risk of HIV infection, screening should only be offered after counselling.

91. T   92. T   93. T

Malaria is commonly due to *Plasmodium falciparum*. It may cause miscarriages, preterm labour and intrauterine growth restriction. Placental infestation occurs in up to 40–50 per cent of cases and when there is severe pyrexia, the mother may present with febrile convulsions.

94. F   95. F

Neonates of addicted mothers may suffer from withdrawal symptoms, which tend to occur within 24–48 hours after delivery. In most cases, breastfeeding reduces the severity of withdrawal symptoms.

96. T   97. T   98. T

Teratogenic drugs in pregnancy include vitamin A, lithium, amphotericin B and thiazide diuretics.

99. T   100. F

Abnormal changes that may be present in women with PET include raised fibrinogen degradation products, thrombocytopenia and abnormal liver function tests. Most of these abnormalities are only present in severe disease. Urinary function is only altered in severe disease.

101. T   102. F

Atosiban, the calcium-channel blocker is associated with reduced maternal pulse pressure and tachycardia but the urinary output is not reduced.

103. T 104. T 105. F

Shoulder dystocia commonly occurs in macrosomic babies, although most of these are of diabetic mothers. Complications include fracture of the long bones, Erb's palsy and fracture of the clavicle. It is one of the important causes of litigation.

106. T 107. T 108. F 109. F 110. T

Sickle cell anaemia, von Recklinghausen's disease and Eisenmenger's syndrome are exacerbated in pregnancy. Pregnancy complications in women with HbSC genotype are less severe than in women with HbSS genotype.

111. F 112. F 113. F

Peripartum cardiomyopathy is associated with a high maternal mortality, especially in the puerperium. It is not a contraindication to epidural analgesia although precautions must be taken, especially with circulatory overload. Prophylactic antibiotics are not required in the management of peripartum cardiomyopathy. Although transplant is not the treatment of choice, it can be performed.

114. T 115. F 116. T

Endometrial ablation should be performed in women who have completed their families because of the complications of pregnancy after this procedure. Some practitioners perform sterilisation at the time of ablation. Endometrial ablation is effective in treating menorrhagia but not the dysmenorrhoea of adenomyosis.

117. T 118. T

Difficulties in waking a patient up from general anaesthesia (GA) may be due to drug reaction, overdose, pulmonary oedema, hypotension and myocardial infarction.

119. F 120. F 121. F 122. F

Visceral injuries occurring at the time of gynaecological surgery should be managed depending on the viscera and the type of injury. If there is a crushing injury to the urethra, an indwelling catheter would be sufficient. All injuries to the bladder involving complete breach of the wall should be repaired with an absorbable material and the bladder rested for 7–10 days. A defunctioning colostomy is required when there is large bowel injury but each case must be assessed on its own merit.

123. T 124. F 125. T 126. T

Transfusions after massive haemorrhage may be complicated by hyperkalaemia, hypothermia and thrombocytopenia.

127. T   128. T   129. T   130. F

Deficiency in 5-alpha-reductase is characterised by masculinisation at puberty and failure of conversion of testosterone to dihydrotestosterone at the target tissues. Testicular regression syndrome is familial and at birth, the testicles are abnormal.

131. F   132. F   133. F

Physiological changes during the ovarian cycle include a luteinising hormone (LH) surge which occurs 24 hours before ovulation. The LH surge does not begin at the same time as the follicle-stimulating hormone surge and ovulation occurs 24–36 hours after the LH surge.

134. T   135. T   136. T   137. T

Precocious puberty is defined as the occurrence of pubertal changes culminating in menstruation before the age of 8 years. Recognised causes include hypothyroidism, craniopharyngioma, neurofibromatosis and McCune–Albright syndrome.

138. F   139. T   140. F

Labial adhesions in a child could be treated with oestradiol cream. They are not usually associated with congenital malformations of the genital tract.

141. F   142. F   143. F   144. F

In a patient presenting with primary amenorrhoea, constitutional factors must be excluded. In this patient, a lower genital tract abnormality is not likely to be the cause as she would most likely have presented with an abdominal mass. Cyclical pains may be due to an obstruction in the vagina or at the level of the cervix rather than from only an imperforate hymen. An ultrasound scan is not as reliable as magnetic resonance imaging in diagnosing a absent uterus as in cases of Müllerian agenesis.

145. T   146. T   147. T

Acceptable treatment options for precocious puberty include gonadotropin-releasing hormone (GnRH) agonists and cyproterone acetate. Although these patients tend be taller for their age, in the long-term, they are shorter because of early closure of the epiphyses.

148. T   149. T   150. T

Hyperprolactinaemia may be caused by phenothiazines, Rauwolfia alkaloids, steroids, cimetidine, metoclopramide, steroids and antidepressant agents.

151. T   152. T

Bromocriptine is a recognised treatment but has several side-effects including hypotension, especially the postural type, dizziness, headaches, nausea and vomiting, and vasospasms of the fingers and toes.

153. T   154. T

Premature ovarian failure, which is associated with a negative progesterone challenge test, occurs in about 10–15 per cent of women presenting with secondary amenorrhoea and treatment is usually ineffective.

155. T   156. T

Spontaneous conception rates up to 80 per cent occur in unexplained infertility of less than 3 years. Treatment with clomifene citrate will improve conception rates.

157. T   158. F   159. F   160. F

Ovarian hyperstimulation syndrome (OHSS) is more likely in women undergoing superovulation induction. Women with polycystic ovary syndrome (PCOS) are at a greater risk and when this occurs treatment should include correction for haemoconcentration. Infertility treatment should not be abandoned because of OHSS. However, when it occurs, the pregnancy should be supported with progestogens rather than human chorionic gonadotropin.

161. T   162. T   163. F   164. F

Male infertility may be associated with antisperm antibodies, which may be identified with either a mixed agglutination reaction or an immunobead test.

165. F   166. F   167. T

Infections with *Ureaplasma urealyticum* are a recognised cause. The administration of testosterone is an ineffective treatment. Cystic fibrosis and bronchiectasis are recognised causes.

168. T   169. T   170. T   171. F

The total number of follicles is related to OHSS since they all produce steroids. The incidence of OHSS is higher with successful pregnancies – reportedly being 2–5-fold higher. Avoidance of sexual intercourse or using a condom is acceptable advice in cases where natural conception is possible. Although treatment is advocated, spontaneous resolution can occur, especially in the mild cases.

172. F   173. T

Missed abortions (failed pregnancies) are associated with a brownish vaginal discharge and disappearing pregnancy symptoms. Most women will report a reduction in breast tenderness. In most cases, an ultrasound scan will reveal an empty gestational sac with no fetal pole.

174. T   175. T   176. F   177. T

Causes of a vaginal discharge in a 4-year-old child include foreign bodies, trauma, infections (especially with parasites, such as threadworms), malignancies and sexual abuse. Clinical examination should be limited to inspection and if there is a need for a more detailed examination, this is best performed with the patient under GA.

178. F   179. T

Patients with PCOS have an elevated plasma oestrone concentration and may be hyperinsulinaemic. Some of them are anovulatory. The diagnosis may be made either by ultrasound scan alone or by biochemistry alone. Weight loss is associated with spontaneous ovulation and for this to be effective, at least 5 per cent of the weight needs to be lost.

180. T   181. T   182. T

Medroxyprogesterone acetate may be used as an effective contraceptive and is also effective in the treatment of endometriosis and endometrial hyperplasia. It is associated with breast tenderness and functional ovarian cysts in about 15 per cent of cases. It is a 17-C progestogen and is therefore not associated with hypertension.

183. T   184. F   185. T

Pelvic abscesses may present with diarrhoea, a throbbing pain in the lower back and a swinging pyrexia. There is usually no associated bacteraemia.

186. T   187. T   188. F   189. F

Carcinoma of the cervix is more common in women with multiple sexual partners, especially in women with human papillomavirus infection. It characteristically starts in the squamocolumnar region and the most common histological type is of the squamous type. Involvement of the ureters would be suggestive of at least stage IIb; however, most cases of stage II do not involve the ureters.

190. T   191. T   192. F   193. F

Premenstrual syndrome is characterised with various psychosomatic symptoms, which are best demonstrated with a symptom diary chart. The diagnosis can be made with a therapeutic GnRH agonist trial.

194. T   195. F   196. F   197. F

Premature menopause is defined as cessation of menstruation occurring before the age of 40 years. During the climacteric there is an increase in gonadotropins in response to increasing resistance of the ovaries to stimulation. Even after menopause the ovary remains an important source of steroids as the stroma continues to produce hormones. Symptoms of menopause are secondary to oestrogen deficiency, although hot flushes are thought to be related to LH surges.

198. T   199. T   200. T   201. T

Risk factors for osteoporosis include cortisol therapy, hypothyroidism, hyperparathyroidism, chronic renal failure, prolonged lactation, early menopause and being underweight.

202. T   203. F   204. F   205. T

Hormone replacement therapy (HRT) increases the risk of VTE 2-fold. Women with an intact uterus would benefit from combined therapy but this is not suitable for every patient. The risk of breast cancer is increased after 5 years on HRT.

206. T   207. T   208. F   209. F

The contraceptive pill may induce breakthrough bleeding and when this occurs within 6 months of starting, reassuring the patient is enough. A change of the pill may correct the complication. When this persists, there may be a need to investigate with a hysteroscopy.

210. F   211. T   212. F   213. T

Female sterilisation is associated with a failure rate of 1:200. This is higher with diathermy than with clips. Gynaecological consultation for menstrual problems after sterilisation is increased and the risk of hysterectomy is higher in women who have been sterilised.

214. T   215. T   216. F

Burst abdomen is a complication that is more common in immunosuppressed patients, those having surgery for malignancy and patients on steroids. Chronic cough and smoking are risk factors for this complication.

217. F   218. F   219. F

Adhesion formation in gynaecological surgery may be reduced by the use of Adept® and Intercede®. Various surgical procedures have been tried unsuccessfully to reduce adhesion formation.

220. F   221. F   222. F   223. T

Cervical intraepithelial neoplasia (CIN) may affect gland crypts. The most important abnormalities are the changes in the nucleus of the cells. Most cases can be treated with large loop excision of the transformation zones (LLETZ).

224. F   225. F

Urethral sphincter incompetence is a synonym for urodynamic (genuine) stress incontinence. The current treatment for this condition is either a colposuspension or tension-free transvaginal vaginal tape. Treatment with anterior colporrhaphy is associated with a 5-year survival rate of 60 per cent.

Section Four
Extended matching questions (EMQs)

1

How to answer EMQs

Extended matching questions (EMQs) should not be considered as simple true and false answers. It is important for the candidates to recognise that several of the options given in the list will be correct answers to the particular question. The issue is whether it is the *best* or *most suitable* or *most appropriate*.

In answering EMQs you should avoid looking at the option list unless you have absolutely no clue as to what the question is all about. A logical approach to answering an EMQ is:

1. First, read the instructions (sometimes referred to as the introduction statement) to the questions. This will give you precisely the task that you are being given. In some case, these instructions may give you a clue as to the theme under which the questions will fall.
2. Read the clinical scenarios or vignettes and decide what you feel is the correct answer, before looking at the option list. It may be wise to consider more than one option but make sure that you have an order (i.e. first, second and third if possible). This is just in case the first option is not in the list of options. In the exams, I would recommend that you write this/these options against the vignette and later refer to this when you must look at the option list.
3. You should repeat one and two above for each of the vignettes/scenarios.
4. Finally, you should look at the list of options and match your chosen option with those on the list.
5. If your options are not on the list, you should look for the one closest to your option. Narrowing your answer is an art that you must learn to master. Some clues to this are provided in (7)
6. If none of the options in the list is close to yours, you should start the process of elimination. It is unlikely that of the 10–25 options that you may have for each question, more than 5–6 will be applicable to the particular scenario or vignette. The only problem with this approach is time constraints.
7. Where you are struggling, you will need to guess. The first step in this process is to narrow down the options. You should initially look at all the information on offer. Use the pointers offered in the vignettes to narrow down the potential answers and return to the modified list for further, more refined thinking. Similarly, do not be caught by the distracters slipped into statements. The difficulty with this approach is time – you only have limited time per question. You should therefore not do this until you have finished all the questions whose answers are quite obvious to you.

2

Sample EMQs

Option list for questions 1–2

A. Aphthous ulcer
B. Bacterial infections
C. Carcinoma of the vulva
D. Condylomata acuminata
E. Chancroid (*Haemophilus ducreyi*)
F. *Entamoeba histolytica* (amoebiosis)
G. *Enterobius vermicularis* (threadworm)
H. Granuloma inguinale
I. Herpes simplex
J. Lichen sclerosus chronicus (neurodermatitis)
K. Lichen sclerosus and squamous metaplasia
L. Lymphogranuloma inguinale
M. Pediculosis
N. Syphilis

Instructions: For each of the following, select from the option list above the SINGLE most likely cause of the ulceration on the vulva. Each option may be selected once, more than once, or not at all.

1. A 27-year-old presents with a progressive swelling of the vulval of 3 years' duration. At the outset, it was a simple ulcer which disappeared very quickly. This was soon followed by a swelling in the groin. This then burst to discharge pus for 3 days. Unfortunately, rather than getting better, her groin started swelling up and this continued to extend to her left labium. On examination, the left labium majorum is found to be hypertrophic and there is evidence of lymphatic obstruction in the left groin.

2. A 20-year-old presents with multiple ulcers on the vulva of 4 days' duration. These ulcers followed rupture of painful blisters. Her last menstrual period was 9 days ago and she is on the combined oral contraceptive pill for contraception. On examination, the vulva is inflamed and contains round tiny ulcers which have a granulated base but the edges are not elevated. There is no associated lymphadenopathy.

Option list for questions 3–4

A. Anterior repair
B. Colposuspension
C. Colpocleisis
D. Diagnostic laparoscopy
E. Hysteroscopy
F. Manchester repair
G. Myomectomy
H. Ovarian cystectomy – laparoscopic
I. Ovarian drilling
J. Polypectomy
K. Posterior repair
L. Radiotherapy
M. Sacrocolpopexy
N. Sacrospinous fixation
O. Salpingectomy – laparoscopic
P. Subtotal hysterectomy
Q. Tension-free transvaginal tape
R. Total abdominal hysterectomy
S. Total abdominal hysterectomy and bilateral salpingo-oophorectomy
T. Trachelectomy
U. Uterine artery embolisation
V. Vaginal hysterectomy
W. Wertheim's hysterectomy

Instructions: For each of the case scenarios described below, select from the option list above the SINGLE most suitable surgical procedure. Each option may be selected once, more than once, or not at all.

3. A 45-year-old G2P2 presenting with stress urinary incontinence and occasional nocturia of 7 months' duration. Urinary frequency is normal and there is no associated urgency or urge incontinence. She is found on examination to have a body mass index (BMI) of 29 kg/m^2, a mild cystocele and a cervix just below the level of the ischial spines. The uterus is bulky but there are no pelvic masses. Urodynamic studies reveal urodynamic severe stress incontinence.

4. A 32-year-old Jehovah's Witness presents with menorrhagia and listlessness of 18 months' duration. She has had three normal vaginal deliveries and following the last one, she was sterilised. Her periods are so heavy that she suffers from giddiness and has to take time off work. On examination, she is pale but is otherwise healthy. There is an abdominopelvic mass extending to the umbilicus which is irregular and firm in consistency. An ultrasound confirms the presence of multiple uterine fibroids, most of which are intramural. The ovaries are normal.

Option list for questions 5–7

A. Antibiotics
B. Bowel anastomosis
C. Drainage
D. Fistulogram
E. Hysterectomy
F. Immediate referral to gynaecological oncologist
G. Immediate transfer to urology unit
H. Indwelling catheter for 48 hours
I. Indwelling catheter for 10 days
J. Indwelling catheter for 10 days and antibiotics
K. Laparotomy and repair
L. Laparotomy and repair by urologist
M. Laparotomy, repair and colostomy
N. Laparoscopic repair
O. Lavage and drainage
P. Nil by mouth for 48 hours
Q. Observe for 24–48 hours
R. Repair and colostomy
S. Retrograde ureteroscopy
T. Transfusion

Instructions: For each of the case scenarios described below, select from the option list the SINGLE most appropriate first line management of the gynaecological surgical complication. Each option may be selected once, more than once, or not at all.

5. A 27-year-old woman is undergoing a laparoscopic resection of rectovaginal endometriosis and during the procedure it is discovered that a small 0.5 × 0.5 cm hole has been made in the ileum close to its junction with the caecum. On closer inspection, this appears to have been secondary to slippage of the laser fibre.

6. A 30-year-old woman is undergoing a laparotomy for a right dermoid cyst. The bowel which is found to be attached to the ovarian cyst is freed from the cyst before cystectomy but the mucosa is breached and there is some anxiety that the breach might have gone into the lumen; on inspection, this was not obvious.

7. A 38-year-old woman is undergoing an abdominal hysterectomy and bilateral salpingo-oophorectomy for large uterine fibroids. During surgery, there is a suspicion that the bladder has been damaged by a clamp (crush injury) although there is no obvious injury seen. At the end of the procedure, an in-and-out catheter drains heavily blood-stained urine.

Option list for questions 8–10

A. A meta-analysis
B. A systematic review
C. Case control study
D. Cohort study
E. Cross-over study
F. Cross-sectional study
G. Experimental study
H. Historical cohort study
I. Longitudinal study
J. Observational study
K. Placebo-controlled study
L. Prospective study
M. Randomised controlled non-blinded study
N. Randomised controlled double-blinded placebo-controlled study
O. Retrospective study
P. Three-arm randomised controlled study

Instructions: For each of the following studies detailed below, select from the options above the SINGLE best description of the type of study. Each option may be selected once, more than once, or not at all.

8. A study in 2005 of 158 women aged 20–29 years who presented between 1996 and 2001 with irregular periods in whom an ultrasound diagnosis of polycystic ovary syndrome (PCOS) was made in the community prior to referral to the gynaecologist.

9. A combination of 14 observational studies published between 2000 and 2005 on the efficacy of intramuscular progestogens in women presenting with threatened preterm labour on inhibiting contractions and prolonging pregnancy.

10. A combination of eight randomised trials to assess the effects of danazol and various gonadotropin-releasing hormone (GnRH) agonists in the symptomatic treatment of endometriosis.

EXTENDED MATCHING QUESTIONS (EMQs)

Options for questions 11–14

A. Amniotic fluid embolism
B. Anaphylactic reaction
C. Cardiomyopathy
D. Cerebrovascular accident
E. Diabetic ketoacidosis
F. Drug reaction
G. Eclampsia
H. Epilepsy
I. Gram-negative septicaemia
J. Mendelson's syndrome
K. Morphine overdose
L. Myocardial infarction
M. Postpartum haemorrhage
N. Pulmonary embolism
O. Ruptured aneurysm
P. Ruptured ovarian cyst
Q. Ruptured spleen
R. Ruptured uterus
S. Thyroid crisis
T. Uterine inversion

Instructions: For each of the patients presented below, selected the SINGLE most likely cause of postpartum collapse. Each option may be used once, more than once, or not at all.

11. A 33-year-old woman collapsed soon after a forceps delivery of her second baby following induction of labour at 42 weeks' gestation. Induction was with a single 3 mg prostaglandin E$_2$ pessary followed by an artificial rupture of fetal membranes (ARM) and Syntocinon®. The total duration of her labour was 10 hours. Prior to delivery there was a bradycardia. Her first baby was delivered by an emergency Caesarean section for fetal distress at 39 weeks' gestation. On examination, her blood pressure (BP) is 70/40 mmHg, pulse 120 bpm but regular and of reasonably good volume. She is very tender in the abdomen but there is no abnormal vaginal bleeding.

12. A 40-year-old primigravida went into spontaneous labour at 38 weeks' gestation. Her pregnancy was uncomplicated but she developed hypertension requiring intravenous labetalol in labour. This was discontinued as her BP started falling after she had an epidural. She had a spontaneous vaginal delivery 3 hours ago and after the epidural catheter was removed, she started complaining of severe headaches and heaviness on her face. She has suddenly collapsed and is unconscious. Her BP is 140/95 mmHg and her pulse is 86 bpm. Her reflexes are normal.

13. Mrs BH was admitted into spontaneous labour at 35 weeks' gestation. She had been feeling unwell prior to admission and also noticed a gush of water from her vagina 2 weeks before admission. An ultrasound scan 2 weeks ago revealed severe oligohydramnios. During labour she felt flustered but was reassured that this was normal. She delivered

7 hours ago and is now complaining of giddiness, abdominal pain or headaches. On examination, her temperature is 35.7°C, pulse is 100 bpm and BP is 80/60 mmHg. Her extremities are cold and clammy.

14. A previously fit 37-year-old women delivered 5 hours ago after an uncomplicated labour at 40 weeks' gestation. Four hours after delivery, she developed a crushing chest pain on the left side associated with a suffocating feeling. She has now collapsed. On examination, she is tachypnoeic, sweaty and hyperventilating. Her BP is 90/50 mmHg and her pulse rate is 108 bpm.

Options for questions 15–16

A. Central venous pressure
B. Diuretics
C. Hydrostatic pressure/Johnson's or O'Sullivan's procedure
D. Inotropes
E. Intravenous diazepam
F. Intravenous ergometrine
G. Intravenous 50 per cent dextrose
H. Intravenous hydrocortisone
I. Internal iliac artery ligation
J. Intravenous labetalol or hydralazine
K. Intravenous line and transfer to intensive care unit
L. Intravenous magnesium sulphate
M. Laparotomy and hysterectomy
N. Lynch's brace suture
O. Oxygen by face mask
P. Pulmonary wedge pressure

Instructions: For each of the following obstetric emergencies, select from the option list above the SINGLE most appropriate immediate management option. Each option may be selected once, more than once, or not at all.

15. A 22-year-old normotensive with an uncomplicated pregnancy delivered 2 hours ago. Following delivery she complained of headaches, jitteriness and visual spots on her eyes. She has not had the classical *grand mal* fit. Her BP is 150/100 mmHg.

16. A 36-year-old teacher is admitted in labour at 39 weeks' gestation. This is her second pregnancy, the first having ended in a neonatal death from Group B haemolytic streptococcus infection. She was given intravenous benzylpenicillin as per the protocol 20 minutes ago. She is now disorientated, irritable, tachypnoeic, cyanosed and complaining of difficulties breathing. Her BP is 120/60 mmHg and her pulse rate is 100 bpm.

Options for questions 17–18

A. Acute cortical renal failure
B. Acute tubular renal failure
C. Adrenal insufficiency
D. Amniotic fluid embolism
E. Cardiac failure
F. Cardiomyopathy
G. Couvelaire uterus
H. Diabetic ketoacidosis
I. Eclampsia
J. Sepsis
K. Septic shock
L. Severe sepsis
M. Systemic inflammatory response
N. Myocardial infarction
O. Pulmonary embolism
P. Respiratory arrest/pulmonary oedema
Q. Urinary retention
R. Vulval oedema

Instructions: The following patients described in the scenarios below developed complications either in labour or soon after delivery. Select from the list of options above the SINGLE most likely diagnosis for each patient. Each option may be selected once, more than once, or not at all.

17. A 33-year-old had a spontaneous vaginal delivery 3 hours ago. Following an uneventful Kielland's forceps delivery she started bleeding and lost in total over 3.5 L of blood. Her urine output over the last 3 hours has been very poor (10 mL). On examination, the uterus is well contracted.

18. A 20-year-old collapsed suddenly after a spontaneous vaginal delivery. This was provoked by the administration of intravenous Syntometrine®. She was healthy throughout pregnancy although noticed that she was increasingly breathless on mild exertion. On examination, her BP is 85/45 mmHg, pulse 98 bpm and respiratory rate is 28 bpm. Her liver is enlarged and there are bilateral crepitations in the lower lungs.

Option list for questions 19–21

A. Abdominal ultrasound scan
B. Amniotomy (ARM)
C. Admit to the antenatal ward
D. Catheterise the bladder
E. Continuous cardiotocography (CTG) with a fetal scalp electrode
F. Continuous CTG with transabdominal transducer
G. Doppler scan of the umbilical artery
H. Emergency Caesarean section
I. Epidural analgesia
J. External cephalic version
K. Fetal blood sampling
L. Group and cross-match
M. Intravenous antibiotics
N. Intravenous cannula
O. Intravenous dextrose saline
P. Intravenous oxytocin
Q. Intravenous Ringer's lactate
R. Intravenous terbutaline
S. Maternal pulse
T. Oxygen by face mask
U. Prostaglandin pessaries
V. Pulmonary wedge pressure catheter
W. Re-examine in 4 hours
X. Turn to left side

Instructions: For each of the following clinical scenarios select from the option list above the SINGLE most appropriate action. Each option may be selected once, more than once, or not at all.

19. A 26-year-old primigravida admitted in spontaneous labour at 40 weeks' gestation was contracting well but could not tolerate the pain. An epidural was therefore sited and she became more comfortable. At vaginal examination (VE), the cervix had dilated to 6 cm (3 cm at the last VE 3 hours ago). Her temperature has risen to 37.4°C on two occasions 30 minutes apart with an associate uncomplicated tachycardia of 170 bpm.

20. A primigravida in labour at 41 weeks' gestation has just had a VE to assess progress of labour which was soon followed by a prolonged bradycardia down to 80 bpm. Prior to the VE, the CTG was reactive and with a normal baseline variability.

21. A 20-year-old primigravida at 37 weeks' gestation was induced for fetal growth restriction. ARM was performed 10 hours ago and meconium-stained liquor was obtained. Intravenous Syntocinon® was commenced immediately after the ARM and an hour later she started contracted regularly and strongly. The cervix was 8 cm at the last VE. The fetal heart rate has risen from a baseline of 144 bpm to 162 bpm with reduced variability and occasional early decelerations.

Option list for question 22

A. Amniocentesis
B. Apt test
C. Biophysical profile
D. Colour Doppler scans of blood vessels
E. Continuous abdominal CTG
F. Cord blood sample
G. Fetal blood sampling
H. Fetal electrocardiogram
I. Fetal echocardiography
J. Fetal haemoglobin estimation
K. Fetal platelet estimation
L. Fetal scalp electrode
M. Fetoscopy
N. Infection screen
O. Pulse oximetry
P. Middle cerebral artery Doppler scan

Instructions: For the case scenario presented below, select from the option list above the SINGLE best investigation you will undertake first. Each option may be selected once, more than once, or not at all.

22. A 30-year-old woman presents in labour at 40 weeks' gestation. During admission, she is found to have an irregular heart rate which is difficult to characterise. On VE the cervix is 5 cm and the membranes are intact.

Option list for questions 23–24

A. Coitus interruptus
B. Condom
C. Copper multiload intrauterine contraceptive device (IUD)
D. Diaphragm
E. 50 µg ethinyl oestradiol combined oral contraceptive pill
F. Levonorgestrel intrauterine system (Mirena®)
G. Medroxyprogesterone acetate
H. Mifepristone
I. Natural family planning
J. Progestogen-only oral contraceptive pill
K. Sequential combined oral contraceptive pill
L. Sterilisation – female
M. Sterilisation – male
N. Subdermal implant Implanon® or Norplant®
O. 30 µg ethinyl oestradiol combined oral contraceptive pill
P. Triphasic combined oral contraceptive pill

Instructions: The patients below are attending for contraceptive advice. Select from the option list above the SINGLE most suitable form of contraception for each patient. Each option may be selected once, more than once, or not at all.

23. A 37-year-old woman attends for contraceptive advice. Her periods are regular and heavy. She has completed her family and was single until recently when a new man entered her life. Her BMI is 25 kg/m².

24. A 20-year-old para 0 + 0 attends for contraceptive advice. She was on the pill 3 years ago but kept forgetting to take them. She feels that she is now more mature and wants something that is reliable. Her BMI is 22 kg/m².

Option list for questions 25–26

A. Adrenal hypoplasia
B. Anorexia nervosa
C. Anxiety
D. Asherman's syndrome
E. Bulimia
F. Congenital adrenal hyperplasia
G. Conn's syndrome
H. Craniopharyngioma
I. Cushing's syndrome
J. Diabetes mellitus
K. Diabetes insipidus
L. Hyperaldosteronism
M. Hyperparathyroidism
N. Hyperprolactinaemia
O. Hyperthyroidism
P. Hypothyroidism
Q. Kallman's syndrome
R. Phaeochromocytoma
S. PCOS
T. Prolactinoma
U. Sheehan's syndrome

Instructions: For each of the following case scenarios described below, select from the option list above the SINGLE most likely diagnosis. Each option may be selected once, more than once, or not at all.

25. A 33-year-old woman presented with primary infertility of 4 years' duration. She also complains of recurrent attacks of throbbing headaches usually accompanied by sweating, palpitations and tremors. She suffers from these episodes almost 2–3 times per month. She has been to see the general practitioner (GP) during the attacks when her BP is found to be raised. The GP ascribes this to her anxiety about her infertility. In between episodes, she is asymptomatic and her BP is normal.

26. A 28-year-old woman presented with a whitish discharge from the breast of 8 months' duration. She experiences occasional headaches but is otherwise normal. On examination, her BMI is $27 \, kg/m^2$ and her BP is 120/67 mmHg. Her hormone profile is as follows: follicle-stimulating hormone (FSH) = 3.0 IU/L, luteinising hormone (LH) = 6.9 IU/L, prolactin = 1790 mIU/L (normal range 0–400 mIU/L), free thyroxine = 14 mIU/L (normal range 0–9 mIU/L), thyroid-stimulating hormone (TSH) = 3.4 mIU/L. An ultrasound of the pelvis shows multiple follicles the largest measuring 14 cm in both ovaries.

Option lists for questions 27–29

A. Adrenalectomy
B. Aromatase inhibitors
C. Bromocriptine
D. Combined oral contraceptive pill
E. Corticosteroids
F. Cyproterone acetate (CPA)
G. Danazol
H. Oestrogens
I. Finasteride
J. GnRH agonist
K. Growth hormones
L. Medroxyprogesterone acetate
M. Neurosurgical excision
N. Ovarian cystectomy
O. Reassurance
P. Separation of fusion
Q. Testicular tumour removal
R. Thyroxine (levothyroxine)

Instructions: For each of the following clinical scenarios, select from the option list above the SINGLE most appropriate first line treatment. Each option may be selected once, more than once, or not at all.

27. A 10-year-old girl presents with an 8-month history of regular menstruation and well-developed secondary sexual characteristics. Her sisters attained menarche at the age of 13 and 14 years. Investigations did not demonstrate any abnormal hormone profile.

28. An 11-year-old girl presented with well-developed secondary sexual characteristics since the age of 7 years. She is investigated and found to have fusion of 'labioscrotal' folds and raised 17-hydroxyprogesterone.

Option list for questions 29–30

A. Adoption
B. Bromocriptine
C. FSH
D. Gamete intrafallopian transfer (GIFT)
E. *In vitro* fertilisation and embryo transfer (IVF-ET)
F. Intrauterine insemination with partner's sperm
G. Intrauterine insemination with donor sperm
H. Intracytoplasmic sperm injection
I. Orchidopexy
J. Percutaneous sperm aspiration
K. Reassurance
L. Salpingotomy
M. Sperm washing and insemination
N. Steroids for antisperm antibodies
O. Testosterone injections
P. Varicocelectomy
Q. Vitamin E

Instructions: For each of the following cases of male infertility, select from the option list above the SINGLE most appropriate initial treatment option. Each option may be selected once, more than once, or not at all.

29. A couple were investigated for infertility and the man was found to have a combination of asthenozoospermia and teratozoospermia. The woman had unilateral tubal blockage at diagnostic laparoscopy and dye test.

30. A couple attended an assisted reproduction unit for investigations for primary infertility. A diagnostic laparoscopy and dye test on the woman showed endometriosis and forced filling and spillage of dye in both tubes. The man was found to have severe oligozoospermia.

Option list for questions 31–32

A. Culture and sensitivity
B. FSH
C. Karyotype
D. LH
E. Mixed agglutination reaction test
F. Orchidometry
G. Photomicrography
H. Serum prolactin
I. Semen analysis
J. Sperm microscopy
K. Testicular biopsy
L. Testosterone
M. Urethral swab
N. Vasoepididymography
O. Zona-free hamster oocyte test

Instructions: For each of the following cases, select from the option list above the SINGLE most important investigation you will perform on the patient to help make a diagnosis of the cause of infertility. Each option may be selected once, more than once, or not at all.

31. A 41-year-old man attends the clinic with his wife for infertility. He is found on examination to be tall, and with small testicles. A semen analysis shows oligozoospermia.

32. A 27-year-old driving instructor presents with infertility and loss of libido. He states that he has never really had an interest in sex. In addition, he has never been able to smell properly, especially coffee and tea.

Option list for questions 33–34

A. Admit into the hospital
B. Administration of Ringer's lactate solution
C. Await spontaneous resolution and providing supporting treatment
D. Central venous pressure line
E. Clotting profile
F. Dialysis
G. Drainage of fluid
H. Drainage of hydrothorax
I. Non-steroidal anti-inflammatory drugs
J. Prolonged bed rest
K. Prophylactic subcutaneous low-molecular-weight heparin
L. Renal and liver function tests
M. Terminate pregnancy
N. Ultrasound examination for ovarian size
O. Withhold administration of human chorionic gonadotropin

Instructions: The following patients underwent superovulation induction and developed the complication of ovarian hyperstimulation syndrome (OHSS). Select from the list above the SINGLE most appropriate medical life-saving first line management option for the patient. Each option may be selected once, more than once, or not at all.

33. A 32-year-old woman is admitted with severe OHSS. She is being given fluids as she is severely dehydrated. An ultrasound scan shows ascites, hydrothorax and ovaries measuring >14 cm in diameter.

34. A 29-year-old woman presented with features of critical OHSS. An ultrasound scan showed ascites and enlarged ovaries (each measuring 17 cm in diameter). She has been commenced on intravenous fluids and thromboprophylaxis with low-molecular-weight heparin.

Option list for questions 35–36

A. Adenomyosis
B. Chronic renal disease
C. Cushing's syndrome
D. Dysfunctional uterine bleeding
E. Endometriosis
F. Endometrial polyps
G. Factor X deficiency
H. Fibroids
I. Hyperthyroidism
J. Hypothyroidism
K. Idiopathic thrombocytopenia
L. IUD
M. Pelvic inflammatory disease
N. PCOS
O. Von Willebrand's disease

Instructions: For each of the following clinical scenarios, select from the option list above the SINGLE most appropriate explanation for the menorrhagia. Each option may be selected once, more than once, or not at all.

35. A 30-year-old woman presented with menorrhagia of 2 years' duration. She had had very heavy bleeding when her tooth was extracted 6 years ago and also noticed that she bruised easily.

36. A 26-year-old woman presented with heavy periods associated with acanthosis nigricans. Examination revealed multiple striae in the lower abdomen and the gluteal region. Her free androgen index was raised but testosterone levels were normal. Sex-hormone binding globulin levels were low but her serum prolactin was 800 mIU/L. However, she had no other symptoms.

Option list for questions 37–38

A. Bacterial vaginosis
B. *Chlamydia trachomatis*
C. Chancroid
D. Genital herpes
E. Granuloma inguinale
F. Human immunodeficiency virus
G. Lymphogranuloma venereum
H. Molluscum contagiosum
I. *Mycoplasma genitalium*
J. *Neisseria gonorrhoea*
K. Pediculosis
L. Syphilis
M. *Trichomonas vaginalis*
N. Tropical ulcer
O. Viral hepatitis
P. *Ureaplasma urealyticum*

Instructions: For each of the clinical scenarios below, select from the option list above the SINGLE most likely sexually transmitted infection (STI) involved. Each option may be selected once, more than once, or not at all.

37. A 22-year-old woman presented with a painful swelling of the right side of her vulva of 2 days' duration. She also complains of a vaginal discharge and dysuria. She had unprotected sexual intercourse 5 days ago after a night out with friends. On examination, she is found to have an inflamed swollen right labium majorum and features of bartholinitis. The external urethra is swollen and inflammed and there is a purulent discharge coming through it.

38. A 20-year-old university student presents to the genitourinary medicine clinic with urinary frequency and dysuria 10 days after sexual intercourse with her regular boyfriend. Although she was generally unwell 3 days ago, she feels well today. On examination, there is nothing abnormal found, either generally or in the pelvis. A urine sample sent for microscopy, culture and sensitivity (M/C/S) was sterile, although it contained pus.

Option list for question 39

A. Bartholinitis
B. Elephantiasis
C. Fitz-Hugh–Curtis syndrome
D. Gonococcal arthritis
E. Interstitial keratitis
F. Liver cell carcinoma
G. Mid-trimester miscarriages
H. Periappendicitis
I. Perihepatitis
J. Reactive arthritis
K. Reiter's syndrome
L. Sensorineural deafness
M. Tabes dorsalis
N. Thoracic aortic aneurysm
O. Tubo-ovarian abscess

Instructions: For the following STI, select from the option list above the SINGLE most appropriate complication ensuing. Each complication may be selected once, more than once, or not all.

39. A 35-year-old woman is diagnosed with an STI for which she is being treated with doxycycline. She develops asymmetrical oligoarthritis affecting mainly the knee joints and the joints of the hands. On examination she is found to have inflamed and swollen knee and hand joints. In addition she has a psoriatic rash on the torso.

Option list for question 40

A. Biopsy for histology
B. Diagnostic laparoscopy
C. Enzyme-linked immunosorbent assay
D. Endocervical swab for Gram stain
E. Enzyme-linked immunoassay
F. Fluid for virology
G. High vaginal swab for Gram stain
H. Ligase chain reaction of urine
I. Rectal swab for Gram stain
J. Stool examination
K. Swab for dark ground microscopy
L. *Treponema* haemagglutination test
M. Urine for M/C/S
N. Urethral swab for a wet preparation
O. Viral serology

Instructions: For the patient described below, select from the option list above the SINGLE best diagnostic test which you will use for identifying the STI involved. Each option may be selected once, more than once, or not at all.

40. A 20-year-old woman presented with upper right abdominal pain and dysuria. On examination, she is mildly pyrexial and the urethral meatus is swollen and there is a discharge coming through it.

3

Explanation of the answers to the sample EMQs

1. E. The features described in the case scenario are typical of those of chancroid caused by *Haemophilus ducreyi*. The other options that might have been considered include aphthous ulcer, granulmoma inguinale, syphilis and lymphogranuloma inguinale. However, the history of purulent discharge distinguishes chancroid from these other options.
2. I. The blisters were painful, suggestive of herpes simplex infection. Syphilitic ulcers are not typically painful.
3. Q. A tension-free transvaginal tape (TVT) is the most suitable surgical procedure. A colposuspension is also suitable but contemporaneously urogynaecologists will recommend a TVT unless there is an associated moderate cystocele. The morbidity and mortality associated with a TVT is less than that with colposuspension. In addition, the success rates are almost similar. A vaginal hysterectomy and an anterior repair are not suitable procedures.
4. U. Uterine artery embolisation is the best option for this patient. She has completed her family, will not accept blood transfusion and has been sterilised. Although a myomectomy and a hysterectomy are other options, uterine artery embolisation has several advantages over these surgical approaches.
5. K. The best option is laparotomy and repair. Although this could be done laparoscopically if the expertise exists, a thorough inspection will be difficult as the injury has been caused by laser and may have penetrated deeper than thought. There is no need for a colostomy as the injury is to the small bowel. Following surgery, she will have to be nil by mouth but this is not the first line management option.
6. P. There is only a suspicion of bowel injury, which is thought to involve only the serosa. If it had involved the mucosa, faeculent material would have been seen. The best approach is to be cautious and in this case, nil by mouth for 48 hours is all that is required. If the injury is more than the serosa, she will develop symptoms. Proceeding to repair and colostomy is not an appropriate option. If one of the options was repair alone, it may be considered.
7. J. The crush injury to the bladder will eventually result in a fistula formation if the bladder is not rested. There is no need to repair it as you will have to resect the crushed area. The best option to ensure that there is no infection is commencing antibiotics and resting the bladder for 10 days.
8. O. This is obviously a retrospective study. The study conducted in 2005 was on polycystic ovary syndrome (PCOS) women investigated between 1999 and 2001. All the other options are unsuitable.

9. B. This is a systematic review rather than a meta-analysis because it is a combination of 'a single tested hypothesis'.

10. A. This is a meta-analysis because the studies combined are addressing a set of related research hypotheses.

11. R. The picture presented is typically that of a ruptured uterus. It is not an amniotic fluid embolism because of the related clinical features (abdominal pain) and no mention of respiratory symptoms. Although a ruptured spleen is possible, there is nothing in the history to make this the most likely diagnosis. Similarly, a ruptured aneurysm is unlikely because of the age of the patient and the features.

12. D. A cerebrovascular accident is the most likely cause of the collapse because of the headaches and heaviness on one side. Eclampsia does not usually cause collapse (tends to cause fits).

13. I. Gram-negative septicaemia is the correct answer because of the history and clinical features (flustered, cold clammy extremities, hypotension and hypothermia). The other options may present in a similar way but the history of prolonged rupture of membranes and abdominal pain should point to chorioamnionitis and sepsis.

14. L. Myocardial infarction, although uncommon, will typically present with a central to left-sided crushing chest pain associated with a suffocating feeling. Pulmonary embolism is the other possibility, but is not the most likely cause of her symptoms.

15. L. The features are typical of those of severe pre-eclampsia and intravenous magnesium sulphate will reduce the risk of progression to eclampsia. Her blood pressure is not high enough to warrant immediate intravenous antihypertensive therapy.

16. H. The features are typical of those of an anaphylactic reaction to benzylpenicillin and the best option is to administer intravenous hydrocortisone. Although oxygen should be administered by face mask, this is not considered the most appropriate immediate action.

17. B. The patient has hypovolaemic renal shut down, which tends to be secondary to acute tubular necrosis and which often recovers completely after fluid replacement therapy. Vulval oedema or urinary retention will cause a poor urinary output but her massive blood loss will make renal failure the most likely diagnosis.

18. E. The most likely option is cardiac failure secondary to circulatory overload following the administration of Syntometrine®. The patient is likely to have had a cardiac problem that was not diagnosed antenatally. None of the other options will present with bilateral crepitations and an enlarged liver.

19. W. The tachycardia in this case is uncomplicated and most likely to be secondary to maternal pyrexia. Administering intravenous antibiotics is perhaps not an appropriate option; neither will it be appropriate to do a fetal scalp blood sample or deliver. She must already be on a cardiotocograph (CTG), hence this should not be considered an option. The best option is therefore to continue monitoring and to reassess in 4 hours. It may be more appropriate to assess the CTG sooner, but this option is not on the list.

20. X. The most likely cause of the prolonged bradycardia is maternal hypotension secondary to supine hypotension syndrome. Turning the patient to the left side will increase venous return to the heart, increase cardiac output and placental perfusion and the tachycardia will recover. There is no need to deliver immediately as the previous CTG was normal.

21. K. The CTG has two abnormal features – reduced baseline variability and early decelera-

tions. In addition, the baseline has risen. This is a growth-restricted fetus being induced and when artificial rupture of fetal membranes was performed, meconium-stained liquor was obtained. Fetal blood sampling should therefore be performed. There is no rush to deliver the baby by Caesarean section.

22. H. A fetal electrocardiogram (ECG) will help in identifying the type of cardiac dysrhythmia; however, this may not be easy to perform antenatally. An ECG may provide information about any structural abnormalities but this is not the best option.

23. F. The Mirena® intrauterine system is the best option for this patient. She has completed her family and has heavy periods. However, she should be offered a reversible form of contraception as she has just recently entered into a new relationship. She may decide to have another baby. The combined oral contraceptive pill is another option but this is not the first choice for this 37-year-old.

24. N. This 20-year-old is unlikely to comply with a contraceptive method that depends on her remembering to take them. The Mirena® is an option which is as effective as Implanon® and this should be considered in nulliparous women only if there is no other option. The combined oral contraceptive pill is not the most suitable option as she has already shown her inability to remember taking them.

25. R. The recurrent nature of her symptoms associated with tremors, palpitations and sweating all point to phaechromocytoma. Thyroid dysfunction may present with some of these features, but not most of them. Cushing's syndrome may present with hypertension but not the features presented in this case.

26. N. The option in this case is quite obvious from the raised prolactin. There are no obvious features to suggest PCOS although the luteinising hormone:follicle-stimulating hormone (LH:FSH) ratio may distract some candidates. The timing of the samples was not indicated and this may well have been taken around the time of ovulation.

27. O. The normal age of menarche in the UK ranges from 10 to14 years. This girl is therefore normal. The only reason why the parents are anxious is because of the timing of menarche in her sisters. Since investigations revealed nothing abnormal, reassurance is all that is needed. In fact, some will argue that she should not have been investigated after a physical examination.

28. E. The most likely diagnosis in this case is congenital adrenal hyperplasia of late onset and the treatment is corticosteroids. Although separating the fused labia is appropriate, it is not the most appropriate option.

29. H. The semen quality is so poor that it is not likely that a pregnancy will be achieved with any other option apart from intracytoplasmic sperm injection.

30. H. Although it could be argued that sperm preparation and artificial insemination by donor or *in vitro* fertilisation and embryo transfer would be acceptable options in this case, the most appropriate one would be ICSI.

31. C. The features in this patient suggest 47XXY, hence a karyotype is the most appropriate option.

32. B. The most likely diagnosis in this patient is Kallman's syndrome and therefore the most appropriate investigation is FSH. The classical diagnostic feature of this syndrome is inability to distinguish between the smell of coffee and tea.

33. K. Severe ovarian hyperstimulation syndrome (OHSS) is an important risk factor for venous thromboembolism (VTE) because of haemoconcentration. She should be

rehydrated with intravenous fluids and drainage of various fluid only embarked upon after stabilising the patient and reducing the risk of VTE.

34. L. Amongst the complications of severe OHSS are renal and hepatic failure, which could eventually be fatal. It is therefore important to establish the status of these organs once rehydration and thromboprophylaxis have been initiated.

35. G. The history of bleeding easily after a tooth extraction and easily bruising suggest a coagulation/clotting factor defect. The most likely one in this case is factor X deficiency.

36. N. The most likely option in this case is PCOS. This is supported by the high free-androgen index, low sex-hormone-binding globulin and raised testosterone levels. The multiple striae and acanthosis nigricans can also be found in women with Cushing's syndrome, but there are no other features of this syndrome.

37. J. Gonococcal infections will typically present 4–5 days after unprotected sexual intercourse with vaginal discharge and dysuria. In most women, this is asymptomatic. The other sexually transmitted infections do not present with purulent discharge. *Chlamydia trachomatis* is more like to be asymptomatic in women and does not usually present with a purulent discharge.

38. B. The interval between exposure and presentation with symptoms (10 days) excludes gonococcal infection. By the time most women with *C. trachomatis* infections are seen, they have no clinical features. The feeling of being unwell is related to the mild pyrexia that some of the patients may experience.

39. K. The features described are those of a reaction to the treatment offered. Reiter's syndrome is therefore the most appropriate complication. The other options are highly unlikely.

40. H. The patient has features of *C. trachomatis*. The abdominal pain is most likely to be perihepatitis. The most accurate test for this infection from the list of options is the ligase chain reaction test from urine. The polymerase chain reaction is also very reliable. Although endocervical swabs appropriately collected are likely to provide a diagnosis, this is not as accurate as the ligase chain reaction test.

Section Five

The objective structured clinical examination (OSCE)

1

Sample OSCE questions

Station 1

Candidate's instructions

Despite the increased awareness of the possible consequences of improperly managed extrauterine pregnancy, it remains an important cause of maternal morbidity and mortality in the UK. You have been requested to produce a protocol on how to manage this condition in your unit and to demonstrate the success of your protocol.

Station 2

Candidate's instructions

Mrs B is 40 years old. She has been referred for contraceptive advice. You are required to take a history and offer her the most appropriate contraceptive advice. You may wish to ask the examiner for additional information.

Station 3

Candidate's instructions

You are undertaking a preoperative ward round and the following patients are on the list for surgery. Discuss how you will undertake your ward round including the counselling you will offer the patients.

1. A 29-year-old woman listed for a laparoscopically assisted vaginal hysterectomy for heavy periods that failed to respond to medical treatment.
2. A 60-year-old woman with hesitancy, frequency and stress urinary incontinence listed for a cystoscopy.
3. A 36-year-old nulliparous woman listed for a diagnostic laparoscopy for deep dyspareunia and dysmenorrhoea.
4. A 19-year-old woman listed for a surgical termination of pregnancy at 8 weeks' gestation.

Station 4

Candidate's instructions

You are the junior doctor in the consultant's clinic and have been asked by your consultant to see and plan the management of the patient whom she first saw 2 months ago. A summary of the patient is given below.

> Mrs T is a 67-year-old woman who attended the gynaecology clinic 2 months ago complaining of stress urinary incontinence. A pelvic examination in the clinic was described as unremarkable. She was sent for urodynamic investigation which revealed urodynamic stress incontinence (USI). She has returned to the clinic for the results of the investigation and a discussion on her management.

Station 5

Candidate's instruction

You are the specialist registrar/specialist trainee in a unit and are about to see Mrs AHP, a 51-year-old woman who had a total abdominal hysterectomy and bilateral salpingo-oophorectomy by your team 5 days ago for atypical hyperplasia of the endometrium, having presented with postmenopausal vaginal bleeding. The histology report is available but she is yet to be informed of its contents. The histology report is enclosed.

> **Histopathology report on Mrs AHP**
> Specimen: uterus, Fallopian tubes and ovaries
>
> *Clinical history*
> Complex hyperplasia on biopsy of endometrium from endometrial biopsy. Total abdominal + bilateral salpingo-oophorectomy done; appears to be a malignancy of endometrium with involvement of the cervix.
>
> *Macroscopic*
> Opened uterus and cervix and both tubes and ovaries $115 \times 95 \times 80$ mm. Macroscopic tumour 100 $\times 40 \times 35$ mm, maximum depth 15 mm, involving endometrial cavity and invading into cervix. Left ovary $35 \times 25 \times 10$ mm with cystic areas. Left Fallopian tube 55 mm. Right ovary $30 \times 20 \times 10$ mm, with cystic areas. Right Fallopian tube 15 mm. The uterus was received opened with resulting contamination of the fixative with multiple pieces of tumour. This has led to problems with interpretation of the histology detailed below.
>
> *Microscopic*
> The endometrium is almost completely replaced by tightly packed abnormal endometrial glands forming a trabecular pattern with some villiform areas, set in a fibrous stroma. The epithelium is pseudostratified and consists of columnar cells with vesicular oval nuclei showing a low degree of nuclear pleomorphism. This endometrioid adenocarcinoma is intramucosal in some areas, but in others invades into the inner half of the myometrium. The serosa is not breached, although there are probable contaminant tumour deposits on the surface. In multiple endometrial blocks there is evidence of tumour invasion into small and large blood vessels. The cervix is invaded by tumour.

The right and left cornua are not involved with tumour. In the left and right parametria, there are multiple areas of tumour deposits between tissue planes. This is difficult to interpret, but the appearance is suggestive of postoperative contamination rather than true spread of tumour. The left ovary contains a luteinised follicle. Peripheral contamination with tumour is noted in the left Fallopian tube. A Müllerian inclusion cyst is noted in the connective tissue between the right ovary and Fallopian tube. Again, probable contaminant tumour is noted in tissue planes in this region.

Conclusion
Well-differentiated endometrioid carcinoma of the endometrium, grade 1, invading cervix, inner half of the myometrium and blood vessels.

Station 6

Candidate's instructions

Mrs Jones had *in vitro* fertilisation and had a twin pregnancy. She went into spontaneous labour at 39 weeks' gestation and is now fully dilated. The first twin is cephalic with the vertex at the introitus. How will you conduct the delivery?

Station 7

Candidate's instruction

A general practitioner has referred a patient to the gynaecology clinic with the following letter. Read the letter below and then obtain the relevant history from the patient. You are expected to discuss the management options with her. The examiner will provide you with additional information should you require it.

> Holly Tree Surgery
> Wooden House Lane
> Thorpes Beast Village
> Walthome WN2 SU7
>
> Dear Dr –
>
> Would you be kind enough to see this 38-year-old woman who has been suffering from very heavy periods for the past 4 years. When I examined her, I noted that her uterus was 24 weeks' size and an ultrasound scan confirmed the presence of uterine fibroids. Her haemoglobin was 7.5 g/dL and I therefore placed her on iron tablets. She has recently been diagnosed with human immunodeficiency virus and is currently on triple antiviral therapy. Her CD4 count has improved significantly since she was commenced on this therapy by the genitourinary medicine physicians.
>
> Thank you for your help.
>
> Yours sincerely
>
> Peter Bowels DRCOG, MRCGP, MBCHB (LEIC)

Station 8

Candidate's instructions

The following patients are on the waiting list of a consultant in your hospital. You task is to review the list and classify the patients' surgery into routine (within 3 months), soon (within 4 weeks) and urgent (within 2 weeks). In addition, you should state whether the proposed surgical procedure is appropriate and what additional precautions/steps may be taken.

1. A fit 54-year-old diabetic with focal atypical endometrial hyperplasia listed for insertion of the levonorgestrel intrauterine system.
2. A 17-year-old girl who presented with severe dysmenorrhoea and heavy periods of 12 months' duration listed for a diagnostic laparoscopy.
3. A 67-year-old woman with a painless ulcer on her right labium majorum listed for an excisional biopsy.
4. A 38-year-old woman with a diagnosis of severe endometriosis which failed to respond to medical treatment, listed for an abdominal hysterectomy and bilateral salpingo-oophorectomy
5. An 8-year-old girl with a bloody vaginal discharge of 2 weeks' duration listed for examination under anaesthesia.
6. A 77-year-old widower living on her own on the list for a vaginal hysterectomy and pelvic floor repair, having been diagnosed with a large cystocele and USI.
7. A 26-year-old woman with a diagnosis of primary infertility placed on the list for a diagnostic laparoscopy and dye test.
8. A 49-year-old severely asthmatic woman on Ventolin® and steroids on the list for a Wertheim's hysterectomy for carcinoma of the cervix stage 1A.
9. A 30-year-old nulligravid woman with a diagnosis of multiple uterine fibroids and severe menorrhagia for myomectomy.

Station 9

Candidate's instructions

You are about to see Mrs B, a lawyer, and her husband, a business executive, who had an unexplained stillbirth at 40 weeks' gestation 3 months ago. They are attending for a postnatal follow-up. The results of the various investigations performed after the delivery, are as follows:

- Glycosylated haemoglobin (HbA1c) – 5 per cent (normal 5–7 per cent)
- Thyroid function test – normal
- Infection screen – normal
- Autopsy – normal external and internal structures
- Placenta – fibrinoid areas scattered within the placenta with some areas of vascular occlusion
- Anticardiolipin IgG antibody – 16 IU/mL (normal (0–14 IU/ml)

- Lupus anticoagulant – 1.16 (normal 0.1–1.09)
- Heterozygous for the prothrombin gene mutation
- Protein S – 60 (normal 80–110)
- Other thrombophilias – normal

Could you conduct her postnatal visit?

Station 10

Candidate's instructions

You arrive on the delivery suite for the morning shift and have been handed the 10 patients shown on the board. The sister-in-charge quickly runs through the problems, telling you that it is busy and she is short of staff. There are six midwives (SM, MD, BG, ST, MM and TT) on duty. SM and MD are capable of siting Venflon®, BG and ST are able to suture episiotomies and MM and TT are newly qualified midwives. On duty with you are an experienced anaesthetic registrar and a General Practitioner Vocational Scheme trainee. You are required to identify the task(s) that need to be done for each patient, the priority in which these patients should be seen and managed, and the member of staff who will be allocated to do these tasks. The 10 patients are as follows:

- Room 1: A 27-year-old woman with a previous Caesarean section for failure to progress in the second stage, in labour for 12 hours and complaining of abdominal pain
- Room 2: Mrs JT – a primigravida at 35 weeks' gestation with premature rupture of fetal membranes and having variable decelerations
- Room 3: Mrs James with uncomplicated twins in early labour at 37 weeks' gestation
- Room 4: A primipara who has been fully dilated and pushing for 2 hours
- Room 5: A 32-year-old primigravida with an undiagnosed breech in labour at 39 weeks' gestation
- Room 6: Mrs PJ with abdominal pains at 26 weeks' gestation
- Room 7: A 42-year-old primigravida at 38 weeks' gestation presenting with vaginal bleeding
- Room 8: Primigravida who delivered 1 hour ago and is awaiting repair of her episiotomy
- Room 9: Uncomplicated primigravida at 41 weeks in normal labour
- Room 10: A 28-year-old woman who delivered 4 hours ago and is being observed for a postoperative pyrexia of 37.6°C

You have 15 minutes to prepare this station and to discuss your answer with the examiner at the next station.

Station 11

Candidate's instructions

A primigravida attended for her anomaly scan at 20 weeks' gestation and the fetus was found to have a diaphragmatic hernia and bilateral talipes equinovarus. She has been informed of the abnormalities by the radiographer. How will you set about managing this patient?

Station 12

Candidate's instructions

Mr B and his wife attended the gynaecology clinic with primary infertility. The couple were investigated and the following results were obtained from a semen analysis, which was repeated twice:

- Time of production   0930
- Time of examination   1015
- Volume   3 mL
- Count   500 000/mL
- Motility   50 per cent
- Morphology   50 per cent
- Cells   1–3/mL

The investigations on Mrs B revealed mild endometriosis, predominantly on the posterior peritoneum and the uterosacral ligaments. How will you counsel the couple on the cause of their infertility and what management will you recommend?

2

Marking schemes

Station 1

Candidate's instructions

Despite the increased awareness of the possible consequences of improperly managed extrauterine pregnancy, it remains an important cause of maternal morbidity and mortality in the UK. You have been requested to produce a protocol on how to manage this condition in your unit and to demonstrate the success of your protocol.

Structured mark sheet

Protocol group – representatives from various stakeholders (general practitioner (GP), nurse – ward/theatre, radiology/ultrasound, haematology and consultant gynaecologist – preferably someone with an interest in emergency gynaecology)

MedLine® search/literature review – sources (National Institute for Health and Clinical Excellence (NICE) and Royal College of Obstetricians and Gynaecologists (RCOG) guidelines, Cochrane reviews, and others)

- Definition of extrauterine pregnancies
- Prevalence of ectopic pregnancies
- Causes of ectopic pregnancy
- Management of ectopic pregnancies

0   1   2   3   4   5

High-risk groups – defining them

- Previous *Chlamydia trachomatis* or *Neisseria gonorrhoea* infection
- Previous ectopic pregnancies
- Single and promiscuous/multiple sexual partners
- Intrauterine contraceptive device (IUD) use
- Tubal surgery
- Infertility treatment

0   1   2   3   4   5

Pro forma for identification of patient with a possible ectopic pregnancy (history and physical examination)

- History – pain, irregular vaginal bleeding, vaginal discharge
- Amenorrhoea
- Shoulder-tip pain
- Features of anaemia
- Cardiovascular system
- Tenderness (abdomen and cervical, especially excitation tenderness)
- Adnexal mass; fullness in the pouch of Douglas

0   1   2   3   4   5

Investigations

- Urinary pregnancy test
- Beta-human chorionic gonadotropin (βhCG) – quantification – important cut-off levels for the identification of an intrauterine gestational sac
- Full blood count (FBC)
- Group and save/cross-match
- Serial measurements of βhCG
- Ultrasound – transvaginal/abdominal

0   1   2   3   4   5

Treatment

- Expectant management
- Surgery:
  - Laparotomy/laparoscopy
  - Salpingectomy, salpingotomy, milking
- Medical, e.g. methotrexate (intramuscular)
- Follow-up after conservative (tube-preserving) management

0   1   3   4   5

Dissemination of protocol and implementation

- Circulate protocol for comments
- Collate comments, modify as appropriate, insert date of implementation and of possible revision
- Implement with support of clinical director
- Communicate protocol to all users including GPs, accident and emergency
- Make protocols available to all units and GP surgeries

0	1	2	3	4	5

Demonstration of success of protocol – audit (retrospective or prospective) after a period of implementation (determined by the number of cases required for an effective audit – liaise with audit unit) and look at the following outcome measures

- Diagnosis
- Treatment – tubal conservation and non-tubal removal
- Missed cases
- Ruptured ectopics
- Blood transfusion
- Admission into hospital
- Mortality
- Audit outcome to members of the unit and discussion of recommendations
- Dissemination and implementing changes identified

0	1	2	3	4	5	6

Global score

Excellent	4
Good	3
Average	2
Below average	1
Poor	0

Reckoner

In the table below, the 1st and 3rd rows represent the total mark awarded from the various sections above and the 2nd and 4th rows are the marks to be awarded for the performance at this station out of 20.

0–2	3–4	5–6	7–8	9–10	11–12	13–14	15–16	17–18	19–20
1	2	3	4	5	6	7	8	9	10
21–22	23–24	25–26	27–28	29–30	31–32	33–34	35–36	37–38	39–40
11	12	13	14	15	16	17	18	19	20

Total mark is out of 20

Comments

It is important to remember that there are two parts to the question. Most candidates will go straight to the audit part. The protocol part actually carries more marks and failure to address this will result in failure. Although audit and drawing up of protocols have always been important aspects of good clinical practice, the advent of clinical governance has made it mandatory for any unit to demonstrate that these components are routinely undertaken. Such a demand means that all trainees must understand the concepts involved and, indeed, must have taken part in either activity. It is therefore only right that the MRCOG examination assesses candidates' ability in this aspect of clinical practice. Most revision courses will, no doubt, go through the routine of audit and how to conduct one. It is important to remember that examiners are aware of this and you should therefore not go into the exams prepared to regurgitate everything you know about audit without relating it to the context of the examination.

How to approach the question

A good starting point is to do a literature/MedLine® search. You should be familiar with sources of information and their drawbacks. Sources include the Cochrane reviews, RCOG guidelines, randomised controlled trials, case-controlled studies, case reports, retrospective reviews, etc. Also remember that NICE produces guidelines. When undertaking this search, you need to focus on the relevant aspects for your protocol. For example, when drawing up a protocol for the identification and management of fetal growth restriction (FGR), your search will focus on the known causes of FGR and the populations at risk, the incidence, diagnosis and management (monitoring and timing of delivery).

You would then like to produce a pro forma on how to identify at-risk groups and how to monitor them to diagnose FGR when it develops, how to monitor the fetuses, and when and how to deliver. Obviously, any protocol must demonstrate a benefit to the unit and this can only be done from data on outcome. This must be built into the protocol.

For any audit, the starting point is to define the standards to be used as benchmark for comparison. Identifying these standards can sometimes be difficult but you should once again consider the following sources:

- Cochrane reviews
- Meta-analyses
- RCOG guidelines
- NICE guidelines
- Randomised controlled trials
- Other types of studies
- Other units
- Textbooks
- Opinions of respected colleagues

Candidates must be aware of the limitations of the different types of evidence.

Once the standards have been defined, a pro forma should be designed to enable information to be gathered. There are two types of audit – prospective and retrospective. The advantages and disadvantages of each type should be familiar to candidates. It is often advisable to consult the audit unit to help with the design of the pro forma and also to calculate the power for the audit. This ensures that the outcome measures are statistically acceptable and may therefore alter practice. Once the information gathering is complete, data should be analysed and presented to all stakeholders. Recommendations should be discussed and agreed upon. Once everyone has bought into these recommendations, they should be implemented and a time frame after which they are re-audited defined.

Candidates should be aware of the following questions:

- How will you ensure that everyone in the unit buys into the recommendations?
- What if one of the consultants refuses to accept the recommendations?
- What if there is nothing in the literature to provide standards for the audit?
- How to disseminate the results of the audit to the stakeholders?
- How to implement the protocol without marginalising colleagues (especially as there is often great anxiety about change)?

Further reading

Saving Mothers' Lives: Reviewing maternal deaths to make motherhood safer – 2003–2005. CEMACH Report, December 2007.

Station 2

Examiner's instructions

At this station, the candidate will be assessed on his/her ability to take a history and offer contraceptive advice. Use the structured mark sheet to assess the candidate.

Candidate's instructions

Mrs B is 40 years old. She has been referred for contraceptive advice. You are required to take a history from her and offer her the most appropriate contraceptive advice. You may wish to ask the examiner for additional information.

Role-player's instruction

You are a 40-year-old housewife and mother of three. Your last child was 3 years ago. You developed high blood pressure (BP), which required hospitalisation and treatment with methyldopa in your last pregnancy. You were on the combined oral contraceptive pill from the age of 24–30, when you got married. Your mother died from a stroke and your weight has been increasing. You are fit and well, and do not smoke, but drink alcohol socially. You consider yourself to be generally well informed about women's issues and have read a lot of information from the internet and in women's magazines about contraception. You believe that you are very clear in your mind as to what is the most effective contraception for you, and indeed, what you want (the combined oral contraceptive pill). In general, your periods are regular and the last menstruation was 3 weeks ago. In your past medical history, you had your gallbladder removed 3 years ago.

Structured mark sheet

Communication

- Introduction and putting the patient at ease
- Communicating at an appropriate level
- Encourages questions and provides suitable answers

History

- Menstrual history
- Obstetric history
- Previous contraception
- Past medical history
- Drug history
- Family history
- Gynaecological and sexual history
- Social history

0   1   2   3   4   5   6   7

Physical examination (the examiner will provide this information but must only do so when the candidates says he/she would like to examine the patient)

- Obese – weight 95 kg
- BP = 145/85 mmHg (with a large cuff)
- Essentially normal pelvic organs
- No breast lumps

0   1   2   3   4

Advice on contraception

- Combined oral contraceptive pill – not suitable (obese, hypertensive, mother died of stroke)
- Alternatives – IUD, sterilisation, Implanon®, the mini-pill – discuss each and the complications
- Vasectomy as an option
- Consider referral to family-planning centre
- May require screening for thrombophilia

0   1   2   4   5

Global score

Excellent	4
Good	3
Average	2
Below average	1
Poor	0

Total mark is out of 20

Station 3

Examiner's instructions

At this station, the candidate is expected to discuss how they will undertake a preoperative ward round on four cases on the list for surgery. You must not give them any clues. Use the reckoner to determine the total score out of 20 for the station.

Candidate's instructions

You are undertaking a preoperative ward round and the following patients are on the list for surgery. Discuss how you will undertake your ward round, including the counselling you will offer the patients.

1. A 29-year-old woman listed for a laparoscopically assisted vaginal hysterectomy for heavy periods that failed to respond to medical treatment.
2. A 60-year-old woman with hesitance, frequency and stress urinary incontinence listed for a cystoscopy.
3. A 36-year-old nulliparous woman listed for a diagnostic laparoscopy for deep dyspareunia and dysmenorrhoea.
4. A 19-year-old woman listed for a surgical termination of pregnancy at 8 weeks' gestation.

Structured mark sheet

Case	Review notes	Enquire after symptoms – have they changed?	Does she understand what is going to be done? What of alternatives – have these been considered?	Explain surgery in layman's terms including complications and postoperative course – stay in hospital and recovery to work	Examine if appropriate	Last menstrual period, pregnancy test and consent
1	√	√	Mirena® discussed? Endometrial ablation?	√	√	√
2	√	√	√	√	√	Consent only
3	√	√	√	√	√	√
4	√	Inappropriate	√	√	√	Consent only

Each of the cases should be answered according to this structure. Each case must be answered separately and not as a generic process. Each case should be marked out of 9 marks and the total including the global score should be out of 40 marks but the overall score for the station should be out of 20 marks determined from the reckoner.

Review

- The patient's notes
- Enquire after her symptoms to ensure that they have not changed
- Confirm that she is having the surgery for which she is scheduled
- Does the patient understand what is going to have done?

0   1   2   3   4

Explain the surgery in layman's terms – some details of what is to be done

- Complications of surgery
- Haemorrhage
- Injury to viscera if applicable
- Other complications and how they will be managed
- Alternatives to surgery if any (e.g. ablation and Mirena® for case 1)
- Complication of anaesthesia
- Recovery, including stay in hospital and time off work

0   1   2   3   4   5

Global score

Excellent	4
Good	3
Average	2
Below average	1
Poor	0

Reckoner

In the table below, the 1st and 3rd rows represent the total mark awarded from the various sections above and the 2nd and 4th rows are the marks to be awarded for the performance at this station out of 20

0–2	3–4	5–6	7–8	9–10	11–12	13–14	15–16	17–18	19–20
1	2	3	4	5	6	7	8	9	10
21–22	23–24	25–26	27–28	29–30	31–32	33–34	35–36	37–38	39–40
11	12	13	14	15	16	17	18	19	20

Total mark is out of 20

Station 4

Examiner's instructions

Use the structured mark sheet for the assessment of this station. You may ask the candidates direct questions aiming to ascertain whether they understand the surgical procedure and post-operative management.

Candidate's instructions

You are the junior doctor in the consultant's clinic and have been asked by your consultant to see and plan the management of the patient whom she first saw 2 months ago. A summary of the patient is given below.

> Mrs T is a 67-year-old woman who attended the gynaecology clinic 2 months ago complaining of stress urinary incontinence. A pelvic examination in the clinic was described as unremarkable. She was sent for urodynamic investigation which revealed urodynamic stress incontinence (USI). She has returned to the clinic for the results of the investigation and a discussion on her management.

Structured mark sheet

Explanations

- The diagnosis to the patient
- Ensuring that the symptoms have not changed:
  - Must exclude symptoms of prolapse – will need to examine patient prior to surgery to ensure that this is not an associated complication that may require treatment
- Discussion of the treatment options:
  - Physiotherapy should be discussed – may require referral to physiotherapy
  - Medical treatment – discuss the options and success rate
  - Surgery – definitive treatment

0   1   2   3   4   5

Description of the surgical procedure – in detail, but not to frighten the patient

- Surgical approaches – tension-free transvaginal tape (TVT), trans-obturator tape (TOT), colposuspension
- Details of the preferred surgical procedure
- Advantages and disadvantages:
  - Anaesthesia morbidity, success rate
- Colposuspension:
  - Abdominal incision under adequate anaesthesia (usually general anaesthesia)

- Surgery in the retropubic area and around the urethra
- Indwelling catheter – suprapubic or urethral
- Drain if necessary
- Success rate of the procedure (approx. 85 per cent 5-year cure rate)
- TVT and TOT:
  - Advantages and disadvantages
  - Success rates – similar to those of colposuspension

| 0 | 1 | 2 | 3 | 4 | 5 |

Postoperative management and course

- Stay in hospital
- Management of the catheter – if any
- Need for thromboprophylaxis
- Follow-up in the gynaecology clinic
- Complications and how they will be managed:
  - Haemorrhage
  - Damage to the bladder
  - Difficulties with voiding after removal of the catheter
- Duration of stay in the hospital
- Return to work
- Support at home

| 0 | 1 | 2 | 3 | 4 | 5 | 6 |

Global score

Excellent	4
Good	3
Average	2
Below average	1
Poor	0

Total mark is out of 20

Station 5

Examiner's instructions

Use the structured mark sheet for the assessment of this station. You may ask the candidate direct questions about chemotherapy and why the need for adjuvant therapy.

Candidate's instruction

You are the specialist registrar/specialist trainee in a unit and are about to see Mrs AHP, a 51-year-old woman who had a total abdominal hysterectomy and bilateral salpingo-oophorectomy by your team 5 days ago for atypical hyperplasia of the endometrium, having presented with postmenopausal vaginal bleeding. The histology report is available but she is yet to be informed of its contents. The histology report is enclosed.

Histopathology report on Mrs AHP
Specimen: uterus, Fallopian tubes and ovaries

Clinical history
Complex hyperplasia on biopsy of endometrium from endometrial biopsy. Total abdominal + bilateral salpingo-oophorectomy done; appears to be a malignancy of endometrium with involvement of the cervix.

Macroscopic
Opened uterus and cervix and both tubes and ovaries $115 \times 95 \times 80$ mm. Macroscopic tumour 100 $\times 40 \times 35$ mm, maximum depth 15 mm, involving endometrial cavity and invading into cervix. Left ovary $35 \times 25 \times 10$ mm with cystic areas. Left Fallopian tube 55 mm. Right ovary $30 \times 20 \times 10$ mm, with cystic areas. Right Fallopian tube 15 mm. The uterus was received opened with resulting contamination of the fixative with multiple pieces of tumour. This has led to problems with interpretation of the histology detailed below.

Microscopic
The endometrium is almost completely replaced by tightly packed abnormal endometrial glands forming a trabecular pattern with some villiform areas, set in a fibrous stroma. The epithelium is pseudostratified and consists of columnar cells with vesicular oval nuclei showing a low degree of nuclear pleomorphism. This endometrioid adenocarcinoma is intramucosal in some areas, but in others invades into the inner half of the myometrium. The serosa is not breached, although there are probable contaminant tumour deposits on the surface. In multiple endometrial blocks there is evidence of tumour invasion into small and large blood vessels. The cervix is invaded by tumour. The right and left cornua are not involved with tumour. In the left and right parametria, there are multiple areas of tumour deposits between tissue planes. This is difficult to interpret, but the appearance is suggestive of postoperative contamination rather than true spread of tumour. The left ovary contains a luteinised follicle. Peripheral contamination with tumour is noted in the left Fallopian tube. A Müllerian inclusion cyst is noted in the connective tissue between the right ovary and Fallopian tube. Again, probable contaminant tumour is noted in tissue planes in this region.

Conclusion
Well-differentiated endometrioid carcinoma of the endometrium, grade 1, invading cervix, inner half of the myometrium and blood vessels.

Structured mark sheet

Explanation of the diagnosis and its implications

- Explanation
- Non-medical language
- Endometrial cancer spreading to the cervix
- Implications for diagnosis:
    - Need for further treatment
    - Need for further investigations:
        - Chest X-ray (CXR)
        - Ultrasound scan/magnetic resonance imaging/computerised tomography
        - Urea and electrolytes
        - Liver function tests
    - Long-term follow-up
    - Referral to multidisciplinary oncology team

0   1   2   3   4   5   6   7   8

Adjuvant therapy and its complications

- Radiotherapy
- External and vault
- Complications of radiotherapy:
    - Diarrhoea
    - Nausea and vomiting
    - Cystitis
    - Skin burns

0   1   2   3   4   5

Follow-up

- Radiotherapist/clinical oncologists
- Gynaecological oncologist/joint clinics
- Involvement of other care experts if necessary

0   1   2   3

Global score

Excellent	4
Good	3
Average	2
Below average	1
Poor	0

Total mark is out of 20

Station 6

Examiner's instructions

Score the candidate on the structured mark sheet. Candidates are expected to describe their conduct of delivery of the twins, including the management of any complications. You are at liberty to ask specific questions, especially about the retained second twin and the need for a breech extraction.

Candidate's instructions

Mrs Jones had *in vitro* fertilisation (IVF) and had a twin pregnancy. She went into spontaneous labour at 39 weeks' gestation and is now fully dilated. The first twin is cephalic with the vertex at the introitus. How will you conduct the delivery?

Structured mark sheet

Ensure

- Intravenous (i.v.) line
- Paediatrician is available
- Anaesthetist is available
- Ultrasound machine is available

0   1   2   3

Delivery

- Twin 1 as normal
- Abdominal examination – lie and presentation of twin 2 – if uncertain, perform an ultrasound scan
- Exterior cephalic version if necessary
- Ensure contractions; may require Syntocinon®
- Await for the descent of presenting part
- Artificial/spontaneous rupture of membranes?
- Conduct of delivery:
  - Cephalic – delivery as normal
  - Breech – assisted delivery

0   1   2   3   4

If fetal distress

- Breech extraction
- Caesarean section
- Internal podalic version and breech extraction
- Ventouse/forceps delivery

0   1   2   3

Third stage

- Syntometrine® with delivery of the anterior shoulder of the second twin or if breech, with delivery of the baby
- Prevention measures against postpartum haemorrhage – Syntocinon® in drip (if any anxiety about uterine tone)

0   1   2   3

Consider Caesarean section if

- Fetal distress (abnormal cardiotocography (CTG)/pH in the first stage)
- Transverse lie of second twin with ruptured membranes
- Fetal distress in second stage with high head and potential difficult delivery – this should be a rare option in twin deliveries

0   1   2   3

Global score

Excellent	4
Good	3
Average	2
Below average	1
Poor	0

0   1   2   3   4

Total mark is out of 20

Station 7

Examiner's instructions

At this station, you should use the structured mark sheet to assess the candidate as he/she takes a history and discusses the management of the clinical problem with the role-player. You should only provide the additional information on examination if it is requested for.

Examination findings

- General examination – pale but not jaundiced
- Looks generally healthy
- Abdominal examination – uniformly distended, obvious mass arising from the pelvis to the size of a 26-week gestation. Irregular and firm in consistency. No ascites. Pelvic examination – no lower genital tract abnormality. Abdominal mass appears to be uterine in origin

Candidate's instruction

A general practitioner (GP) has referred a patient to the gynaecology clinic with the following letter. Read the letter below and then obtain the relevant history from the patient. You are expected to discuss the management options with her. The examiner will provide you with additional information should you require it.

> Holly Tree Surgery
> Wooden House Lane
> Thorpes Beast Village
> Walthome WN2 SU7
>
> Dear Dr –
>
> Would you be kind enough to see this 38-year-old woman who has been suffering from very heavy periods for the past 4 years. When I examined her, I noted that her uterus was 24 weeks' size and an ultrasound scan confirmed the presence of uterine fibroids. Her haemoglobin was 7.5 g/dL and I therefore placed her on iron tablets. She has recently been diagnosed with human immunodeficiency virus (HIV) and is currently on triple antiviral therapy. Her CD4 count has improved significantly since she was commenced on this therapy by the genitourinary medicine (GUM) physicians.
>
> Thank you for your help.
>
> Yours sincerely
>
> Peter Bowels DRCOG, MRCGP, MBChB (Leic)

Role-player's instruction

You are a 38-year-old happily married woman with very heavy periods of 4 years' duration. Your periods are regular, occurring every 28–30 days and lasting for 6–8 days. Four years ago they were only lasting for 3–4 days. You have to change your heavy-duty pads every 2 hours on days 1–5 of your periods. You pass clots, and commonly bleed through the pads. At the end of each period, you feel very weak and listless. You are currently on iron tablets as your iron level was low. The bleeding is very embarrassing and you have to stay home during the heavy periods. Your GP has offered you various drugs, including Ponstan®, norethisterone and Cyklokapron® to no avail. You have no children and have been trying for a family for the past 3 years. You would very much like to have a child. Your last menstrual period was 3 weeks ago and you started menstruating at the age of 12 years.

Past medical history

- Had been an i.v. drug user (sharing needles) for 6 years but stopped last year
- Recently diagnosed as HIV positive and receiving three different drugs from the GUM clinic
- Had appendix removed at the age of 17 years

Social history

- Drinks alcohol occasionally but smokes 20 cigarettes per day

Structured mark sheet

History

- Symptoms
- Duration
- Menstrual history
- Period before onset of menorrhagia
- Infertility/obstetric history
- Past medical history – HIV and treatment
- Social history – previous drug abuser and smoking

0   1   2   3

Investigations

- FBC and film
- Ultrasound scan
- Thyroid function test – this is only indicated if there are symptoms of thyroid dysfunction

- 21-day progesterone
- Semen analysis
- Explanation of tests

0   1   2   3

Treatment

- Medical: gonadotropin-releasing hormone (GnRH) analogues; danazol
- Surgery: myomectomy; hysterectomy; uterine artery embolisation
- Explanation of the treatment options

Medical treatment

- GnRH agonists – effective in controlling periods and fibroid size but not permanent (will be associated with anovulation and therefore pregnancy not possible during treatment)
- Advantage of medical treatment – will allow time for haemoglobin to improve and HIV control to be maximised before embarking on further surgery or pregnancy
- Danazol – temporary but will reduce periods and maybe size of fibroids (will affect fertility and not advisable if pregnancy is planned – risk of virilising female fetus). This is not a drug recommended for use in the UK because of potential side-effects

Surgical

- Myomectomy – risk of progression to hysterectomy, risk of needle injury to surgeon
- Hysterectomy – option most unlikely to be acceptable

Interventional radiological

- Uterine artery embolisation

0   1   2   3   4   5   6   7

Other issues

- HIV – fertility (need counselling on HIV and fertility treatment)
- Counselling about chances of success

0   1   2   3

Global score

Excellent	4
Good	3
Average	2
Below average	1
Poor	0

0   1   2   3   4

Total mark is out of 20

Station 8

Examiner's instructions

At this station, the candidate is expected to go through a surgical waiting list and categorise the patients into routine, soon or urgent; indicate the venue of the surgery (inpatient or day case) and discuss any additional procedure that is required.

Candidate's instructions

The following patients are on the waiting list of a consultant in your hospital. You task is to review the list and classify the patients' surgery into routine (within 3 months), soon (within 4 weeks) and urgent (within 2 weeks). In addition, you should state whether the proposed surgical procedure is appropriate and what additional precautions/steps may be taken.

1. A fit 54-year-old diabetic with focal atypical endometrial hyperplasia listed for insertion of the levonorgestrel intrauterine system.
2. A 17-year-old girl who presented with severe dysmenorrhoea and heavy periods of 12 months' duration listed for a diagnostic laparoscopy.
3. A 67-year-old woman with a painless ulcer on her right labium majorum listed for an excisional biopsy.
4. A 38-year-old woman with a diagnosis of severe endometriosis which failed to respond to medical treatment, listed for an abdominal hysterectomy and bilateral salpingo-oophorectomy.
5. An 8-year-old girl with a bloody vaginal discharge of 2 weeks' duration listed for examination under anaesthesia.
6. A 77-year-old widower living on her own on the list for a vaginal hysterectomy and pelvic floor repair, having been diagnosed with a large cystocele and USI.
7. A 26-year-old woman with a diagnosis of primary infertility placed on the list for a diagnostic laparoscopy and dye test.
8. A 49-year-old severely asthmatic woman on Ventolin® and steroids on the list for a Wertheim's hysterectomy for carcinoma of the cervix stage 1A.
9. A 30-year-old nulligravid woman with a diagnosis of multiple uterine fibroids and severe menorrhagia for myomectomy.

Structured mark sheet

Use the table below to score each candidate.

Case no.	Appropriateness	Category	Venue	Additional procedures	Score
1.	Inappropriate	Urgent	Inpatient	Hysterectomy and bilateral salpingo-oophorectomy, first on the list and by gynaecological oncologist, insulin on sliding scale	0 1 2 3 4
2.	Inappropriate	–	–	Medical treatment – e.g. combined oral contraceptive pill	0 1 2 3 4
3.	Appropriate	Urgent	Inpatient	Surgery by gynaecological oncologist	0 1 2 3 4
4.	Appropriate	Routine	Inpatient	Counsel about hormone replacement therapy, consider procedure to identify course of ureters	0 1 2 3 4
5.	Appropriate	Urgent	Day case	Ensure bed on paediatric ward, local anaesthetic cream for drip	0 1 2 3 4
6.	Appropriate	Routine	Inpatient	ECG, urinalysis, arrange social support after surgery	0 1 2 3 4
7.	Appropriate	Routine	Day case	Semen analysis and 21-day progesterone, pregnancy test of day of surgery	0 1 2 3 4
8.	Appropriate	Urgent	Inpatient	Physician review and lung function test, surgery by gynaecological oncologist, group and cross-match blood	0 1 2 3 4
9.	Appropriate	Routine	Inpatient	Group and cross-match/ consent for hysterectomy	0 1 2 3 4

Global score

Excellent	4
Good	3
Average	2
Below average	1
Poor	0

0   1   2   3   4

Reckoner

In the table below, the 1st and 3rd rows represent the total mark awarded from the various sections above the 2nd and 4th rows are the marks to be awarded for the performance at this station.

0–2	3–4	5–6	7–8	9–10	11–12	13–14	15–16	17–18	19–20
1	2	3	4	5	6	7	8	9	10
21–22	23–24	25–26	27–28	29–30	31–32	33–34	35–36	37–38	39–40
11	12	13	14	15	16	17	18	19	20

Total mark is out of 20

Station 9

Examiner's instructions

Candidates have 15 minutes to conduct the postnatal visit of this patient. Award marks for thoughtfulness in approach, clarity of explanation and ability to gain the patient's confidence. You may ask the patient what she thinks of the candidate. Use the structured mark sheet to score the candidate.

Candidate's instructions

You are about to see Mrs B, a lawyer, and her husband, a business executive, who had an unexplained stillbirth at 40 weeks' gestation 3 months ago. They are attending for a postnatal follow-up. The results of the various investigations performed after the delivery, are as follows:

- Glycosylated haemoglobin (HbA1c) – 5 per cent (normal 5–7 per cent)
- Thyroid function test – normal
- Infection screen – normal
- Autopsy – normal external and internal structures
- Placenta – fibrinoid areas scattered within the placenta with some areas of vascular occlusion
- Anticardiolipin IgG antibody – 16 IU/mL (normal (0–14 IU/mL)
- Lupus anticoagulant – 1.16 (normal 0.1–1.09)
- Heterozygous for the prothrombin gene mutation
- Protein S – 60 (normal 80–110)
- Other thrombophilias – normal

Could you conduct her postnatal visit?

Structured mark sheet

Introduction

- Enquiry after problems since delivery:
  - How coping
  - Menstrual problems
  - Non-medical language
- Eye contact
- Sympathy/empathy

0   1   2   3

Explanation of the results

- Inform about the normal results and then the abnormal results
- Need to repeat some of the investigations (protein C unreliable)
- Relevance of abnormal results and the implications
- Appropriate interpretation in relation to loss

0   1   2   3   4

Plan for subsequent pregnancy

- Monitoring (ultrasound and Doppler scans)
- Combined care with haematologist/refer to centre with expertise
- Treatment (aspirin and low-molecular-weight heparin)
- Duration of treatment – throughout pregnancy and for 6 weeks after delivery, stop aspirin at 34 weeks
- Timing of delivery – induction at 38–39 weeks

0   1   2   3   4   5

Counselling

- Support groups
- Menstrual cycle
- Lifestyle modifications in view of abnormal thrombophilia
- Other problems

0   1   2   3   4

Global score

Excellent   4
Good   3
Average   2
Below average 1
Poor   0

0   1   2   3   4

Total mark is out of 20

Station 10

Examiner's instructions

The candidates have had 15 minutes to prepare this station. They are expected to discuss the tasks to be performed for each patient, the order in which these tasks will be undertaken and how they will allocate the staff available to each task.

Candidate's instructions

You arrive on the delivery suite for the morning shift and have been handed the 10 patients shown on the board. The sister-in-charge quickly runs through the problems, telling you that it is busy and she is short of staff. There are six midwives (SM, MD, BG, ST, MM and TT) on duty. SM and MD are capable of siting Venflon®, BG and ST are able to suture episiotomies and MM and TT are newly qualified midwives. On duty with you are an experienced anaesthetic registrar and a General Practitioner Vocational Scheme trainee. You are required to identify the task(s) that need to be done for each patient, the priority in which these patients should be seen and managed, and the member of staff who will be allocated to do these tasks. The 10 patients are as follows:

- Room 1: A 27-year-old woman with a previous Caesarean section for failure to progress in the second stage, in labour for 12 hours and complaining of abdominal pain
- Room 2: Mrs JT – a primigravida at 35 weeks' gestation with premature rupture of fetal membranes and having variable decelerations
- Room 3: Mrs James with uncomplicated twins in early labour at 37 weeks' gestation
- Room 4: A primipara who has been fully dilated and pushing for 2 hours
- Room 5: A 32-year-old primigravida with an undiagnosed breech in labour at 39 weeks' gestation
- Room 6: Mrs PJ with abdominal pains at 26 weeks' gestation
- Room 7: A 42-year-old primigravida at 38 weeks' gestation presenting with vaginal bleeding
- Room 8: Primigravida who delivered 1 hour ago and is awaiting repair of her episiotomy
- Room 9: Uncomplicated primigravida at 41 weeks in normal labour
- Room 10: A 28-year-old woman who delivered 4 hours ago and is being observed for a postoperative pyrexia of 37.6°C

You have 15 minutes to prepare this station and to discuss your answer with the examiner at the next station.

Tasks

- Room 1: Any vaginal bleeding? Assess maternal vital signs, reasons for failure to progress (e.g. adequacy of contractions or disproportion) and fetal wellbeing – CTG
- Room 2: Need to exclude cord prolapse or compression
- Room 3: Ensure Venflon® is sited, blood for group and save serum, notify anaesthetist, assess fetal health
- Room 4: Need to assess reasons for failure to deliver and fetal health (CTG)
- Room 5: Need to discuss options of delivery and assess suitability for a vaginal delivery. Inform anaesthetist
- Room 6: Assess CTG, more information about pain and associated bleeding
- Room 7: Assessment of the bleeding, state of the fetus and additional information, e.g. contracting?
- Room 8: Needs suturing of episiotomy – midwife
- Room 9: Normal labouring patient – no action – to be managed by midwife
- Room 10: Assess, after history and examination, consider antibiotics

0	1	2	3	4	5	6	7	8	9	10
11	12	13	14	15	16	17	18			

Priority of tasks and staff allocation

- Urgent review of patients in rooms 3, 1 and 8
- A quick vaginal examination (VE) of patient in room 2 will exclude cord prolapse. Turn patient to side to see effect. If CTG normal, consider as cord compression. Will need delivering
- Patient in room 1 requires an urgent assessment to rule out imminent rupture. Urgently assess the state of fetus and vital signs of mother. Quick abdominal and VE for signs of rupture and evidence of disproportion
- Patient in room 8 requires urgent exclusion of abruption. Quick VE to assess state of the cervix
- Senior house officer (SHO) to see patient in room 7 and exclude abruption and ensure fetal health is satisfactory
- Midwife to continue monitoring patient with twins in room 3 until assessed
- Semi-urgent review of patient in room 5 by registrar. Needs a VE to determine why not delivered. If good contractions and head low enough, expedite delivery with forceps or ventouse. If vaginal delivery not possible, for Caesarean section. May require Syntocinon® if head is high and contractions are poor
- Semi-review of patient in room 6 by registrar
- SHO to review patient in room 10 and start on antibiotics

0	1	2	3	4	5	6	7	8	9	10
11	12	13	14	15	16	17	18			

Global score

Excellent	4
Good	3
Average	2
Below average	1
Poor	0

0	1	2	3	4

Reckoner

In the table below, the 1st and 3rd rows represent the total marks awarded from the various sections above and the 2nd and 4th rows are the marks to be awarded for the performance at this station out of 20.

0–2	3–4	5–6	7–8	9–10	11–12	13–14	15–16	17–18	19–20
1	2	3	4	5	6	7	8	9	10
21–22	23–24	25–26	27–28	29–30	31–32	33–34	35–36	37–38	39–40
11	12	13	14	15	16	17	18	19	20

Total mark is out of 20

Station 11

Examiner's instructions

At this station, the candidate is expected to offer counselling on prenatal diagnosis. Marks should be awarded for candidate's ability to communicate in a language that a lay person will understand.

Candidate's instructions

A primigravida attended for her anomaly scan at 20 weeks' gestation and the fetus was found to have a diaphragmatic hernia and bilateral talipes equinovarus. She has been informed of the abnormalities by the radiographer. How will you set about managing this patient?

Structured mark sheet

Introduction

- Does she want her partner/relative to be called to come and join her?
- Explanation of the diagnosis to the patient
- Putting patient at ease and empathising
- Implications of abnormalities
- Need to exclude other associated subtle structural and chromosomal abnormalities

0   1   2   3

Investigations

- Although other structural and chromosomal abnormalities may be excluded, baby may still be syndromic
- Further scanning at tertiary level – fetomaternal medicine unit

Prenatal karyotyping

- Amniocentesis + fluorescent *in situ* hybridisation (FISH) – advantages/disadvantages (only for specific probes, therefore other uncommon karyotypic abnormalities not excluded) – early result – 24–48 hours. Standard amniocentesis – 2–3 weeks for results
- Chorionic villus sampling (CVS) (placental biopsy) – FISH – 24–48 hours (only five chromosomal abnormalities can be identified):
  - Direct preparation – results within 48–72 hours (more chromosomal abnormalities will be identified). Risk of mosaicism
- Miscarriage risk with both tests – 0.5–1 per cent with amniocentesis; 1 per cent with CVS

0   1   2   3   4   5   6

Options

- Karyotypye abnormal – termination of pregnancy/continue
- If termination, gestational age more than 21 weeks, consider feticide with KCl, etc.
- If before 21 weeks, prostaglandins and mifepristone (RU486)
- Other abnormalities severe enough to affect outcome – termination option

0   1   2   3   4

Others

- No karyotypic abnormality or decision to continue with pregnancy
- Counselling by geneticists
- Plastic surgeon to discuss management after of the cleft and talipes (photographs may be helpful)
- Neonatologist involvement – feeding difficulties, vocalisation and complications of aspiration pneumonia
- Serial follow-up ultrasound scans for growth and complications, such as polyhydramnios

0   1   2   3

Global score

Excellent	4
Good	3
Average	2
Below average	1
Poor	0

0   1   2   3   4

Total mark is out of 20

Station 12

Examiner's instructions

At this station, the candidate is expected to conduct a postnatal follow-up visit for a couple who had a stillbirth. Use the structured mark sheet to assess each candidate.

Candidate's instructions

Mr B and his wife attended the gynaecology clinic with primary infertility. The couple were investigated and the following results were obtained from a semen analysis, which was repeated twice

- Time of production   0930
- Time of examination   1015
- Volume   3 mL
- Count   500 000/mL
- Motility   50 per cent
- Morphology   50 per cent
- Cells   1–3/mL

The investigations on Mrs B revealed mild endometriosis, predominantly on the posterior peritoneum and the uterosacral ligaments. How will you counsel the couple on the cause of their infertility and what management will you recommend?

Structured mark sheet

Explanation of the results

- Of the semen analysis
- Of the diagnostic laparoscopy
- Implications of laparoscopic findings – minimal disease recognised to be associated with infertility
- Male factors needs to be rechecked – oligozoospermia needs to be confirmed
- Evidence now favours surgical treatment of minimal to mild endometriosis in women with infertility – RCOG guidelines

0   1   2   3   4   5   6   7

Options

- Assisted reproduction techniques – explaining the difference and implications of each of the techniques:
  - Artificial insemination by donor
  - Artificial insemination by husband
  - IVF with husband or donor – spermatozoa

| 0 | 1 | 2 | 3 | 4 | 5 | 6 | 7 |

Others

- Adoption

| 0 | 1 | 2 |

Global score

Excellent	4
Good	3
Average	2
Below average	1
Poor	0

| 0 | 1 | 2 | 3 | 4 |

Total mark is out of 20

Index

For the EMQs, MCQs and OSCEs, entries appear in the form '471(481)' indicating page numbers for both the question and (answer).

hepatic failure, ovarian hyperstimulation
    syndrome 511(519)
hepatitis B 28–30
hernia
    congenital diaphragmatic 89–91, 528(555–6)
    inguinolabial 304, 305
herpes, genital (predominantly HSV-2) 496(516)
    maternal 31–3
hirsutism 314–17
history-taking in prenatal screening 75–6, 77
HIV (human immunodeficiency virus)
    pregnant woman 38–40, 472(482)
        universal vs selective screening 26–7
    uterine fibroid management and 281–3
home delivery 177–9
hormonal long-acting reversible contraceptives
        (LARCs incl. subdermal implants) 245,
        350–2, 506(518)
    older women 353, 354, 506(518)
    post-abortion 258, 259
hormone replacement therapy 368–70, 479(490)
    contraception and 355
    post-gynaecological surgery in protein S
        deficiency 447, 448
    post-radiotherapy 413
hospital
    admission in pregnancy
        for bed rest in preterm labour prevention
            129
        in previous emergency CS for transverse lie
            189
        unstable lie 120, 121
    discharge see discharge
HPV (human papilloma virus)
    cervical cancer and 401
    vaccination 403
HSV see herpes
human chorionic gonadotropin (hCG incl. βhCG)
    in gestational trophoblastic disease, levels
        choriocarcinoma 437, 438
        hydatidiform mole 439, 442
    for ovulatory induction 336, 337
        hyperstimulation risk 340
human immunodeficiency virus see HIV
human menopausal gonadotropin (hMG) for
        ovulatory induction 336
    hyperstimulation risk 340
human papilloma virus see HPV
hydatidiform mole 439–43
hydralazine 47
hydrops, fetal 474(484)
hyperprolactinaemia 252, 321–2, 507(518)
hypertension
    in PCOS 318

in pregnancy 41
hypoglycaemia, neonatal 217
    feeding refusal due to 224
hypotension, intrapartum 71, 72
    in epidural analgesia 207
hypothermia, neonatal 218–19
    feeding difficulties and 224
hypotonia, uterine, postpartum 196
hypovolaemic shock after vaginal hysterectomy
    455–6
hysterectomy 475(486)
    and bilateral salpingo-oophorectomy see
        salpingo-oophorectomy
    cervical cancer 410, 424
    difficulties in waking up from general
        anaesthesia 476
    dysmenorrhoea 250
    endometrial atypical hyperplasia 419
    endometrial cancer 421, 422
        prognosis and its improvement 145–7
    endometriosis 288
    fibroids 247, 275
        HIV-positive woman 283
    menorrhagia 247
    ovarian cystic malignancy in adolescent 434
    ovarian cystic mass discovery 449–50
    postpartum haemorrhage 196
        Caesarean 191, 194
    shock following 455–6
    ureteric damage in 451–2
    vaginal see vaginal hysterectomy
hysterosalpinography (HSG)
    in cervical weakness 128
    in infertility 331
hysteroscopy, outpatient, postmenopausal
        bleeding 376–7
hysterosonography, fertility investigations 331,
        332

iatrogenic injury see trauma
iliac artery ligation, internal
    post-CS 191
    post-vaginal delivery 196
imaging (incl. radiology)
    cervical cancer 409, 410
    menarchal delay 324, 325
    ovarian cancer screening 430
    ovarian cyst 294–5
    PCOS 315
    tubal, in fertility investigations 331–3
    see also specific modalities
immune thrombocytopenia, maternal 474(484)
immunisation (active) see vaccination
Implanon, post-abortion 258, 259

COCP in *see* combined oral contraceptive pill
mental subnormality and intrapartum care 169–71
meshes, genital prolapse 396–7, 398, 398–9
meta-analysis 499(516)
metabolic complications of maternal diabetes, neonatal 217
methotrexate, ectopic pregnancy 270, 271
mifepristone 263, 265
Mirena *see* levonorgestrel intrauterine system
miscarriage (spontaneous abortion) 471(482), 478(489)
  hydatidiform mole 439–43
  incomplete septic 260–2
misoprostol, induction of labour 161
molar pregnancy 435–43
  advice on/management of subsequent pregnancy 436, 438, 439, 440, 442, 443
monitoring
  fetal *see* fetus
  maternal, premature rupture of membranes 133, 134–5
monozygotic pregnancy, intrauterine death and complications in surviving twin 474(484)
mortality *see* death
Müllerian agenesis 306–7
multiple pregnancy (incl. twins) 525(542–3)
  cord prolapse 176
  death of one monozygotic twin, complications in surviving twin 474(484)
  preterm labour 131
  reducing number of fetuses 462
myocardial infarction, postpartum 501(517)
myomectomy 247, 274, 276, 279
  adhesion formation following, risk reduction 480(491)
  HIV-positive woman 282, 283
  polypectomy and 276

National Health Service, infertility treatment 464–5
Neisseria gonorrhoeae 513(519)
neonates (newborns) 215–24
  diabetes and *see* diabetes
  Down syndrome 230–2
  in fetal growth restriction
    complications 114, 115–16, 473(484)
    management 101, 103
  hepatitis B and 29, 30
  HIV and 39, 40
  HSV-2 and 33
  mentally-subnormal mother and care of 171
  septicaemia *see* septicaemia
  smoking and 17

TB and 63
neoplasm *see* malignancy; tumours
neovagina 307
neural tube defects 472(483)
newborns *see* neonates
NHS, infertility treatment 464–5
nicotine replacement therapy 18
nifedipine 47
non-absorbable meshes 398
non-accidental injury, maternal 20–2
non-steroidal anti-inflammatory drugs (NSAIDs), menorrhagia 244–5
norethisterone, menorrhagia 245
Norplant, post-abortion 258, 259
NSAIDs, menorrhagia 244–5
nuchal translucency (NT) 75, 76, 77
  Down's syndrome diagnosis 85, 86
nutritional management, neonatal 224

obesity *see* weight
obstetric history, past
  home delivery and 178
  in prenatal screening 75, 77
oestradiol implants and patches, severe premenstrual syndrome 255
oestrogen
  deficiency symptoms with cervical cancer radiotherapy 413
  therapy
    atypical endometrial hyperplasia risk 419
    PCOS 316
    stress incontinence 383
  see also combined oral contraceptive pill; hormone replacement therapy
oligohydramnios 473(484)
oligospermia 342–3, 509(518), 510(518)
omphalocele (exomphalos) 79–81
oncogenes and ovarian cancer prognosis 428
oophorectomy
  bilateral
    endometriosis 288
    endometriosis, pregnancy desire and 288
    severe premenstrual syndrome 255
  ovarian cyst 295
  see also salpingo-oophorectomy
operative obstetrics *see* Caesarean section
oral contraceptive pill
  combined *see* combined oral contraceptive pill
  progestogen-only, following abortion 257, 259
oral glucose tolerance test 65
osteoporosis 479(490)
  postmenopausal risk 378–80
ovaries
  cysts *see* cyst; polycystic ovarian syndrome